recovery

Library Alliance

and mental illness

Personal recovery and mental illness

A guide for mental health professionals

Mike Slade

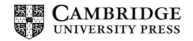

CAMBRIDGE UNIVERSITY PRESS
Cambridge, New York, Melbourne, Madrid, Cape Town, Singapore,
São Paulo, Delhi, Dubai, Tokyo, Mexico City

Cambridge University Press
The Edinburgh Building, Cambridge CB2 8RU, UK

Published in the United States of America
by Cambridge University Press, New York

www.cambridge.org
Information on this title: www.cambridge.org/9780521746588

First published 2009
3rd printing 2011

Printed in the United Kingdom at the University Press, Cambridge

A catalogue record for this publication is available from the British Library

Library of Congress Cataloging-in-Publication Data

Slade, Mike.
Personal recovery and mental illness : a guide for mental health
professionals / Mike Slade.
    p. ; cm.
  Includes bibliographical references and index.
  ISBN 978-0-521-74658-8 (pbk.)
1. Mental health services.   2. Mental health.   I. Title.
  [DNLM: 1. Mental Disorders–rehabilitation.   2. Mental Health
Services. WM 400 S631p 2009]
  RA790.5.S484 2009
  616.89–dc22
                                                                    2009008944

ISBN 978-0-521-74658-8 paperback

Additional resources for this publication at www.cambridge.org/
9780521746588

for Charlotte

Contents

Section 3–Recovery-focussed mental health services

Section 4–Challenges

List of case studies

	Case study	Location
1	Peace Ranch	Ontario, Canada
2	Family peer support workers	Melbourne, Australia
3	Sharing Your Recovery Story	Philadelphia, USA
4	Developing a peer support specialist infrastructure	Scotland
5	Youth peer support workers	Melbourne, Australia
6	Warmline	Wellington, New Zealand
7	Rethink garden project	Salisbury, England
8	The Light House	Napier, New Zealand
9	In-patient psychodrama group	Melbourne, Australia
10	Collaborative Recovery Model	New South Wales, Australia
11	Person-centred planning	Connecticut, USA
12	The Golden Ducky award	Los Angeles, USA
13	The Strengths Model	Melbourne, Australia
14	The Living Room	Phoenix, USA
15	Key We Way	Kapiti Coast, New Zealand
16	IPS for young people	Melbourne, Australia
17	Education for well-being	Boston, USA
18	The MHA Village approach to employment	Los Angeles, USA
19	Mental Health at Work	Australia
20	*Like Minds, Like Mine* campaign	New Zealand
21	Implementing the Collaborative Recovery Model	Victoria, Australia
22	Implementing pro-recovery policy	New Zealand
23	Implementing the Strengths Model	Melbourne, Australia
24	Recovery Innovations	Phoenix, USA
25	Recovery Devon	Devon, England
26	Trialogues	German-speaking Europe

Acknowledgements

The streetlights and signposts on my journey down the recovery road have been provided by many people, including Allison Alexander, Retta Andresen, Bill Anthony, Janey Antoniou and Pippa Brown (who contributed Case Study 7), Paul Barry, Chyrell Bellamy, Pat Bracken, Simon Bradstreet, Michael Brazendale, Peter Caputi, Laurie Davidson, Pat Deegan, Bob Drake, Marianne Farkas, Cheryl Gagne, Helen Gilburt, Helen Glover, Sonja Goldsack, Courtenay Harding, Ruth Harrison, Nick Haslam, Mark Hayward, Nigel Henderson, Dori Hutchinson, Gene Johnson, Lucy Johnstone, Levent Küey, Martha Long, Jenny Lynch, Pat McGorry, Chris McNamara, Graham Meadows, Lorraine Michael, Steve Onken, Rachel Perkins, Debbie Peterson, Vanessa Pinfold, Shula Ramon, John Read, Julie Repper, Priscilla Ridgway, Sally Rogers, Marius Romme, Diana Rose, Alan Rosen, Joe Ruiz, Zlatka Russinova, Beate Schrank, Geoff Shepherd, Greg Teague, Phil Thomas, Heidi Torreiter, Eric Tripp-McKay, Bill White, David Whitwell, Paul Wolfson, Gina Woodhead and Sam Yeats. This book has been influenced by them all.

Many experts generously commented on chapter drafts: Neal Adams, Piers Allott, Michaela Amering, Janey Antoniou, Jonathan Bindman, Jed Boardman, Derek Bolton, Mike Clark, Sunny Collings, Mike Crawford, Trevor Crowe, Larry Davidson, Pete Ellis, Alison Faulkner, Bridget Hamilton, Dave Harper, Corey Keyes, Eóin Killackey, Elizabeth Kuipers, Rob MacPherson, Paul Moran, Kim Mueser, Lindsay Oades, Mary O'Hagan, Ingrid Ozols, Dave Pilon, Stefan Priebe, Glenn Roberts, Jörg Strobel, George Szmukler, Graham Thornicroft, Janis Tondora, Tom Trauer and Rob Whitley. Their insightful suggestions led to the correction of a host of errors and mis-statements – those that remain (and the overall views expressed in the book) are of course my responsibility.

This book was written during a leave of absence from my normal duties, for which I sincerely thank the Institute of Psychiatry, the South London and Maudsley NHS Foundation Trust, and colleagues who generously covered my responsibilities: Tom Craig, Neil Hammond, Louise Howard, Morven Leese, Paul McCrone and Sara Tresilian. My visiting appointment with the Melbourne clinical service headed by David Castle was organised by Tom Trauer, who provided consistently wise advice. I was fortunate to have excellent administrative support from Kelly Davies, Natalie Knoesen and Joe Mirza. Katie James and Richard Marley at Cambridge University Press provided consistently constructive guidance.

Acknowledgements often recognise the contribution of family, but perhaps I have more to thank mine for than most authors. Writing this book involved living abroad for a year. To make this possible, my family left work, school and home for life on the road. Their unfailing love and support has helped me to learn more about life as well as work during the writing of the book. I am supremely grateful to Charlotte, Emily and Isabel.

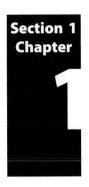
Mental illness and recovery
Overview of the book

This book is about mental health services – what they currently do, and how they would need to change if their goal is to promote 'personal recovery'. What does this term mean? Different understandings of recovery are considered in Chapter 3, but personal recovery is defined in this book as meaning[1]:

> a deeply personal, unique process of changing one's attitudes, values, feelings, goals, skills, and/or roles. It is a way of living a satisfying, hopeful, and contributing life even within the limitations caused by illness. Recovery involves the development of new meaning and purpose in one's life as one grows beyond the catastrophic effects of mental illness.

Focussing on personal recovery will require fundamental changes in the values, beliefs and working practices of mental health professionals. Why is this necessary?

What's the problem?

People using mental health services lie on a spectrum.

At one end of the spectrum are people who benefit from mental health services as currently structured. Typically, this group contains people who are progressing well in life, and are then struck down by mental illness. The application of effective treatments helps the person to get back to normal – to come to view the mental illness experience as a bump in the road of their life, which they get over and move on from. For this group, mental health services as currently configured promote recovery (because clinical recovery, which we define in Chapter 3, is the same as personal recovery).

In the middle of the spectrum are a group of people for whom mental health services promise much but do not fully deliver. This group find that the impact of the mental illness does lessen over time, but it is not clear how much this is because of the treatment and how much because of other influences – the passing of time, learning to reduce and manage stress better, developing social roles such as worker and friend and partner, making sense of their experiences in a way that offers a hopeful or better future, etc. For this group, mental health services as currently configured are insufficient – they provide effective treatments but personal recovery involves more than treatment.

At the other end of the spectrum are a group of people for whom the mental health system, with its current preoccupations, imperatives and values, is harmful. This group find that the impact of the mental illness increases over time, to the point where their whole identity is enmeshed with the mental patient role. The more treatments and interventions are provided, the further away a normal life becomes. The horizons of their life increasingly narrow to a mental health (i.e. illness) ghetto. In previous generations, these people would have lived in a visible institution. Nowadays they are increasingly likely to reside in a virtual institution[2] – a life lived exclusively in dedicated buildings and social networks containing mental health patients and staff. For this group, mental health services as currently configured are toxic – they provide treatments with the promise of cure, but in reality they hinder personal recovery.

This book will identify how this situation has come about, identify the elements of mental health services which can be either insufficient or toxic, and chart a way forward. The central thesis is that if the primary aim of mental health services is to promote personal recovery, then the values, structure, workforce skills and activities of the service should all be oriented towards this end.

Aims of the book

This book is written primarily for mental health professionals, and has three aims in relation to personal recovery: convincing, crystallising and catalysing.

The first aim is to **convince** that a focus on personal recovery is a desirable direction of travel for mental health services. Five broad reasons are proposed. The epistemological rationale is that the experience of mental illness is most helpfully understood from a constructivist perspective, which necessarily involves giving primacy to the values and preferences of the individual. The ethical rationale is that an emphasis on professionally judged best interests has inadvertently done harm, and a better approach would involve support oriented around the individual's goals rather than around clinical imperatives. The effectiveness rationale is that the benefits of the most common treatment (medication) have been systematically exaggerated, and a broader approach is needed. The empowerment rationale is that a focus on clinical recovery has consistently involved the interests of the individual person with a mental illness being subordinated to the interests of other dominant groups in society – 'their' life has not been safe in our hands. Finally, the policy rationale is quite simply that, in many countries, public sector mental health professionals have been told to develop a focus on personal recovery. Chapters 24 and 25 also contribute to this aim, by providing potential responses to some concerns expressed by clinicians and consumers about personal recovery.

The second aim is to **crystallise** exactly what personal recovery means. This is addressed in two ways. First, in Chapter 9 a Personal Recovery Framework is proposed. I was hesitant about developing a theoretical framework, since one impetus for writing this book was a belief that the recovery world needs a little less theory and ideology, and a bit more of a focus on concrete implications and working practices. However, the recovery support tasks identified for mental health professionals are implicitly based on an underpinning theory of personal recovery, so it seemed better to make this explicit and hence more amenable to debate and improvement. Second, the book is written from the perspective that there are different types of knowledge. Evidence which comes from group-level scientific designs is currently valued in the scientific literature more than evidence that comes from individuals. It will be argued in Chapter 4 that the pendulum has swung too far, and what is needed is a blending of group-level and individual-level evidence. The optimal balance involves attaching importance to both the individual perspective of the expert-by-experience and the training, knowledge and (occasionally) personal views of the professional expert-by-training. The style of writing is intended to model what this means in practice: arguments are made using both empirical study data (e.g. clinical trials and systematic reviews) and insightful quotes from individuals, sprinkled with a few personal observations. More authoritative statements can be made where there is concordance between different types of knowledge, e.g. in the content of consumer accounts of recovery and the scientific focus of positive psychology (explored in Chapter 14).

The third aim is to **catalyse** – to provide a response to the mental health professional who is convinced about the values, has crystallised beliefs and knowledge about personal recovery, and wants to know where in practice to start. Case studies of best practice from around the world are included. These provide a resource of innovative, established strategies which increase the organisational and clinical focus on personal recovery. They also serve as a bridge between the worlds of theory and practice. The coherence of a good theory is seductive – it makes the world simpler by ignoring its complexity. In reality, no theory is universally applicable, and the case studies serve to illustrate the challenge of turning theory into practice. Web resources listed in the Appendix give further pointers to some recovery resources.

New goals, values, knowledge and working practices

We will argue that the primary goal of mental health services needs to change, from its current focus on treating illness in order to produce clinical recovery, to a new focus on supporting personal recovery by promoting well-being.

Supporting personal recovery requires a change in values. The new values involve services being driven by the priorities and aspirations of the individual, rather than giving primacy to clinical preoccupations and imperatives. This will involve mental health professionals **listening to and acting on what the individuals themselves say**. Although, as Henry Mencken cautioned, 'There is always an easy solution to every human problem – neat, plausible, and wrong'[3] (p. 443), this simple suggestion is in fact both necessary and revolutionary, with deep implications for how mental health services are provided.

Why is a values shift needed? Because many constructs held by clinicians as incontestable revealed truths are in fact highly contested, although those contesting them – service users – have until recently not had a voice. Repper and Perkins[4] note that there has been a systematic denial of this voice. For example, media reporting on mental health issues disseminates the views of clinical experts, family members, politicians, indeed anyone other than the people actually experiencing the difficulties[5]. The evidence-based response to this diversity of views is to show modesty in the claims made for the scope and applicability of any individual clinical model. A term used in this book is being tentative – applying professional knowledge competently but humbly to support people in their recovery journey. Professionals who recognise that their world-view is built on sand work very differently to those who believe that their own world-view is true. This is why values and relationships are central – it's not just what you do, it's how you do it.

New knowledge will be needed, because the treatment of illness and the promotion of well-being require different, though overlapping, actions. The science of illness provides only limited levers of change. For the clinician, treating illness in order to promote well-being is like fighting with one hand tied behind their back. Furthermore, mental health services can be toxic in relation to personal recovery where the trade-off between short-term and long-term effects is not recognised. Avoidance of illness is a clinical preoccupation, and has a short-term horizon. Development of well-being is a long-term process, and involves different tasks. For example, being relieved of employment demands has short-term benefits for treating illness, but chronic unemployment hinders wellness. Having responsibility for your life taken by others can allow stabilisation in the short term, but long-term leads to dependence and disengagement from your own life. Being given a mental illness diagnosis brings the short-term relief of understanding, but if it becomes a dominant identity then it creates an engulfing role which can destroy hope for a normal life.

Some of the new knowledge comes from the lived experience of people with mental illness. Their authentic and clear voice is becoming heard throughout the system, and has deep consequences for mental health services. Their voice is given prominence in Chapters 3 and 9. Some of the new knowledge comes from positive psychology: the science of well-being. This emerging science involves empirical investigation of what is needed for a good life, and is applied to mental health services in Chapter 14. It is a central assumption in this book that people with mental illness are fundamentally similar to people without mental illness in their need for life to be pleasant, engaged, meaningful and achieving. A sophisticated and balanced perspective on the trade-off between actions to treat illness and actions to promote well-being places the clinician in a better position to contribute beneficially to people's lives.

What does this mean in practice? We propose in Chapter 9 a theory-based Personal Recovery Framework, which is based on four key processes involved in the journey to recovery: hope, identity, meaning and personal responsibility. On the basis of this Personal Recovery Framework, recovery support tasks for mental health services are identified and elaborated in Chapters 10 to 23.

So this book is arguing for fundamental shifts in clinical practice:

- A change of goal, from promoting clinical recovery to promoting personal recovery
- A values-based shift to give the patient perspective primacy
- The incorporation of scientific knowledge from the academic discipline of positive psychology into routine clinical practice
- A focus by mental health professionals on tasks which support personal recovery.

The profound ethical, behavioural and professional implications of these shifts are considered.

Structure of the book

The book has four sections. Section 1 provides an overview of where mental health services are now, and different understandings of recovery. The aim is to show that clinical recovery and personal recovery are not the same thing, and to raise the question of which should be the primary goal for mental health services.

Section 2 outlines five rationales for giving primacy to personal recovery. This section contains the more detailed discussions of, sometimes, esoteric theory. The goal is to provide a range of arguments in favour of personal recovery.

Section 3 puts meat on the bones of the idea of a mental health service focussed on personal recovery, both in terms of what personal recovery means, and envisaging what recovery-focussed services look like. Some of it is speculative, involving comment on current practice with un-evaluated suggestions about how this could be different. Some of it is already implemented, and reported as case studies from innovative recovery-focussed sites internationally.

Section 4 looks to the future, in two ways. First, by addressing the potential concerns of clinicians and consumers. Second, by suggesting concrete actions for the mental health system, with illustrative case studies.

Many references are cited, partly to provide a response to the 'What's the evidence for recovery?' question, and partly to acknowledge where the ideas presented here have come from others. The book is therefore intended to signpost some of the many resources in the large and growing world of recovery.

The book is written to be dipped into. Readers new to the field of recovery might start with Section 1, and then read Chapter 22 for indicators of a recovery-focussed service.

Knowledgeable but unconvinced readers might start with Chapters 24 and 25, and then pick from Section 2 as per their personal tastes for different types of argument. Readers wanting to crystallise their understanding of what personal recovery means might read Section 1 followed by Chapter 9. Finally, readers looking to change their own practice might read Section 3 and Chapter 26, and to influence the practice of others will find Section 2 and Chapters 24 and 25 relevant.

Collective nouns

This book is about the group of people whose lives are lived in actual or potential contact with mental health services. What to call these people, and their defining characteristic? Existing suggestions range along a spectrum, and each contains implicit assumptions.

At one end of the spectrum, the problem (and therefore the label) is seen as internal to the person. This finds expression in calls to use the term brain illness instead of mental illness[6], and for schizophrenia to be re-named as dopamine dysregulation disorder[7].

In the middle lie perspectives which are sensitive to the implications of locating the problem either entirely internally or entirely externally. For example, clinical psychology literature is often somewhat antagonistic towards the underlying assumptions of discontinuity embedded in descriptive taxonomies, yet diagnostic categories are nevertheless routinely adopted as the best available organising framework[8]. At this point on the spectrum, the validity issues with diagnosis are recognised[9;10], and addressed by seeking to develop more valid categories, such as a disaggregation of schizophrenia into Sensitivity-, Post Traumatic Stress-, Anxiety- and Drug-related psychosis[11].

At the other end of the spectrum, the problem is seen as external, and so described by the person's relationship to or history in mental health services. Labelling suggestions from this perspective include[12]:

- Mental health consumer
- Psychiatric survivor
- Person labelled with a psychiatric disability
- Person diagnosed with a psychiatric disorder
- Person with a mental health history
- Person with mental health issues
- Consumer/Survivor/eX-inmate (CSX)
- Person who has experienced the mental health system
- Person experiencing severe and overwhelming mental and emotional problems, such as 'despair'
- Person our society considers to have very different and unusual behaviour, such as 'not sleeping'.

From this end of the spectrum, there is a call for the term schizophrenia to be abandoned altogether[13].

In this book, the term **mental illness** will be used to describe the experience itself. This term places the experience in the domain of medicine, despite arguing for the limitations of this frame of reference. However, any euphemism for a person with a mental illness cannot easily escape this implication. For example, in relation to the phrase 'person with mental health problems', Repper and Perkins ask, 'What is a "health problem" if not an "illness"?'[4] (p. viii). Their solution is to adopt alternative and less value-laden terminology, such as unshared perceptions and unusual experiences, which are intended to avoid the assumptions embedded in psychiatric terms such as delusions and hallucinations. However, these terms are too specific for the trans-diagnostic focus of this book.

What about the person with the mental illness? The international shift from talking about psychiatric services to mental health services has highlighted the need to find a more neutral term than patient. Certainly, language is important – how you say it is how you see it. But a preoccupation with language can be all too easily dismissed as political correctness, and provides a convenient excuse to ignore the real epistemological, ethical and clinical challenges. Therefore, the standard terms **consumer, peer, patient, client** and **service user** are used to describe the person. They are used interchangeably, with the most appropriate term chosen for the particular context.

This book is written for people working in mental health services who are employed on the basis of their professional training and skills. Most multidisciplinary mental health teams routinely include occupational therapists, mental health / psychiatric nurses, social workers, psychiatrists and clinical or counselling psychologists, and can also include art therapists, benefits advisors, dance therapists, dieticians, drama therapists, employment advisors, housing advisors, music therapists, physiotherapists and psychotherapists, among others. All these professional groups will be referred to collectively as **professionals, mental health professionals** or **clinicians**. Much inter-professional jostling for position takes place (normally) behind the scenes in multidisciplinary teams, and this book tries to side-step these issues by using these generic terms for all varieties of professional. This is not of course meant to imply that all professional groups are the same, or that the nomenclature is accepted by all groups (e.g. in the UK many social workers do not see themselves as clinicians), but rather that this book is focussed on the emergent properties of the mental health system as a whole.

Author perspective

I write as a clinical academic, working in both the scientific world which values particular types of knowledge and the clinical world which involves individuals struggling to find a way forward in their life, and creating complex ethical and practice dilemmas for professionals.

Personally, I think mental illness is real in the sense of being a meaningful phenomenon. That said, strong statements such as 'schizophrenia is a brain disease' seem to me to go beyond the available evidence[9;10;14], and are as unhelpfully simplistic in understanding human experience as 'love is a brain condition'. In this I am influenced by my professional identity as a clinical psychologist, which socialises into a multiple-model view of the world. This is a good antidote to rigidity of thinking, but creates the vulnerability of being unable to say anything with clarity and certainty. I have tried to overcome this disability by communicating as clearly as possible what a mental health service which is focussed on personal recovery might look like. No doubt this makes visible my own beliefs, including tribal loyalties to my profession, a therapeutic orientation towards cognitive behavioural therapy and away from long-term psychological therapies, and my perspective on the diverse views of people using mental health services.

This book aims to highlight discrepancies between some aspects of current practice and what is needed to support personal recovery. It is not intended to be a comprehensive text-book on mental health care – excellent text-books already exist[15;16], and omission of a topic does not imply unimportance. Furthermore, presenting alternatives necessarily involves depicting current mental health services somewhat negatively. The danger is that some individual professionals may feel criticised, which is far from the intention. The clinical reader who thinks 'But I don't do that' may well be right. There is much to value in mental health services, and this book has emerged from seeing skilled, caring and recovery-promoting mental health professionals in action. Current mental health values and working practices which hinder recovery, insofar as they exist, are emergent system properties rather than resulting from the practice of individuals.

I do not write from the perspective of a consumer. However, many of the ideas on which this book is based have emerged from consumer rather than professional thinking about mental illness. My goal is to be a messenger: translating the consumer notion of recovery into the language and mindset of professionals. Inevitably, my own opinions (e.g. that recovery is at its heart an issue of social justice) may lead to translation errors. My hope is that the reader, whether consumer or professional, will choose to look past these biases and errors, and be challenged instead to create mental health services which focus on well-being more than illness, and are based on the priorities of the consumer rather than of the professional.

We turn now to the nuts-and-bolts of what mental illness is, and is not.

The nature of mental illness

What is mental illness?

The centre of gravity of mental illness is subjective experience. All branches of medicine require a combination of signs (observable indicators) and symptoms (subjective report of the patients) to reach a clinical explanation, but psychiatry is the only branch in which illnesses are primarily diagnosed and treated on the basis of the patient's self-report. There is no test which demonstrates that mental illness exists where neither the affected person nor the people in their life were aware of any problems. A central proposition then is that the start point for understanding mental illness is as an experience.

In this regard, mental illness differs from physical illness. Indeed, examples such as syphilis and epilepsy suggest that once a physical marker or cause is found, it moves to another branch of medicine and ceases to be viewed as a mental illness. The debate about the dividing line is of course ongoing, with calls for depression to be viewed as a neurological condition[17]. Overall, the pragmatic meaning of mental illness is a disorder with no established physical cause: a functional illness. The *emphasis* in understanding mental illness should be on the subjective experience.

What approaches have been developed to make sense of these experiences? Three broad ways of understanding mental illness have developed, which we call Clinical, Disability and Diversity models. We start with Clinical models, which are the dominant explanatory framework used in mental health services[18].

Clinical models

Clinical models are ways of seeing the world which have been developed by the various mental health professions, and which inform day-to-day clinical practice. The dominant professional group in mental health care has been psychiatry, and so inevitably many of the issues that will be raised relate to the ideas of psychiatry. However, the intention is not to criticise medical approaches specifically. Other groups have their models too, and if they were more dominant then the limitations of their models would become all too apparent. Indeed, at a personal level, one driver for writing this book was a recognition that psychological models do not always help individuals to make sense of their experiences. Rather, the intent is to raise cross-cutting issues with all clinical models used by mental health professionals, such as their emphasis on the role of the expert, privileged knowledge, best interests, and the central role expectation of intervening and treating.

One term we deliberately avoid is medical model, which is usually used pejoratively by non-medical people[19;20] to imply either a reductionist focus on biology to the exclusion of human experience or a general critique of the dominance of psychiatry[21;22]. Most mental health professionals are extremely aware of the suffering and the social challenges experienced by people with mental illness. However, since professionals often feel they can do little to directly influence the environment, they tend to focus on the individual. We will later argue that the social and environmental context of the person is too influential to be simply ignored.

Clinical models of mental disorder use evidence from clinical science, with a focus on accurate assessment of the individual followed by application of the evidence base to identify the most effective treatment. We will consider the three most commonly used models of mental disorder: biomedical, biopsychosocial and cognitive.

Clinical model 1: biomedical

The biomedical model of illness involves two key assumptions: an illness has a single underlying biological cause (a disease), and removal of this disease will result in a return to health[23]. Neither assumption is universally true in relation to mental illness. For example[23]:

> many patients present with symptoms that are not attributable to any underlying pathology or disease. Nevertheless, such patients are often given a medical diagnosis, implying an underlying structural cause and reflecting cultural expectations . . . Most healthcare systems also assume that treatment after diagnosis is brief and acts quickly. Indeed, the medical model might more accurately be termed the surgical model, given the pre-eminence of surgery in popular culture and health organisation.
>
> (p. 1399)

The biomedical model has been incorporated into medical understanding of mental illness, especially through the influence of the German philosopher and psychiatrist Karl Jaspers[24]. He emphasised the importance of understanding (*verstehen* in German) over causal explanation (*erklaren*). This leads in his phenomenological approach to the use of empathy and intuitive understanding by the clinician to establish meaningful connection with the inner world of the patient, through careful listening[24]: 'the phenomenological approach involves painstaking, detailed and laborious study of facts observed in the individual patient at the conscious level' (p. vi). This listening allows the clinician to see what the patient really means, and indeed to amplify or elaborate aspects which connect with or fit for the patient. However, this listening is not neutral – it is done to fit the patient's report into a predefined theoretical framework.

A key feature of Jasperian phenomenology is a belief in a universal *form* over a context-specific *content*: a third-person auditory hallucination is viewed as the same form for anyone who hears a voice talking about them, whether the voice is of an ancestor, a father, a childhood abuser, or an alien. Jaspers's phenomenology gives primacy to psychopathology in the individual (expressed in the form of diagnosis or symptoms) over the epiphenomenon of its socioculturally influenced expression in the environment. The purpose of the phenomenological approach is therefore to obtain a 'precise description of psychopathology'[25].

The biomedical model of mental illness is then a model of psychopathology, in which listening is used to elicit phenomena of psychopathology. Pat Bracken and Phil Thomas note that this focus on systematic examination of conscious mental phenomena is held up as a clear advance[26]:

> Most contemporary psychiatrists would argue that their assessments involve a detached, factual listing of the patient's symptoms accompanied by a clear analysis of the person's mental state . . . In this process, the experiences that trouble the patient . . . are taken out of the patient's own language and reformulated in psychiatric

> terminology . . . This process is carried out in an attempt to render psychiatric practice more scientific, the idea being that if we are to have a science of psychopathology, we need a clearly defined language through which a scientific discourse can proceed. Without this, we are 'limited' to a level of interpretation that is based only on personal narrative and locally defined meanings. A science of psychopathology demands concepts that are universally valid and reliable. In other words, it demands a concern with the 'forms' of psychopathology.
>
> (p. 108)

They go on to highlight the implicit assumption: 'Psychiatry has never really doubted the idea that a science of psychopathology is needed or even possible . . . It has never been in doubt that there *are* forms, diagnostic entities 'out there' awaiting identification and clarification' (p. 108). An assumption they challenge:

> Meaning involves relationships and interconnections; a background context against which things show up in different ways . . . The world of psychiatry, involving emotions, thoughts, beliefs and behaviours, is a world of meaning and thus context. Indeed, it is the centrality of these twin issues of meaning and context that separates the world of the 'mental' from the rest of medicine . . . psychiatry is precisely delineated by the fact that its *central* focus is the 'mental world' of its patients. Meaning and context are thus essential elements of the world of mental health and simply cannot be regarded as 'inconvenient limitations', issues that can be ignored or wished away.
>
> (pp. 109–110)

The interested reader is referred to their detailed discussion of the evolution of thinking about phenomenology. (Summarising, they argue that Jaspers's distinction between form and content reflects a Cartesian duality, and leads to a view that investigating phenomenology of form and hermeneutics – interpretation – of content are different activities. Heidegger's critique of this duality is that human reality is always embodied and encultured.) However, the point here is a pragmatic rather than philosophical one. The approach of eliciting features of psychopathology through mental state examination is a core feature of the biomedical model of mental illness. The problem with this is expressed by Lucy Johnstone[27]: '*Personal meaning is the first and biggest casualty of the biomedical model*' (p. 81). She elaborates:

> Psychiatry not only fails to address emotional and relationship problems, but actually reinforces them, for lack of a whole-person, whole-system way of understanding them. By using a medical label to 'Rescue' people, it takes responsibility away from them, encouraging them to rely on an external solution which is rarely forthcoming, and then blaming them for their continuing difficulties and powerlessness. The personal meaning of people's distressing experiences and the psychological and social origins of their difficulties are obscured by turning them into 'symptoms' of an 'illness' located within one individual.
>
> (p. 201)

The result of filtering human experience through the psychopathological sieve is an impoverished and decontextualised version of meaning. This ignores other approaches to understanding the experience of mental illness. For example, Simon Heyes has written an articulate guide for other consumers to recovery[28], and the resulting media coverage reported[29]:

> In Heyes view, people with mental health problems provide a sort of 'early warning system' for society. 'If dolphins start getting washed up on the beach, people start to

think there might be something wrong with the environment, they don't blame the dolphins for their lifestyle. Living in a constant state of flux places huge pressure on individuals. There is a perception of almost limitless choice combined with a sense of personal responsibility, while at the same time things that might have once given grounding have broken down.'

(p. 5)

How can the loss of meaning arising from Jasperian phenomenology be addressed? The approach used in the biopsychosocial model of mental illness is to more explicitly include consideration of psychological and social factors.

Clinical model 2: biopsychosocial

Most mental health professionals now align, at least in rhetoric, with a biopsychosocial model[30]. This model proposes that mental illness does not exist in a biological vacuum, and recognises that interpersonal, contextual and societal factors impact on the interpretation, onset, course and outcome of mental illness[31]. The model is based on a stress-vulnerability diathesis – that an internal vulnerability interacts with an aversive environment to produce psychotic experiences[32].

However, biopsychosocial models have been criticised for being disguised reincarnations of a biomedical model. As Repper and Perkins put it[4]:

It is a perspective which suggests that a person's thoughts and behaviour can be explained by physical malfunctioning, usually of neurotransmitters within the brain. Since it is clear that social and environmental factors have an impact on physical processes, an organic approach does not discount these influences, but views physical malfunctioning as the underlying cause of problems.

(p. 23)

This critique has an empirical basis. The anthropologist Robert Barrett found that the biopsychosocial model in reality gives primacy to the bio-[33]. His analysis of Australian psychiatric hospital casenotes indicated that schizophrenia is constructed as a disease process located externally to the person, which fragments the individual as an entity. The casenote structure divides the account of the person into segments, which are 'ambiguously connected elements including "history," "presenting complaint," "appearance," "insight," etc., based upon ideas such as . . . [the] "biopsychosocial" model of mental illness'[34]. In other words, and not surprisingly, the structure of the mental state examination influences the results obtained. If the questions implicitly locate the problem as an illness in the person, then the responses probably will as well.

In reality the biopsychosocial model is far more closely aligned with a biologically focussed biomedical model than with either psychological or social models. We illustrate this in relation to schizophrenia (Box 2.1).

This call for modesty in not over-extending what we know is a central value in this book.

The bio- in biopsychosocial

Lucy Johnstone points out that the biopsychosocial model has two meanings[35]. In a weak sense, it is of course true that biology and psychology and social all interact, but by explaining everything the model explains nothing. In a strong sense, the model gives primacy to the bio-part as the primary causal factor, hence preserving the assumption that psychological and social factors are merely triggers of an underlying illness, and do not have any inherent meaning. The key indicator of a biomedical model of illness – diagnosis – remains central to the biopsychosocial model, rather than one of three equally valued components. This has led even its adherents to reduce their ambitions for the model[36]: 'the value of the biopsychosocial model has not been in the discovery of new scientific laws, as the term 'new paradigm' would suggest, but rather in guiding parsimonious application of medical knowledge to the needs of each patient' (p. 576). Why does the biopsychosocial model give primacy to the bio-? One reason is that research is complex, needing to integrate biological (e.g. symptoms, genetic influence), psychological (e.g. interpersonal coping skills, resilience, cognitive stages of change), environmental (e.g. access to effective psychosocial rehabilitation programmes and supportive social networks) and sociopolitical (e.g. impact of stigma from the community, attributes of the treatment system, impact of consumer advocacy) levels[37]. Faced with this complexity, it is easy to understand why clinicians and researchers focus their efforts on the 'low-hanging fruit' of specific intrapsychic deficits.

Box 2.1 The causes of schizophrenia

The example of schizophrenia: what do we know about its causes?
Psychiatric epidemiology has identified many risk factors for schizophrenia[a]:
Odds ratio 8.0–10.0
  Family history
Odds ratio 6.0–7.9
  Obstetric central nervous system damage. Prenatal bereavement
Odds ratio 4.0–5.9
  Rubella. Central nervous system infection
Odds ratio 1.1–3.9
  Obstetric (hypoxia, Rh incompatibility, pre-eclampsia, low birth weight). Birth (winter, urban). Infection (influenza, respiratory, poliovirus). Prenatal (famine, flood, unwantedness, maternal deprivation)
Non-genetic sources of vulnerability have also been identified:
- Higher rates of childhood trauma in people who subsequently experience symptoms of psychosis than those who do not, with the possibility of a causal relationship shown by a dose–effect relationship[b,c].
- Reasonable[d] (though not undisputed[e]) evidence that cannabis is causal for schizophrenia, e.g. a study of 50 000 Swedish conscripts showing a dose–effect relationship, with the odds ratio for incident schizophrenia rising from 1.2 in those who had used cannabis at all before conscription to more than 6 in frequent cannabis users[f].

Current evidence indicates that the strongest effect is genetic. This is certainly a dominant element of psychoeducational programmes and information leaflets[g]. However, a comprehensive review of genetic evidence in schizophrenia concluded[h]:

> At present, the data for schizophrenia are confusing, and there are two broad possibilities. The first possibility is that the current findings for some of the best current genes are true. This implies that the genetics of schizophrenia are different from other complex traits in the existence of very high degrees of etiological heterogeneity: schizophrenia is hyper-complex, and we need to invoke more complicated genetic models than other biomedical disorders. The alternative possibility is that the current findings are clouded by Type 1 and Type 2 error. Schizophrenia is similar to other complex traits: it is possible that there are kernels of wheat, but it is highly likely that there is a lot of chaff . . . At present, we cannot resolve these possibilities.

(p. 617)

Box 2.1 (cont.)

Indeed, the largest study to date found no significant association between the strongest 14 candidate genes and schizophrenia[i]. What we know for sure is limited, even in highly researched conditions such as schizophrenia. Yet the presentation of schizophrenia research systematically over-emphasises the evidence that mental illness is a brain disease[j], and ignores alternative explanations[k,l,m,n]. Especially given the huge disparity in funding for biological versus other ways of understanding schizophrenia, current evidence does not support giving absolute primacy to biology in understanding schizophrenia. The mechanism of interaction between identified risk factors remains unclear, with credible proposals covering biology (e.g. phenotypic expression[o], dopaminergic dysregulation[p]), psychology (e.g. bias against disconfirmatory evidence[q], jumping to conclusions[r]) and social (e.g. economic systems[m]). Since biological, psychological and social factors are all potentially implicated, a truly biopsychosocial model of schizophrenia – rather than one giving primacy to biological explanations – is indicated.

Notes:

[a]Murray RM, Jones PB, Susser E, van Os J, Cannon M. *The Epidemiology of Schizophrenia*. Cambridge: Cambridge University Press; 2003.

[b]Read J. Childhood trauma, psychosis and schizophrenia: a literature review with theoretical and clinical implications. *Acta Psychiatrica Scandinavica* 2005; 112:330–350.

[c]Raine A, Mellingen K, Liu J, Venables P, Mednick S. Effects of environmental enrichment at ages 3–5 years on schizotypal personality and antisocial behavior at ages 17 and 23 years. *American Journal of Psychiatry* 2003; 160:1627–1635.

[d]Henquet C, Murray R, Linszen D, van Os J. The environment and schizophrenia: the role of cannabis use. *Schizophrenia Bulletin* 2005; 31:608–612.

[e]Hall W, Degenhardt L, Teesson M. Cannabis use and psychotic disorders: an update. *Drug and Alcohol Review* 2004; 23:433–443.

[f]Zammit S, Lewis G. Exploring the relationship between cannabis use and psychosis. *Addiction* 2004; 99: 1353–1355.

[g]Read J. Schizophrenia, drug companies and the internet. *Social Science and Medicine* 2008; 66:99–109.

[h]Sullivan PF. The genetics of schizophrenia. *PLoS Medicine* 2005; 2(7):e212 0614–0618.

[i]Sanders AR, Duan J, Levinson DF, et al. No significant association of 14 candidate genes with schizophrenia in a large European ancestry sample: implications for psychiatric genetics. *American Journal of Psychiatry* 2008; 165:497–506.

[j]Boyle M. It's all done with smoke and mirrors. Or, how to create the illusion of a schizophrenic brain disease. *Clinical Psychology* 2002; 12:9–16.

[k]Read J, Mosher L, Bentall RP (eds). *Models of Madness: Psychological, Social and Biological Approaches to Schizophrenia*. Hove: Brunner-Routledge; 2004.

[l]Boyle M. *Schizophrenia, a Scientific Delusion? 2nd edn*. London: Routledge; 2002.

[m]Warner R. *Recovery from Schizophrenia: Psychiatry and Political Economy*, 3rd edn. New York: Brunner-Routledge; 2004.

[n]Ross CA, Pam A (eds). *Pseudoscience in Biological Psychiatry: Blaming the body*. New York: John Wiley; 1995.

[o]Tsuang MT. Schizophrenia: genes and environment. *Biological Psychiatry* 2000; 3(1):210–220.

[p]Murray R. Phenomenology and life course approach to psychosis: symptoms, outcome, and cultural variation. *Psychiatric Research Report* 2006; 22(3):13.

[q]Woodward T, Moritz S, Cuttler C, Whitman J. The contribution of a cognitive bias against disconfirmatory evidence (BADE) to delusions in schizophrenia. *Journal of Clinical and Experimental Neuropsychology* 2006; 28(4):605–617.

[r]Colbert SM, Peters E. Need for closure and jumping-to-conclusions in delusion-prone individuals. *Journal of Nervous and Mental Disease* 2002; 190(1):27–31.

A second reason may be professional. If what is currently understood to be a mental illness moves to being understood as primarily a psychological or social phenomenon, then this has potential implications for the status and power of existing professional groups. For example, it is unclear how this will fit with the struggle of psychiatry to position itself as a legitimate branch of medicine, with equal status and credibility. This struggle finds expression in the neo-Kraepelinian (i.e. following Emil Kraepelin) movement towards an emphasis on reliable diagnosis and application of evidence-based medicine in psychiatry. Nancy Andreasen predicted in her influential book 'The Broken Brain' that future psychiatric consultations would last for no more than 15 minutes, to allow the optimal medication to be chosen[38]. Clearly, such a consultation has no room for the messiness of meaning.

Whatever the reason, the emphasis on biology in biomedical and biopsychosocial models has not been without its critics. Concern has been expressed by many psychiatrists, including Duncan Double[39], Ronnie Laing[40], Joanna Moncrieff[41], Marius Romme[42], Thomas Szasz[43] and Pat Bracken and Phil Thomas[26]. Nonetheless, these models remain dominant[44]: 'At present, almost all of health care spending is directed at biomedically oriented care. As George Engel[30] stated 30 years ago ". . . nothing will change unless or until those who control resources have the wisdom to venture off the beaten path of exclusive reliance on biomedicine as the only approach to health care"' (p. 2). Biomedical and biopsychosocial models have many strengths. They are systematised bodies of knowledge, amenable to testing and amendment in the light of new knowledge. They are transferable across time and space – an intervention developed in one country can at least in theory be transferred to another, and new generations of health professionals can be trained into the models of the previous. Clinical models lead to action – they provide guidance for expert practitioners about what to do. Finally, and most importantly, the testimonies of individuals show that many patients have benefited from the treatments based on these clinical models.

However, the goal of this book is to argue for a transformation *within* mental health services, so it is helpful to map out problems as a precursor to arguing for this change. Therefore we now review some of the negative implications of these models. A central argument is that the imposition or use without reservation of any clinical model is unjustified in almost all circumstances.

What's the problem?

To understand why there is a problem, it is helpful to illuminate the core assumptions and evolved working practices of the biomedical and the biopsychosocial clinical models. These are shown in Table 2.1.

Any characterisation is necessarily limited by outliers. Clinicians working with mentally disordered offenders might view their primary role as protection of the public. Clinicians working with people experiencing early psychosis or long-term mental illness may have a more nuanced rhetoric about recovery than 'getting back to normal'. However, these assumptions and working practices are found in most mental health services. The problem is that they do not fit reality, in four ways:

Mismatch 1: mental illness is not (only) *caused* by disturbed homeostasis
Mismatch 2: diagnosis does not 'cut nature at its joints'
Mismatch 3: assessment processes create stigma
Mismatch 4: treatment does not cure
We now consider each mismatch.

Mismatch 1: mental illness is not (only) caused by disturbed homeostasis

The Jasperian distinction between understanding and explaining is crucial. Understanding is an *interpretation* or a partial view of a phenomenon. Since there are always many possible interpretations, no single understanding is intrinsically superior – they cannot be ranked a priori. We can certainly construct methods of ranking different understandings. The degree

Table 2.1 Working practices in the biomedical and biopsychosocial models

Domain	Dominant concept/approach
Responsibilities and relationships	
Ethical imperatives on clinicians	Acting in best interests, responsibility for the patient
Clinician's primary responsibility	To diagnose and treat the mental illness
Patient's primary responsibility	To take treatment as prescribed
Clinician's relationship with patient	Expert and authoritative
Assessment	
Basic understanding of mental illness	Psychopathology resulting from disturbed homeostasis
Assessment focus	Intrapsychic deficits and problems
Meaning attributed by the patient	Peripheral
Assessment goal	To identify the mental illness and hence make a diagnosis
Action	
Driver for clinical and patient action	Avoidance motivation – the avoidance of symptoms or suffering
Focus of action	Clinicians treating the patient
Proximal aim of treatment	Symptom reduction, functional improvement
Distal aim of treatment	Cure the illness
Evaluation of treatment success	By the clinician, through objective outcome assessment
Meaning of recovery	Restoration of disturbed homeostasis – getting back to normal

of consensus and the implications for specific stakeholder groups are common approaches. But these are post hoc constructions – there is nothing intrinsically better about one interpretation over another. Therefore the usefulness of a particular understanding should be judged in relation to whether it is helpful, not whether it is true (i.e. measurably more accurate than other understandings).

By contrast, an explanation reveals something of the *essence* of a phenomenon. Explanations can be ranked – the best explanations most closely fit current observable data and are a better predictor of the future. At any point in time, it is reasonable to treat an explanation as the closest available approximation to a true picture of what is going on. This revelatory aspect justifies primacy over descriptive accounts.

The centre of gravity of the biomedical and biopsychosocial models is diagnosis. But there is a key difference between diagnoses of physical and mental illness. A diagnosis of a physical illness provides an explanation. The statement *'Inflammation of the meninges causes meningitis'* is an explanation, and more true than the descriptive lists of the signs and symptoms of meningitis (each of which may be present in a specific patient to a differing amount). It tells us something of what is going on (aetiology) and how things will unfold (prognosis), irrespective of what the patient believes or the social context of the patient.

A diagnosis of a mental illness, on the other hand, is an understanding. The statement *'Bereavement causes depression'* is an understanding, which may or may not apply or be helpful for different patients with depression. Its utility depends crucially on the beliefs and context of the patient and whether they find it a useful way of making sense of the experience. It is descriptive, not explanatory. Hence the axiom that *diagnosis is prognosis*[45] is true in physical illness (because explanations predict) but does not apply within mental illness. As the creators of DSM-IV-TR (www.dsmivtr.org) put it:'Patients sharing the same diagnostic label do not necessarily have disturbances that share the same etiology nor would they necessarily respond to the same treatment.' A conceptual framework for identifying the implications of this distinction is provided by Ray Pawson and Nick Tilley, in their seminal book *'Realistic Evaluation'*[46]. They identify two theories of causation: generative and successionist[47]. **Successionist theory** holds that causation is unobservable, and observational data are the only mechanism for inferring causality. This theory leads to the methods of experimental manipulation and pre-post-comparison of experimental and control groups. **Generative theory**, by contrast, holds that there is an observable connection between causally connected events, and that internal features of the thing being changed are central to understanding causality.

Within this framework, a successionist notion of causality underpins the statement *Gravity causes an apple to fall to Earth*. The word 'causes' could be prefaced with 'always'. A statement underpinned by a generative notion of causality would be *Rising house prices cause consumer confidence to fall*. The word 'cause' cannot here be prefaced by 'always'. In a health context, the statement *'Inflammation of the meninges causes meningitis'* is successionist, whereas *'Bereavement causes depression'* is generative.

Pawson and Tilley apply this distinction to social programmes, which they define as 'the interplays of individual and institution, of agency and structure, and of micro and macro social processes' (p. 63). They argue for a move from a successionist to a generative model of causation, in which 'causal outcomes follow from mechanisms acting in contexts' (p. 58). Prediction can then be made through an understanding of the causal mechanisms linking input with outcome and of the contextual factors influencing these processes.

This distinction allows an unpicking of two meanings of the term 'mental illness is caused by disturbed homeostasis'. One meaning is that mental illness is observable in the biological substrate. This is true but uninteresting. All human feelings and behaviours can be observed at the level of biology – consider the experiences of savouring, being in love, sexual arousal, aggression, etc. These experiences can clearly also be understood as psychological or social phenomena. It may of course be helpful to understand the biological correlates of mental illness, since these may provide points of remedial intervention, but they do not explain mental illness.

The second meaning is that mental illness occurs as a result of disturbed homeostasis – all would be well if it were not for the imbalance in these internal processes, and mental illness exists and can be explained in isolation from psychological and social context. It is this explanatory meaning which is explicitly rejected by taxonomists. Identification of invariant final common pathways which are biological (e.g. dopamine dysregulation) or effective treatments targeting restoration of homeostasis (e.g. pharmacotherapy) only impacts on how useful the understanding is – it does not provide an explanation. Mental illness is not *essentially* biological. This is concordant with the emphasis on context in *Postpsychiatry*[26]:

> A key element of what we call postpsychiatry is the view that modernist psychiatry has been built on what some commentators have called 'methodological individualism', the assumption that different psychological states can be examined in isolation from the world around them. Postpsychiatry seeks to overcome this orientation by bringing contextual issues centre stage. By contextual issues, we are referring to the fact that human psychology is always embodied (wrapped up in the complex biology of a

human body), encultured (involved in the linguistic, cultural and political reality of the society in which it exists) and temporal (never fixed, but constantly in flux and always involved in a journey from past to future).

(p. 170)

The experience and interpretation of mental illness occurs within this complex social vortex of biology, culture and time. This is depicted in the model of the person shown in Figure 2.1.

Figure 2.1 is not of course meant to be a grand theory of the person, so it is deliberately left unelaborated. (I would include existential and spiritual as other important dimensions – others would have different preferences.) Rather, the diagram is intended to make the simple point that increasing understanding at any modality (e.g. biological, psychological, etc.) is a welcome scientific advance, but does not – and cannot – provide *the* explanation of experience. This interconnectedness of levels of explanation is beginning to be discussed in mainstream psychiatric literature[48].

A generative model of causation is more helpful to understand why bereavement causes depression in some people but not in others. This would involve moving away from the decontextualised invariant understanding exemplified by diagnosis, and instead seeking to understand the meaning and context of mental illness. For some people, their experience is most helpfully understood in terms of a mental illness diagnosis. For others, it is not. This is why the invariant use of a biomedical or biopsychosocial model is sometimes helpful, sometimes insufficient, and sometimes toxic. This issue is often apparent in clinical practice. For example, I was asked to provide psychological therapy for a woman with 'treatment-resistant depression'. The referral letter detailed her depressive symptomatology and the various pharmacological approaches which had been tried with the patient, none of which had successfully treated her depression. When I met the lady, she disclosed that she was being regularly beaten by her husband. Although she clearly was depressed as a consequence, the use of depression as an explanation for her experiences was toxic.

A mental illness diagnosis should therefore not be treated *as if* it is an explanation. If diagnosis is one of many ways of understanding, what does this mean for clinicians? A truly evidence-based clinician (i.e. one who recognises the limitations of their world-view) would offer their expertise as a resource, which may or may not be helpful to or utilised by the patient. This clearly will involve a role transition. It may be reasonable to state to a patient '*You have meningitis*', if this is the best available explanation. The statement '*You have depression*' is a different animal – it should more precisely be stated as '*Your experience can be understood as depression*'. This then becomes an informed suggestion about how it might

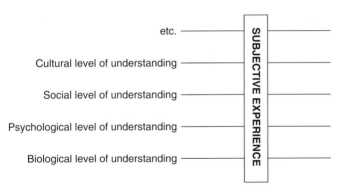

Figure 2.1 A model of subjective experience.

be helpful to understand the experience, rather than an authoritative pronouncement about what is really going on.

This will be challenging for professionals trained to believe they are being taught how things really are. Diagnosis does not reveal truth – it has a different purpose[49]: 'The primary purpose of the DSM is to facilitate communication among mental health professionals.' Viewing diagnosis as primarily an inter-professional communication aid rather than a revealed truth would lead to a tentative attitude towards diagnostic categories. This tentativeness would occur not because of a desire to withhold the awful truth from the patient, but because of a recognition that diagnosis no more captures what is really going on than a book can be described by listing all the words it contains. Beyond a certain point, headcounts (of words or symptoms) have no information content. Knowing the number of times that depression-related words occur in a book may say something about what the book is about, but knowing the number of times the letter 'e' occurs adds virtually nothing. Similarly, each taxonomic iteration has diminishing returns. At the time of writing, great effort and debate is going into the development of DSM-V. What is striking is that this edifice of descriptive psychopathology will probably have no impact whatsoever on clinical practice. Beyond a certain level of granularity, all people with symptoms of psychosis are (literally and clinically) treated the same. Again, this is recognised by the leaders of DSM-V (www.dsm5.org/planning.cfm): 'limitations in the current diagnostic paradigm embodied in the current DSM-IV suggest that future research efforts that are exclusively focused on refining the DSM-defined syndromes may never be successful in uncovering their underlying etiologies.' In this regard a certain humility is called for. The semantic groupings which were used to make sense of difference 200 years ago are unrecognisable from the diagnostic categories in use today. Without doubt, in another 200 years the way we conceptualise subjective experiences will be similarly different. To make categorical pronouncements that a disorder exists and that the patient has it does not reflect this changing reality. We now explore this point further.

Mismatch 2: diagnosis does not 'cut nature at its joints'

A consequence of viewing diagnosis as a partial understanding rather than as a revelatory explanation is that there cannot be stable, invariant (over time and culture) psychopathological diagnostic categories. Therefore we would expect debate about diagnostic categories to be based on non-empirical considerations. This is exactly what we find.

The history of how diagnostic categories have come and gone from DSM is salutary reading for anyone who views diagnosis as objective descriptions of discrete disorders. The battle between neo-Kraepelinians and psychoanalysts over 'neurosis', successive gay rights demonstrations eventually leading to the removal of 'homosexuality' as late as 1974, and debates about paraphilia as a mental illness[50] are simply some of the more interesting tips of the diagnostic iceberg. The issue can again be illustrated in relation to schizophrenia.

Box 2.2 captures some of the debate about the diagnosis, but the point to note is that this is not a scientific debate – the absence of a disease marker for schizophrenia means that arguments for and against it relate to its clinical and social consequences, rather than its empirical basis as a discrete disorder.

The diagnostic endeavour is out of control. The Diagnostic and Statistical Manual (DSM) I contained 112 mental disorders when published in 1952. This has risen incrementally: 182 in DSM-II (1968); 265 in DSM-III (1980); and 374 in DSM-IV (1994). The only obvious hindrances to introducing new diagnostic categories are the views of existing stakeholders (e.g. psychoanalysts) or 'patient' groups (e.g. gay and lesbian people). These

Box 2.2 The diagnosis of schizophrenia

The example of schizophrenia: should the diagnosis be retained?
The validity of the diagnostic category of 'schizophrenia' has been repeatedly challenged[a,b,c]. This has led to the suggestion from some consumer groups, such as the Campaign for the Abolition of the Schizophrenia Label (www.asylumonline.net), to abolish the label 'schizophrenia'. Even from within psychiatry there are calls to discontinue the term as stigmatising, not scientifically valid and unhelpfully focussing on a biological explanation of what is a heterogeneous and context-influenced disorder[d].

One response has been to argue that we should keep the status quo, because changing the name may foster a belief that the person rather than the illness is to blame for their symptoms[e].

Another approach has been used in Japan, where the previous term for schizophrenia (*Seishin Bunretsu Byo* – a disease of a split and disorganised mind) has been replaced with *Togo-Shicchou-Sho* (a transient state of loosened association)[f]. However, this approach has been criticised on the grounds that stigmatising associations are not reduced simply by changing the name[g].

A third response is to propose 'better' categories. For example, David Kingdon proposes to replace Schizophrenia with Sensitivity Psychosis, Post Traumatic Stress Psychosis, Anxiety Psychosis, Drug-related Psychosis. He showed that whereas 63% of service users were negative about the term schizophrenia, this proportion dropped to 16% with these new terms[h], and in a study of 241 medical students there was a much greater likelihood of generating positive views about the potential of recovery with these new categories[i].

Notes:
[a]Read J, Mosher L, Bentall RP (eds). *Models of Madness: Psychological, Social and Biological Approaches to Schizophrenia.* Hove: Brunner-Routledge; 2004.
[b]Maddux JE. Stopping the "madness". Positive psychology and the deconstruction of the illness ideology and the DSM. In: Snyder CR, Lopez JS, eds. *Handbook of Positive Psychology.* New York: Oxford; 2002. 13–24.
[c]Boyle M. *Schizophrenia, a Scientific Delusion?* 2nd edn. London: Routledge; 2002.
[d]Kingdon D. Down with schizophrenia. *New Scientist* 2007; **2625**:22.
[e]Penn DL. Politically correct labels and schizophrenia. A rose by any other name? *Schizophrenia Bulletin* 2001; **27**:197–203.
[f]Kim Y, Berrios GE. Impact of the term schizophrenia on the culture of ideograph: the Japanese experience. *Schizophrenia Bulletin* 2001; **27**(2):181–185.
[g]Lieberman J, First MB. Renaming schizophrenia. *BMJ* 2007; **334**:108.
[h]Kingdon D. Down with schizophrenia. *New Scientist* 2007; **2625**:22.
[i]Kingdon D, Kinoshita K, Naeem F, Swelam M, Hansen L, Vincent S et al. Schizophrenia can and should be renamed. *BMJ* 2007; **334**:221–222.

are an insufficient buttress against the two powerful forces which have led to this avalanche of diagnostic categories – 'a kaleidoscope of putative disorders'[51]. The first force is a consequence of Enlightenment values. As Bracken and Thomas put it[26]:

> One important promise of the Enlightenment was that human pain and suffering
> would be overcome by the advance of rationality and science. To this end, psychiatry
> has attempted to replace spirituality, moral, political and folk understandings of
> madness with the framework of psychopathology. The culmination of this was the
> 'decade of the brain' when it was firmly asserted that the causes of madness are to be
> found in neurotransmitter abnormalities.
>
> (p. 9)

The second spur to this 'development' has been a confluence of commercial and professional interests. The greater the spread of diagnostic categories, the more money is to be made in treating these conditions, and the more influence can be obtained by mental health professions. One in eight adults in the USA are now prescribed anti-depressants each year[52]. The opening up of new markets by pharmaceutical companies through disease marketing[53] is discussed in Chapter 6.

This increase in diagnostic categories is not science – it is colonisation of the human condition. It is also not a neutral activity – it directly impacts on social understandings of human experience[54]: 'DSM is a guidebook that tells us how we should think about manifestations of sadness and anxiety, sexual activities, alcohol and substance abuse, and many other behaviours. Consequently, the categories created for DSM reorient our thinking about important social matters and affect our social institutions' (p. 11). This issue is particularly germane to psychiatry, given the centrality of diagnosis to professional practice. David Whitwell, a psychiatrist, notes and apparently agrees with the concerns about diagnosis expressed by clinical psychologist Richard Bentall[14], but then concludes:

> Bentall is able to do this because he is a psychologist. For a psychiatrist the fact remains that having a diagnosis is still central to medical ways of understanding people with mental health problems. If I, as a psychiatrist, were to say to a court or a tribunal that after assessing someone's condition . . . that they had serious problems, but I did not choose to make a diagnosis, it would call into question whether I was acting as a psychiatrist at all . . . It is a bit like asking the church to consider the claims of atheism. There is a whole world of psychiatric literature, and much of it only makes sense on the assumption that there are separate mental illnesses.[22]
>
> (p. 30)

If clinical practice is to match reality, then it needs to be recognised that diagnosis is one of many ways of making sense of experience. This is important, because giving a diagnosis is a powerful act. Some people find a diagnosis to be positively helpful in making sense of their experiences[55]:'Getting a diagnosis helped. It at least gave me the chance to say "I agree with this diagnosis", and it gave me a starting point to work forward from' (p. 54). Whereas for others, it is a hindrance to recovery[56]: 'Certainly to my self-esteem, to the people I go to church with, the people that I've worked with, to my family, to former friends, [being given a diagnosis of schizophrenia has] been a big disadvantage' (p. 29). It is this aspect of diagnosis to which we now turn.

Mismatch 3: assessment processes create stigma

As we will discuss more in Chapter 16, clinical assessment should cover four dimensions[57]:

Dimension 1: deficiencies and undermining characteristics of the person
Dimension 2: strengths and assets of the person
Dimension 3: lacks and destructive factors in the environment
Dimension 4: resource and opportunities in the environment

However, to make a diagnosis only Dimension 1 need be considered. Since assessment in biomedical and biopsychosocial models is oriented towards making a diagnosis, clinical interactions tend to focus on Dimension 1. This focus leads to three problems[57]:

Problem 1. Deindividuation

The process of labelling leads to perceptions of diminished within-group differences and exaggerated between-group differences[58]. This creates a toxic cocktail with the *optimal distinctiveness theory*[59], which suggests that identification with a group simultaneously meets the need for similarity (through within-group comparisons) and difference (through between-group comparisons). People who are made to believe that they are very different from others will assert their similarity by identifying with large, inclusive and indistinctive groups. The resulting genuine lack of distinctiveness then provides confirmatory evidence for the belief that people with mental illness are fundamentally similar. Social psychology experiments show that within-group deindividuation (attenuation of differences) has consequences for how the person is seen. For example, more 'librarian-like' behaviour is remembered about a person when they are presented as a librarian than as a waitress[60]. The issue is recognised in caveats attached to DSM-IV[61]:

> Individuals sharing a diagnosis are likely to be heterogeneous even in regard to the defining features of the diagnosis
>> There is a need to . . . capture additional information that goes far beyond diagnosis
>> A common misconception is that a classification of mental disorders classifies people, when actually what are being classified are disorders that people have.

This subtlety is not, however, evident in research[62], public perception[63] or clinical practice[33]. For example, a review of how diagnosis is used in research studies showed a decline in the proportion of people-categorising instances (e.g. 'schizophrenic', 'borderline patients') from 94%–100% (across diagnoses) in 1975–9 to approximately 50% in 2000–4. The authors conclude[62]: 'Terminology categorizing patients continues to be used and is still used equally as often as terminology categorizing disorders among people who are supposed to be the most educated about this important human rights issue' (p. 103). Labelling with a diagnosis emphasises similarity with others from the same group. The huge amount of financial and human resource put into establishing the reliability of categorising increasingly fine-grained slices of human experience cannot disguise the essentially impoverished (i.e. lacking ecological validity) picture that results. People with the same mental illness are fundamentally different from each other. A key problem with diagnosis is that it ignores these differences.

Problem 2. Neglect of environment

The neglect of environment in diagnostic taxonomies is *almost* total. The exception is Axis IV 'Psychosocial and environmental problems'. However, the influence of this axis on current clinical practice is virtually nil, and in any event the Axis focus is on problems (i.e. Dimension 3), not resources (Dimension 4). Indeed, the advice is to avoid listing 'so-called positive stressors, such as a job promotion' unless they 'constitute or lead to a problem'[61] (p.29). This focus on individual over environment is discordant with the experiences of people with mental illness, with the result that 'many of them find biomedical interpretations limited – at best unhelpful, and at worst harmful'[64].

Problem 3. Negative bias

The concepts of saliency, value and context combine in toxic ways in mental illness to lead to a negative bias. If something about the person stands out sufficiently (i.e. with sufficient **saliency**, such as a diagnostic label presented as an explanatory fact) and is regarded as having a negative **value** (i.e. has stigmatising associations), and if the **context** is vague or sparse (i.e. nothing else is known about the person), then this will adversely influence views about the person[65]. Use of diagnosis as an explanation accompanied by neglect of the environment leads directly to a negative perception about the person.

This negative bias is then maintained through a learned clinical discourse which systematically elicits risk factors, problems and deficits, and substantially ignores protective factors, strengths and abilities. For example, protective developmental factors associated with good psychosocial resilience are shown in Table 2.2[66].

Table 2.2 Protective developmental factors associated with psychosocial resilience

Level	Type	Protective factor
Child	Cognitive	Intelligence; problem-solving skills; attentional skills; easy temperament (infant) and adaptability (later)
	Personality	Positive self-perceptions; self-efficacy; faith/sense of meaning in life; positive outlook; good sense of humour; sociability/attractiveness to others
	Emotional	Ability to self-regulate emotions; self-esteem; values own talents
Family	Caregiver	Close relationship with adult caregivers; authoritative parenting (high warmth, structure, monitoring and expectations); parental involvement in child's education; parents with protective factors listed for child (above)
	Environmental	Positive family climate; low parental discord; organised home environment; close relationships with other prosocial, competent, supportive adults; connections to prosocial and rule-abiding peers
	Social	Post-secondary education of parents; socioeconomic advantages
Community	Educational	Effective schools; ties to prosocial organisations (e.g. clubs, scouts)
	Environmental	High 'collective efficacy' in neighbourhood; high public safety; good emergency services; good public health care availability

These factors are not elicited during clinical assessment. Indeed, they are not taught in most professional training. By contrast, the risk factors for schizophrenia (shown earlier in Box 2.1) will all be assessed during a 'good' history-taking. Current assessment procedures are guaranteed to show up some deviation or other, such as a breakdown experienced by your great-aunt ('family history of mental illness'), a forceps delivery ('perinatal complications'), taking longer than typical to learn to walk ('delayed developmental milestones'), finding it hard to make friends ('schizoid personality'), and being naughty ('conduct disorder') – all of which become evidence for the validity of a diagnosis. The confirmation bias that results further reinforces the belief that patients have deficits and problems, but few intrinsic strengths. As Peter Chadwick puts it[67]:

> Deficit-obsessed research can only produce theories and attitudes which are disrespectful of clients and are also likely to induce behaviour in clinicians such that service users are not properly listened to, not believed, not fairly assessed, are likely treated as inadequate and are also not expected to be able to become independent and competent individuals in managing life's tasks.

Sometimes the absurdity of the resulting assessment discourse is highlighted, as by the woman with a diagnosis of schizophrenia who exasperatedly exclaimed during an interview[68]: 'Why don't you ever ask me what I do to help myself?' (p. 182). It is also parodied, as in Chadwick's call to add Pathologically Middle-of-the-Road Personality Disorder (MORPID) and Totally Colourless Personality Syndrome (TOCOLOPS) to DSM-V[69]. Chadwick was one of the first writers to write from the perspective of a consumer academic[67]:

> Rather than concentrating on those aspects of the psychology and physiology of schizophrenic people that reveal *deficits*, this [book] attempts to turn the coin over and seek what has become known as the 'schizophrenic credit'. In the context of this endeavour it is legitimate to ask, for example, whether . . . schizophrenia-prone people . . . have areas of enhanced functioning compared to 'standard-minded' people.
>
> (p. xii, references omitted)

This focus on deficits has several implications. It creates an assessment mentality in which the patient is a holder of a mental illness, and the illness can be identified through a mental state examination. By emphasising difference, it maintains stigmatising views within mental health professionals[70]. It supports the belief that the clinician's job is to treat the illness, not the person's job to recover their life. It fosters dependency – the good patient is compliant with treatment. Finally, since the treatment doesn't actually cure the person, a role as a person with mental illness can become an engulfing role[71]. Rapp and Goscha identify the implications of this last process[72]:

- These engulfing roles – bag lady, junkie, schizophrenic – are viewed in a highly negative way by others
- People in these roles increasingly associate only with others in the same group, leading to impoverished social networks
- The person is defined by others exclusively in terms of their engulfing role
- There are no established routes of gaining status in, or exiting from, the role
- There are therefore few incentives to set or work towards realistic longer-term goals, leading to impoverished expectations of a good future
- There is an absence of natural processes that lead people to recognise and amend their unrealistic perceptions or attributions
- Poverty is common and opportunities to become economically productive are limited, which creates further stress and, in some, the desire to seek reinstitutionalisation.

A deficit-focussed assessment process aimed at establishing diagnosis creates stigma. Lucy Johnstone illustrates the impact on people following diagnosis[35]:

> I walked into (the psychiatrist's office) as Don and walked out a schizophrenic . . . I remember feeling afraid, demoralised, evil.
>
> The diagnosis becomes a burden . . . you are an outcast in society. It took me years to feel OK about myself again.
>
> The killing of hope . . . it almost feels like, well, your hands are tied, your cards laid and your fate set.
>
> I think schizophrenia will always make me a second class citizen . . . I am labelled for the rest of my life.
>
> Once it was known that I had spent time in the 'nutters' hospital, my neighbours gave me hell.

This diagnostic frame of reference is in marked contrast to how most individuals make sense of their problems[73]: 'Being treated in a medicalised way, as if they had physical illnesses, formed the basis of negative evaluations and complaints on the part of most users in every aspect of their management . . . In summary, the professional discourse and the lay discourse about personal distress are incompatible.' This discordance persists in public explanations[63]: 'The public, internationally, continues to prefer psychosocial to biogenetic explanations and treatments for schizophrenia.' This tension is not present to the same degree in physical illness. Even in chronic conditions, people do not self-label as a diabetes service avoider, or an asthma clinic survivor, or a renal unit ex-inmate. I have heard DSM-IV described by consumers as *The Book Of Insults*. Peter Chadwick notes that[67]: 'even the briefest perusal of the current literature on schizophrenia will immediately reveal to the uninitiated that this collection of problems is viewed by practitioners almost exclusively in terms of dysfunction and disorder. A positive or charitable phrase or sentence rarely meets the eye' (p. xii). The acceptance of a deficit-saturated reality has profound consequences for role expectations. Since patients are not seen as having any self-righting capacity, and since few environmental strengths and supports are identified, the person needs to be 'righted' through treatment by others. We therefore turn now to treatment.

Mismatch 4: treatment does not cure

The need to treat has been described by David Whitwell as 'the curse of psychiatry'[22]:

> The professionals know that they can be judged to be negligent if they fail to use the powers [of compulsion] available to them. The psychological effects of this are profound on both sides. The effects have become more intense in recent years due to high profile cases where professionals have been blamed for failing to prevent disasters. The message that has come from such cases is that members of staff are responsible for the outcome; – that if only they did their jobs properly, tragedies would not happen.
>
> (p. 171)

He identifies naïve psychiatric practice as based on a belief that treatment makes people recover, and so the job of medical professionals is to deliver treatment. This is true not only of psychiatry. In the UK, care plans set out the planned intervention elements, and are written by the care manager (generally nurses, occupational therapists or social workers). An audit of 1732 care plan entries for 244 patients found that 74% of actions involved staff doing something *to* the patient, with only 14% involving doing something *with* the patient and 11% the person doing something for themselves[74]. Treatment involving the clinician doing something to the patient is the norm.

The problem with this approach is that the promise of treatment leading to cure is not delivered. Each new round of treatment (e.g. insulin coma therapy, psychosurgery, electro-convulsive therapy) has heralded a 'revived cult of curability'[75]. Invariably, some patients benefit (reinforcing clinician's beliefs about the effectiveness of the treatment). But some partially or temporarily benefit, and some seem to decline despite (or, perhaps, because of) aggressive treatment. The initial optimism soon fades, and the limitations of the treatment for both staff and patients become apparent. Creating an expectation that the expert clinician will treat and cure the patient is actively unhelpful. As Whitwell puts it[22]: 'It is unfair to give treatment saying that it will bring about recovery – yet knowing it will not; saying that the treatment is enough to make an average person better – so if it doesn't work for you, then it must be your fault. Giving directions, yet knowing that nobody reaches the destination' (p. 15). The biopsychosocial model contains a double bind[35]: the message about responsibility is both 'you have a medical illness with primarily biological causes' and 'your problems are a meaningful and understandable response to your life circumstances'. This creates unresolvable contradictions: you have an illness which is not your fault BUT you retain responsibility for it and must make an effort to get better BUT you must do it our way because we are the experts in your illness. This leads to some of the 'problem behaviours' which are evident in mental health services: not taking medication (non-compliance) versus keeping asking for medication (too dependent); not accepting they're ill (lacks insight) versus sitting around on the ward not getting better (sick role behaviour); being too demanding of services (leading to a borderline personality disorder diagnosis) versus not engaging with services (leading to assertive outreach team involvement). Within this parody is a serious reality: services often inadvertently end up replicating the very problem that brought the person into contact with services.

A focus on treatment as something done to the patient has two specifically damaging effects. First, it locates the primary responsibility for change in the wrong place – with the clinician rather than with the patient. This assumption is imported from health contexts where patient passivity is an advantage (e.g. surgery), although even in physical health settings the debate about the role of lifestyle (e.g. patient behaviours such as smoking or over-eating) is unresolved.

Second, the assumption that treatment involves the clinician doing something to the patient constrains possible solutions. For example, protective factors for resilience were described in Table 2.2, and it was noted that these are not in general assessed when taking a history. Their absence means that interventions to promote resilience are unlikely to be considered, which (drawing from Table 2.2) might include community programmes to reduce teenage substance misuse, easy access to emergency housing, community policing to reduce crime levels, individual tuition to improve academic attainment, building skateboard parks, funding and supporting attendance at youth clubs, teaching effective coping strategies, developing mentoring relationships with prosocial older children, providing extra-curricular activities to foster relations with prosocial peers, and supporting cultural traditions that provide opportunities for bonds with prosocial adults[66]. It is no coincidence that the majority of these interventions are environmental rather than individual.

Pragmatism versus consistency

Do these mismatches between biomedical/biopsychosocial models and reality really matter? Clinical work is pragmatic: patients, often in desperate situations, ask for support and treatment. Surely it's our job as clinicians to help? Perhaps these inconsistencies are clever academic points to make, but simply irrelevant to day-to-day practice?

Four pragmatic arguments might justify the unreserved and invariant use of a clinical model to make sense of a person's experience:

Justification 1:   the model is the only way of understanding the experience
   OR
Justification 2:   the benefits always outweigh the costs
   OR
Justification 3:   the model predicts prognosis
   OR
Justification 4:   the resulting actions cure the patient.

It can be argued that all four justifications are present for many physical illnesses. The biomedical model has generated important advances for physical illness, from abdominal aneurysm to zyomycosis. In these cases, authoritative and unreserved use of a biomedical model may be justified.

However, none of the conditions is satisfied for mental illness. For Justification 1, we have already noted the existence of multiple credible (and incompatible) models of understanding mental illness. More generally, the meaning attributed to mental illness has varied over time, as we discuss in Chapter 7. For example, in relation to psychosis, Rachel Perkins argues that[76]: 'Different models of madness derive from different constructions of the world and events within it, but none is "true" in any absolute sense. There is nothing "truer" about assorted neurotransmitters than there is about intrapsychic processes, inner children or various deities.' The apparently dispassionate statement in Justification 2 is actually a statement of values, since comparing costs and benefits involves putting value on each. Placing more value on the experiences, aspirations and preferences of patients would significantly change the cost–benefit analysis away from the imposition of a clinical model.

We have specifically considered Justifications 3 and 4, and concluded that neither accurate prognosis nor consistent cure follows from the use of biomedical/biopsychosocial models.

Biomedical and biopsychosocial models have been evaluated. These are of course not the only clinical models. At present, there are two putative cure-alls: pharmacotherapy and cognitive behaviour therapy (CBT). Evidence for pharmacotherapy is reviewed in Chapter 6. For now, we turn to the third clinical model, which underpins CBT.

Clinical model 3: cognitive

Early psychological efforts to explain mental worlds and developmental changes through clinical observation underpinned Freudian, Kleinian and Jungian theories. These core insights were then stretched into general theories, applicable across time and culture. By the 1950s the limitations in the ability of these theories to be applied to, and fix, problems of mental distress became apparent.

Psychology as an academic discipline (equally as keen as psychiatry to demonstrate scientific credibility) retrenched into experimental and information-processing approaches – the former involving rats in mazes, the latter esoteric cognitive processing tasks. These provided some clinically important insights. You can make a rat (and so, perhaps, a person) depressed by inducing learned helplessness – a sense that there is no order to the chaos of life, and no pattern of behaviour which consistently leads to a desired reward or avoidance of punishment. People with a diagnosis of schizophrenia (and so, perhaps, the patient sitting in front of you) tend to jump to conclusions in the absence of the typical amount of evidence, and to hold those conclusions with unusually high levels of conviction.

These approaches culminated in the cognitive revolution in the 1960s. Cognitive therapy developments were led by the American psychiatrist Aaron Beck. The central insight of the cognitive model of mental disorder is that cognitions (beliefs) matter. The way we see the world, the interpretations we put on events, the expectations we have about how things will turn out, and our self-image all influence what experiences we have. Expecting the day to go badly, staying in bed because there is no reason to get up, having no sense of agency to change one's situation, coping with feeling low in ways that bring short-term relief but cause long-term damage – these all both create and maintain depression. This is not a new insight – Epictetus stated 'We are disturbed not by events, but by the views which we take of them'. More recently, the Personal Construct Theory of George Kelly proposed that people do not experience reality directly, but interpret or construe their experiences in the world[77]. The importance of behavioural as well as cognitive change has become evident over time, and since the 1990s the dominant cognitive model has been CBT. CBT has been embraced by the profession of clinical psychology, which has developed considerable empirical evidence of effectiveness for many conditions, and with many modes of therapy delivery (e.g. group, individual, computerised).

The key distinction from the biomedical model is the emphasis on interpretation mediating experiences. However, although this approach has the potential to work out-wards from the individual's meaning, in practice the CBT movement has gone in a different direction. For example, the practice of clinical psychology in the USA has been characterised as based on four traditional assumptions[78]:

1. Clinical psychology is concerned with psychopathology – deviant, abnormal and maladaptive behavioural and emotional conditions
2. Psychopathology, clinical problems and clinical populations differ in kind, not just degree, from normal problems in non-clinical populations
3. Psychological disorders are analogous to biological or medical diseases and reside somewhere *inside* the individual

4. The clinician's task is to identify (diagnose) the disorder (disease) inside the person (patient) and to prescribe an intervention (treatment) that will eliminate (cure) the internal disorder (disease).

Not much has changed for clinical psychology since its inception as a profession[79]:

> the language of clinical psychology remains the language of medicine and pathology – what may be called the language of the illness ideology. Terms such as *symptom*, *disorder*, *pathology*, *illness*, *diagnosis*, *treatment*, *doctor*, *patient*, *clinical* and *clinician* are [used]. These terms emphasize abnormality over normality, maladjustment over adjustment, and sickness over health. They promote the dichotomy between normal and abnormal behaviors, clinical and nonclinical problems, and clinical and nonclinical populations. They situate the locus of human adjustment and maladjustment inside the person rather than in the person's interactions with the environment, or in sociocultural values and sociocultural forces such as prejudice and opposition. Finally, these terms portray the person who is seeking help as passive victims of intrapsychic and biological forces beyond their direct control who therefore should be passive recipients of an expert's 'care and cure'.
>
> (p. 14)

CBT is individualised in the sense that it is based on a person-specific formulation rather than a diagnosis, and has the potential to restore meaning and personal responsibility[80]. Formulation is not of course a new idea: its origins include Freud's case studies and the use within therapy of a co-constructed formulation in Cognitive Analytic Therapy[81]. Formulation moves assessment in the right direction – away from the reductionism of diagnostic categories and towards the richness of personal meaning. However, psychological therapies are not free from meaning-diminishing assumptions, such as their focus on the individual[82]: 'Psychoanalysis and humanistic psychology are prone to particular forms of reductionism in their conception of the human condition. This leads to their being conservative-by-default in that they frame socially derived forms of oppression as individual problems.' CBT can certainly be added to the list, with its emphasis on interpretation of phenomenological experience rather than a focus on poverty, abuse, homelessness or other socially and interpersonally toxic life events. CBT remains embedded in a psychopathology framework. It focuses on meaning in the post-Enlightenment sense of rationality, evidenced by its use of techniques such as collaborative empiricism and reality testing, with their embedded philosophical assumptions which we explicate in Chapter 4. For now, the point being made is that CBT as currently practised is congruent with many of the same assumptions about underpinning psychopathology as biomedical and biopsychosocial models.

All three clinical models impose a theoretically based framework which de-emphasises context and gives primacy to professional interpretation. Genuine understanding, by contrast, is contextualised and meaning-rich[83]:

> A young man hears a voice threatening 'I'm going to desecrate your daughter's grave'. Prior to a recurrence of his psychotic illness he heard indirectly that his daughter, living far away with his estranged wife, had died some months earlier and he has missed the funeral. He did not even know where she was buried. There seemed a meaningful connection between his life experience and his current symptoms. We could understand that he felt guilt and bereaved, that this news of loss has rekindled a deep sense of failure and loneliness, that his self-critical and self-punishing feelings had some relationship with the threatening voice – but how could this ever be proven? What kind of experimental method comparing people who had experienced either bereavement or psychosis would give sound evidence of a causal connection?

> Understanding these meaningful connections was very helpful in his care and treatment and unlocked many other meanings besides, but clearly did not explain why he was presenting with a psychotic illness.

We started this chapter by positioning mental illness as, before all else, a type of experience. This has two deep implications, both of which we have identified as key problems with clinical models. First, mental illness exists alongside the rest of phenomenological experience – the inner, subjective world. Therefore to overly focus on the illness part is misplaced. Second, great caution should be exercised in imposing a model of understanding the experience, rather than supporting the person to find their own interpretation.

So what other options are available? We consider two classes of model: disability and diversity.

Disability models

A social disability model for mental illness is a different approach to mental illness[4]. It has been defined by Liz Sayce[84]:

> The social model of disability holds that a person is disabled if he or she is, for example, blind, and experiences barriers and exclusion as a result. The term is not limited to those who 'use' blindness services nor to people who are 'surviving'. It covers everyone affected by discrimination on the grounds of the supposed imperfection of disability. It allows for transforming negative associations into positive ones, through disability pride.

This approach has several advantages. First, it does not presume a particular construction of understanding – medical, psychological, familial, societal, cultural and spiritual constructions can all be accommodated. A social disability model thus side-steps some of the issues of clinical models.

Second, the alignment is increased between mental illness and other, more established, disability groups. This has potential benefits in terms of more benevolent societal attitudes. For example, the success criteria for treatments then become much more focussed on ecologically valid measures of important social roles, rather than myopically fixated on symptom reduction. The effectiveness of a wheelchair is not judged in terms of whether it helps the person to walk, but how much it enables the person to do the things they want to do[4]. A social disability model encourages the use of treatments and support which keep the individual in their life.

Finally, this alignment de-emphasises illness, and the issue moves from 'What's the matter with you?' to 'What do you need to do your job or live your life?'. The focus on adaptation includes both the need for the individual to adapt to the new and changed reality of their life, and (because of the adverse social consequences) the contribution of a socially inclusive and accessible environment. This leads to a more holistic view of the person-in-context. As Rachel Perkins put it[85]: 'Mental health problems are not a full time job – we have lives to lead. Any services, or treatments, or interventions, or supports must be judged in these terms – how much they allow us to lead the lives we wish to lead.' It also leads to a wider role for mental health professionals. Instead of a focus primarily on the direct consequences of the illness itself, at least three levels of impact need to be considered:

1. **The illness**

    The direct impact of the symptoms – people in contact with mental health services often present with high levels of distress caused by their experiences.

2. **The treatment**

A social disability model highlights that treatment is not only about making an 'ill' person 'well'. This brings into view a wider set of questions about the impact of treatment.

Autonomy and responsibility – if I get benefit after an intervention, did I get better because of the pill, the therapist, or the therapy? All locate the source of control externally, rather than enhancing autonomy by generating an internal locus of control.

The centrality of social roles – work and relationships are a cause, not a consequence, of mental well-being. Encouraging a sick role can be toxic, if the cessation of social roles and responsibilities becomes long-term.

The harmful aspects of treatment – the side-effects (note the minimising language) of medication and other treatments can be more important than the intended therapeutic effects. Treatment which marks someone out as different (e.g. by causing them to look odd, or be overly sedated, or be constantly thirsty) reduces the opportunities for the person to be accepted in society.

Hopefulness and hopelessness – the degree to which clinical actions keep people in their lives is vital. Interventions which create dependency or passivity or promote hopelessness are damaging.

3. **The social consequences**

People who are in contact with mental health services experience stigma, defined by Graham Thornicroft as having three elements: problems of knowledge (ignorance), problems of negative attitudes (prejudice) and problems of behaviour (discrimination)[86]. These problems arise from mainstream beliefs about madness. Personal experience of mental health problems remains a taboo among mental health professionals[70], indicating a negative them-and-us view which supports and informs negative public attitudes.

These multiple levels can leave 'many people with mental illness feeling devalued and ignored and [have] resulted in mistrust and alienation from the mental health system'[87]. Repper and Perkins suggest that[4]:

> It is these multiple and interlocking traumas that have such a devastating impact on people's lives, often leaving them disconnected from themselves, from friends and family, from the communities in which they live, and from meaning and purpose in life. Unless mental health workers understand and address this complex range of barriers, we may inadvertently impede recovery by alienating people from the services that are supposed to assist them.

(p. 49)

A particularly important domain of social exclusion is in relation to work and employment. This is an area in which biomedical and biopsychosocial models of mental illness can be harmful, since the focus on treating the illness before returning to work can lead to a loss of established work skills, a reduction in confidence, and internalised low expectations. Jed Boardman identifies several advantages of a social disability model in this domain[88]:

- It offers a more helpful conceptual basis for understanding and promoting employment opportunities for people who use mental health services and offers more hope of recovery of social roles
- It better captures the experience of discrimination and exclusion central to the lives of many mental health service users and addresses the barriers to employment
- It is consistent with current government policy . . .

- It is consistent with the views of users and people with disabilities
- It assists in achieving dialogue with employers

(p. 330)

We all need accommodations at work. For example, office-based workers need light and a chair. The social disability model points to the importance of accommodations at work for people with mental illness, not as an act of charity but because there is a legal right for people with mental illness to be able to work. It also addresses disclosure issues. Expecting job candidates to disclose about their experiences of mental illness is unrealistic when they believe they will be actively discriminated against during the recruitment process[89]. Similarly, expecting employers to provide active accommodations for people with mental illness is unrealistic, where their view of mental illness is informed by highly negative media portrayals and social beliefs, and where they are unaware of their legal responsibilities. The social disability model positions responsibility as shared.

Diversity models

A third type of model is more explicitly challenging about embedded psychopathological assumptions contained in clinical and disability models. Diversity models align with other liberation movements, and focus on emancipatory changes needed in society rather than either treatment of, or adaptation by, the individual. This follows in the tradition of established forms of identity politics, such as civil rights movements, gender politics and disability rights/independent living movements. Diversity models challenge three embedded assumptions: that mental illness is psychopathology, dichotomous and negative.

Assumption 1: mental illness experiences are psychopathological

We saw earlier how anthropological research shows that mental health practice constructs mental illness as an external entity[33]. Diversity models challenge this construction, and instead focus on the need to integrate all aspects of human experience (including those labelled by others as 'mental illness') into a proud and coherent self-identity. Part of this involves challenging the illness-based, and consequently negative, values by re-appropriating language. The term 'madness' is increasingly being used by service users[90] and non-medical mental health professionals[9] over the legal term 'insanity' or the (literally) clinical term 'psychosis'. For example, Mad Pride (www.mindfreedom.org) seeks to directly challenge the value attached to mental illness terminology[91]:

> When people enter mental health services, they assume a role in relation to that service. People become 'consumers', 'clients' and 'service users' . . . The effect of this, though it may be well-meaning, is to disenfranchise and create a stigmatised identity, both internally for the 'consumer', and in the larger culture . . . A key idea behind Mad Pride . . . is to counter stigma and discrimination through celebrating mad culture . . . [This involves] reclaiming of words like 'mad', 'lunatic' and 'psychotic and proud', just as African-Americans reclaimed the word 'black' and lesbian and gay culture reclaimed the word 'gay'.

(p. 138)

One initiative to challenge perceptions was the 'First National Nutters Conference' held in Napier, New Zealand in 2006, which was open to both 'nutters' and 'the chronically normal' (www.lighthousetrust.co.nz). Consumer-led and carer-led groups are forming coalitions to fight stigma (see Appendix). More politically active coalitions, such as Mad Pride and Mad Chicks (www.mad-chicks.org.uk), challenge basic understandings of 'mental illness' experiences.

Assumption 2: mental illness is dichotomous – people are either normal or mentally ill

A related assumption is that mental illness can be constructed as a discontinuous phenomenon. This is embedded in the concept of a psychopathological 'form', yet not empirically validated. Surveys of non-psychiatric populations find that the annual period prevalence of any mental disorder in the adult US population is 22%[92], in Germany is 31%[93], and lifetime prevalence in New Zealand is 40%[94]. Up to what prevalence level is it helpful to view an experience as deviant?

Perhaps only 'severe' mental illness is discontinuous? Not so. The lifetime prevalence of self-reported psychosis symptoms in the National Comorbidity Survey was 28%, compared with a clinician-rated prevalence of psychosis diagnosis of 0.7%[95]. At 15-year follow-up, 25% of the Dunedin birth cohort reported at least one delusional or hallucinatory experience that was unrelated to drug use or physical illness, but only 3.7% fulfilled criteria for schizophreniform disorder[96]. A population-based survey in Australia found that 11.7% of respondents endorsed one or more items designed to identify delusion-like experiences[97]. As Johns and van Os put it[98]:

> disease at the level of the general population generally exists as a continuum of severity rather than as an all-or-none phenomenon. Thus, blood pressure and glucose tolerance are continuously distributed characteristics in the general population, but because the clinical decision to treat is dichotomous, terms such as hypertension and diabetes are used in medicine. This clinical perspective, however, cannot be taken as evidence that these conditions exist as such in nature; they are the extremes of a continuous characteristic.
>
> (p. 1126)

Moving from population-level epidemiological data towards more focussed investigation is revealing. For example, there is no difference in range of, or conviction in, delusional items endorsed from a psychosis check-list between in-patients with psychosis and either Hare Krishna or druidic practitioners[99]. The patients were distinguishable only by their higher levels of distress and preoccupation, which suggests that the distinction between mental illness and other forms of deviation from normality may be subjective rather than objective. This finding has been replicated in other populations[100;101]. Indeed, when 84% of mental health nurses report having experienced an auditory hallucination[102], it is easy to see why service users who feel they are being positioned as fundamentally different from the rest of society may challenge this assumption. Mad Pride has developed an alternative Universal Declaration of Mental Rights and Freedoms:

> **We hold this truth**
> That all human beings are created different. That every human being has the right to be mentally free and independent.
> That every human being has the right to feel, see, hear, sense, imagine, believe or experience anything at all, in any way, at any time.
> That every human being has the right to behave in any way that does not harm others or break fair and just laws.
> That no human being shall be subjected without consent to incarceration, restraint, punishment, or psychological or medical intervention in an attempt to control, repress or alter the individual's thoughts, feelings or experiences.

Assumption 3: mental illness is wholly negative

Many people achieve eminence in their field whilst simultaneously exhibiting symptoms of mental disorder. For example, Felix Post[103] investigated the lives of 291 eminent scientists, writers, politicians, artists, thinkers and writers. He found that 15% had shown no evidence of mental disorder, 25% had shown evidence of mild mental disorder, 30% of marked mental disorder, and 30% of severe mental disorder. He also showed a similar result with mental disorder among 93 of 100 poets, prose fiction writers and playwrights[104]. Lawrence went further, describing the lives of 75 luminaries who achieved greatness not despite but because of their manic depression[105]. Therefore high achievement and mental illness can co-exist, so a severe mental illness label should not, from an empirical perspective, lead to impoverished expectations.

At least as important, and possibly more inspiring, are the first-person accounts of life being deeper, stronger or richer after mental illness has struck. Compilations of these accounts[106–108] make salutary reading for professionals, both in highlighting the disjunction between clinical and self-reported accounts, and in the diversity of what helps people recover. For example, Repper and Perkins[4] include the following quotes:

> I have often asked myself whether, given the choice, I would choose to have manic depressive illness . . . Strangely enough I think I would choose to have it. It's complicated. Depression is awful beyond words or sounds or images . . . So why would I want anything to do with this illness? Because I honestly believe that as a result of it I have felt more things, more deeply; had more experiences, more intensely, loved more, and been loved; laughed more often for having cried more often; appreciated more the springs, for all the winters; worn death 'as close as dungarees', appreciated it – and life – more; seen the finest and the most terrible in people, and slowly learned the values of caring, loyalty and seeing things through.[109]
>
> As I found myself, psychosis – particularly in the early euphoric phase, if it obtains – can be at least the beginning of spiritual enlightenment. It may open doors to such experiences that the person can make productive use of later when they are well.[67]
>
> Because I have faced this pain, I am able to feel more deeply, reach out to others more authentically. To this day, the experience's bewildering array of symbolism involves me in its interpretation. Much of it involved the modern day anxiety towards death: from the stranger who I first met who I thought was death, to the attempt to write the last page of history in black. But the experience also showed me that there is a world on the other side of death.[110]

This has profound implications for how we view the mental illness experience. For example, Peter Chadwick has suggested that whilst madness is a discontinuity, it is still meaningful and not all negative, since over-active pattern recognition enhanced his creativity[67]. He concludes that 'it's a poor show if we can only aim to be sane'. This is succinctly expressed by Susie Crooks[91]: 'There's probably a bit of madness in all of us. I see my condition as actually contributing to who I am as a person. I don't see it as a disability. I just work hard to put a human face on madness' (p. 139).

Implications of a diversity model

Diversity models are overtly challenging to clinical and disability models. For example, rationalism is not given automatic primacy as a superior state. This post-modern rejection of a core Enlightenment value leads consumers to ask why, if it is unacceptable in a liberal democracy to forcibly change the religious beliefs of people, is it acceptable to forcibly change the 'delusional' views of people with mental illness?

The balance of power also changes. For example, the expertise of professionals is subverted by the suggestion from consumer-activist Arana Pearson (www.keepwell.com.au) to encourage consumers to use the letters QBE after their name – Qualified By Experience.

A diversity model also has some need for separatism. If oppression shapes the consciousness of the oppressed such that they internalise their oppression, then only when members of the oppressor group are not present to enforce unjust notions of equality, justice and right can the oppressed begin consciousness-raising. For the oppressed, this separation is a means to the end: liberation defined in their own terms. This is one reason why some user groups are actively opposed to involvement from clinicians, and why even the most liberal clinicians can avoid attempting to involve consumer-activists. Being thought of as an oppressor (from the clinician's perspective) or willingly working with oppressors (from the alienated consumer's perspective) are uncomfortable positions.

Clinical work within a diversity framework is also different, with much greater attention paid to empowerment of the individual, and awareness of sociocultural pressures and assumptions. If someone wants helps on their own terms with their 'mental illness', all well and good – a civilised society will respond to this, in the same way as it will respond to support someone coming to terms with their own sexuality, ethnicity or spirituality. If someone does not want help, then the implications of a diversity approach are that any discomfort arising from this choice is not the individual's problem, but should be located where it belongs – in the microcosm of the mental health system and the macrocosm of society.

Adjudicating between models

We have identified three broad ways of understanding mental illness, summarised in Table 2.3.

Each model has its merits and, in the absence of comparative data, it is not possible to adjudicate between them. What can be said with certainty is that the proponents of each approach should realise that their model is simply a hypothesis – the current reasonable

Table 2.3 Clinical, disability and diversity models

	Clinical model	Disability model	Diversity model
Source of problem	Illness in the person	The combination of mental illness and societal response	Society
Treatment	Necessary and appropriate	Necessary but insufficient	Only if wanted, never if not wanted
Expertise	In the professional	Shared	In the consumer
Central role of the mental health professional	Providing evidence-based treatments	Advocacy	Supporting consumer activism
Role of the mental health service user	Taking treatment	Developing inter-dependence – taking appropriate support and developing self-management skills	Accepting and valuing oneself, losing self-stigmatising beliefs
Strengths	Provides a clear explanatory model, and leads to well-developed treatments	De-emphasises illness Encourages social inclusion Consistent with existing disability discrimination legislation	Doesn't pathologise Places power in the hands of the individual consumer
Weaknesses	Doesn't fit for everyone Promises cure but doesn't deliver	Retains paternalistic approach	How to gate-keep support resources if everyone is 'normal'?

explanation of the facts. Therefore an authentic (rather than simply expressed) tentativeness is needed in applying the model to an individual.

Tentativeness has costs and benefits. Whitwell notes the calming effect of even a novice psychiatrist who applies the clinical model with confidence, and can contain the anxiety of an otherwise chaotic situation[22]. However, as Repper and Perkins note[4], this can lead to over-involvement and blaming:

> It is not uncommon for mental health workers to become 'over-helpful', to make decisions for the person and to do things for him/her rather than supporting him/her to do things unassisted . . . If our sense of worth is dependent on continued improvement, then we all too easily become disappointed and angry when, despite our best efforts, the client does not make the progress we expected. We feel let down and may blame that person for 'lack of motivation', 'non-compliance', 'self-defeating behaviour', and 'failure to follow advice'.
>
> (p. 72)

In mental health crises there is often a need for certainty, but in life there is often a need for uncertainty. The tension between these two needs is a difficult balance, especially given the almost total absence of empirical evidence comparing different approaches.

Having identified that there is more than one reasonable explanatory model of understanding 'mental illness' experiences, we turn now to a cross-cutting theme: recovery. Talking about recovery involves addressing some disputed issues: what does recovery mean and involve, how do we recognise and measure it, and how can it be supported? Addressing these issues is the focus of the remainder of this book.

We start by considering different approaches to understanding recovery.

Chapter 3

What is recovery?

One word, two meanings

The term 'recovery' is at the heart of a debate about the *raison d'être* of mental health services. In Chapter 2 we argued that treatment of mental illness does not always cure the mental illness. We now present empirical research into schizophrenia demonstrating that recovery in the sense of cure – what we will call **clinical recovery** – is indeed lower than 100%, but also higher than consistent with a degenerative course of the disorder. However, some consumers self-report as being recovered, even when they experience ongoing symptoms. This new understanding of recovery – which we call **personal recovery** – would represent a fundamental shift in the values of mental health services if (as we argue it should be) it is embraced as the primary goal of mental health services.

We begin with clinical approaches to operationalising recovery.

Meaning 1: clinical recovery

The first meaning of recovery has emerged from professional-led research. Clinical recovery has four key features:

1. It is an outcome or a state, generally dichotomous
2. It is observable – in clinical parlance, it is objective, not subjective
3. It is rated by the expert clinician, not the patient
4. The definition of recovery is invariant across individuals.

Various definitions of recovery have been proposed by mental health professionals. For example, Torgalsbøen proposes that recovery in schizophrenia be defined as[111]:

- A reliable previous diagnosis of schizophrenia
- Criteria for diagnosis not fulfilled at present
- Out of hospital for at least 5 years
- Present psychosocial functioning within a 'normal' range (e.g. scores > 65 on GAF)
- Not on antipsychotic medication or only on low dosage (less than half 'defined daily doses').

The intention with this definition is that it be operationalisable – suitable for use in empirical research. It contains diagnostic, service use, functioning and treatment elements. Each of these can vary for reasons not related to the individual and whether they are recovered. Diagnostic criteria can (and do – see Chapter 2) change. Hospitals close and home treatment teams operate in the deinstitutionalisation era, so admission thresholds alter. Functioning is dependent on the opportunities in the environment. Medication regimes are influenced by prescriber beliefs.

A more socially focussed definition is proposed by Libermann and Kopelowicz[112]:

- Full symptom remission
- Full or part-time work or education

Table 3.1 Recovery rates in long-term follow-up studies of psychosis

Lead researcher	Location	Year	n	Mean length of follow-up (years)	% Recovered or significantly improved
Huber[a]	Bonn	1975	502	22	57
Ciompi[b]	Lausanne	1976	289	37	53
Bleuler[c]	Zurich	1978	208	23	53–68
Tsuang[d]	Iowa	1979	186	35	46
Harding[e]	Vermont	1987	269	32	62–68
Ogawa[f]	Japan	1987	140	23	57
Marneros[g]	Cologne	1989	249	25	58
DeSisto[h]	Maine	1995	269	35	49
Harrison[i]	18-site	2001	776	25	56

Notes:
[a]Huber G, Gross G, Schuttler R. A long-term follow-up study of schizophrenia: psychiatric course and prognosis. *Acta Psychiatrica Scandinavica* 1975; **52**:49–57.
[b]Ciompi L, Muller C. *The Life-course and Aging of Schizophrenics: A long-term follow-up study into old age*. Berlin: Springer; 1976.
[c]Bleuler M. *The Schizophrenic Disorders*. New Haven, CT: Yale University Press; 1978.
[d]Tsuang MT, Woolson RF, Fleming J. Long-term outcome of major psychosis. *Archives of General Psychiatry* 1979; **36**:1295–1301.
[e]Harding CM, Brooks G, Ashikage T, Strauss JS, Brier A. The Vermont longitudinal study of persons with severe mental illness II: long-term outcome of subjects who retrospectively met DSM-III criteria for schizophrenia. *American Journal of Psychiatry* 1987; **144**:727–735.
[f]Ogawa K, Miya M, Watarai A, Nakazawa M, Yuasa S, Utena H. A long-term follow-up study of schizophrenia in Japan, with special reference to the course of social adjustment. *British Journal of Psychiatry* 1987; **151**:758–765.
[g]Marneros A, Deister A, Rohde A, Steinmeyer EM, Junemann H. Long-term outcome of schizoaffective and schizophrenic disorders, a comparative study, I: Definitions, methods, psychopathological and social outcome. *European Archives of Psychiatry and Clinical Neuroscience* 1989; **238**:118–125.
[h]DeSisto MJ, Harding CM, McCormick RV, Ashikage T, Brooks G. The Maine and Vermont three-decades studies of serious mental illness: II. Longitudinal course. *British Journal of Psychiatry* 1995; **167**:338–342.
[i]Harrison G, Hopper K, Craig T, Laska E, Siegel C, Wanderling J et al. Recovery from psychotic illness: a 15- and 25-year international follow-up study. *British Journal of Psychiatry* 2001; **178**:506–517.

- Independent living without supervision by informal carers
- Having friends with whom activities can be shared
- All sustained for a period of two years.

Their conclusion is that 'it is now realistic to set as a goal the feasibility of recovery from schizophrenia for half or more individuals with first episode'. Does this fit with findings from naturalistic longitudinal studies? Results are difficult to interpret due to differences in participant selection, definition of recovery, use of retrospective versus prospective tracking, frequency of repeated measurement, length of follow-up, location and time period[37]. Perhaps the most meaningful data comes from studies with long follow-up periods. In Table 3.1 we show all 20-year or longer follow-up studies published until 2008.

For example, Courtenay Harding's study in Vermont involved 32-year follow-up of the most difficult-to-place third of people resident in a psychiatric institution[113]. At follow-up she found markedly higher rates of recovery indicators than would be expected from this institutionalised group, with 81% able to look after themselves, and 68% having moderately close to close friendships. Just over half (54%) were still in touch with mental health services. Overall, 25% were fully recovered and 41% showed significant improvement, i.e. 68% of the most dependent third had at least partially recovered, implying that only 11% of people with severe and enduring mental health problems remain unrecovered and deep in the system. This is of course much less than the clinical rule of thirds (i.e. a third recover, a third have fluctuating course and a third will never get better) would suggest.

These empirical data challenge the applicability of a chronic disease model to mental illness, with its embedded assumption that conditions like schizophrenia are necessarily life-long and have a deteriorating course. The most recent collation of all long-term follow-up studies included over 1000 patients between 12 and 26 years after initial assessment[114]. Commenting on the results, Richard Warner concludes[115]:

> What do we learn of the lives of people with schizophrenia from this fascinating study . . .? Most importantly, Kraepelin's view that a deteriorating course is a hallmark of the illness just isn't true. Heterogeneity of outcome, both in terms of symptoms and functioning, is the signature feature . . . bad outcome is not a necessary component of the natural history of schizophrenia; it is a consequence of the interaction between the individual and his or her social and economic world.

Consistent with the issues discussed in Chapter 2, we need to acknowledge that sometimes this recovery has been in spite of, rather than because of, mental health services[116]: 'The psychiatric system far from being a sanctuary and a system of healing was . . . a system of fear and continuation of illness for me. Like so many others recovery was a process that I did not encounter within the system, indeed . . . it was not until I left the system that the recovery process really got underway in my life.' Perhaps this problem arises from treating recovery as an outcome. Although this allows prevalence questions to be addressed, it also implicitly involves deep assumptions about normality. As Ruth Ralph and Patrick Corrigan put it[117]: 'This kind of definition begs several questions that need to be addressed to come up with an understanding of recovery as outcome: How many goals must be achieved to be considered recovered? For that matter, how much life success is considered 'normal'?' (p. 5). The people who use mental health services have called for a new approach[118]: 'The field of psychiatric disabilities requires an enriched knowledge base and literature to guide innovation in policy and practice under a recovery paradigm. We must reach beyond our storehouse of writings that describe psychiatric disorder as a catastrophic life event.' The second meaning of 'recovery' provides this enriched knowledge base.

Meaning 2: personal recovery

People personally affected by mental illness have become increasingly vocal in communicating both what their life is like with the mental illness and what helps in moving beyond the role of a patient with mental illness. Early accounts were written by individual pioneers[116;118–122]. These brave, and sometimes oppositional and challenging, voices provide ecologically valid pointers to what recovery looks and feels like from the inside.

Once individual stories were more visible, compilations and syntheses of these accounts began to emerge from around the (especially Anglophone) world, e.g. from Australia[123], New Zealand[107;124–126], Scotland[55;127], the USA[118;128;129] and England[106;108]. The understanding of recovery which has emerged from these accounts has a different focus from clinical recovery, for example in emphasising the centrality of hope, identity, meaning and personal responsibility[123;130;131]. The translation of these ideas into an action plan for mental health services is the primary goal of this book.

We will refer to the consumer-based understanding of recovery as **personal recovery**, to reflect its individually defined and experienced nature. To note, other distinguishing terms have also been used, including recovery 'from' versus recovery 'in'[132], clinical recovery versus social recovery[133], scientific versus consumer models of recovery[134], and service-based recovery versus user-based recovery[135].

Opinions in the consumer literature about recovery are wide-ranging, and cannot be uniformly characterised. This multiplicity of perspectives in itself has a lesson for mental health services – no one approach works for, or 'fits', everyone. There is no right way for a person to recover.

Nonetheless, some themes emerge. A first clear point of divergence from the clinical perspective is that recovery is seen as a journey into life, not an outcome to be arrived at. As Repper and Perkins put it[4]: 'Recovery is not about "getting rid" of problems. It is about seeing people beyond their problems – their abilities, possibilities, interests and dreams – and recovering the social roles and relationships that give life value and meaning' (p. ix). Many definitions of recovery have been proposed by those who are experiencing it:

> Recovery refers to the lived or real life experience of people as they accept and overcome the challenge of the disability . . . they experience themselves as recovering a new sense of self and of purpose within and beyond the limits of disability[119].
>
> For me, recovery means that I'm not in hospital and I'm not sitting in supported accommodation somewhere with someone looking after me. Since I've recovered, I've found that in spite of my illness I can still contribute and have an input into what goes on in my life, input that is not necessarily tied up with medication, my mental illness or other illnesses [55].
>
> (p. 61)

This book will use the most widely cited definition, by Bill Anthony[1]:

> Recovery is a deeply personal, unique process of changing one's attitudes, values, feelings, goals, skills, and/or roles. It is a way of living a satisfying, hopeful, and contributing life even within the limitations caused by illness. Recovery involves the development of new meaning and purpose in one's life as one grows beyond the catastrophic effects of mental illness.

It is consistent with the less widely cited but more succinct definition proposed by Retta Andresen and colleagues, that recovery involves[123]: 'The establishment of a fulfilling, meaningful life and a positive sense of identity founded on hopefulness and self determination' (p. 588). For those who value succinctness, the definition we use in our local service is[136]: 'Recovery involves living as well as possible'.

One implication of these definitions is that personal recovery is an individual process. Just as there is no one right way to do or experience recovery, so also what helps an individual at one time in their life may not help them at another. If mental health services are to be focussed on promoting personal recovery, then this means there cannot be a single recovery model for services. This is a profound point, and challenging to the concepts of clinical guidelines, evidence-based practice and care pathways. The issue will be explored further in relation to the Apollonian versus Dionysian spectrum, in Chapter 4. For now, we note that a recovery-focussed service is an approach, a way of thinking, a set of attitudes and values put into practice by skilled mental health practitioners. Caution should therefore be exercised about being highly prescriptive about the nature of recovery, and what a recovery-focussed service should look like and how it should work.

Key elements of a recovery approach have been identified by Rachel Perkins and Julie Repper[4] in the UK and Ruth Ralph[137] in the USA, and are summarised in Table 3.2.

Table 3.2 Descriptions of personal recovery

Summary description	Aspect identified by Perkins and Repper	Aspect identified by Ralph
Recovery involves a journey	Recovery is a continuing journey, not an end-product or a result	Recovery is a journey from alienation to a sense of meaning and purpose
from disengagement to engagement,		Recovery is moving from withdrawal to engagement and active participation in life
from surviving to living and growing.	Recovery is about growth	Recovery is active coping rather than passive adjustment
Although awareness of the journey often starts in adversity, such as mental illness,		Recovery is breaking through denial and achieving understanding and acceptance
	A recovery vision is not limited to a particular theory about the nature and causes of mental health problems	
the journey is not about the adversity.	Recovery is not the same as cure	
Although the journey of recovery has many routes,	Recovery can, and does, occur without professional intervention	
and each person's journey is unique,	Everyone's recovery journey is different and deeply personal. There are no rules of recovery, no formula for 'success'	
it often involves finding the courage to hope for a good future and to relate to yourself		Recovery is the reawakening of hope after despair
	Recovery is about taking back control over one's own life	Recovery means no longer viewing oneself as primarily a person with a psychiatric disorder and reclaiming a positive sense of self
and others in beneficial ways.		Recovery is not accomplished alone; the journey involves support and partnership
Setbacks are inevitable, but the challenge is universal	Recovery is not a linear process	Recovery is a complex and nonlinear journey
	Recovery is not specific to people with mental health problems	

Personal recovery has high ecological validity – it emerges from the narratives of people with mental illness who describe themselves as recovered or in recovery. It also removes the unhelpful evaluative element of whether, according to some externally defined criteria, someone has achieved recovery.

A disadvantage of personal recovery is that it makes operationalisation of the concept and empirical investigation problematic. If recovery is an ongoing, idiosyncratic and sometimes cyclical process, how can we get a reliable snapshot or show positive change? This does not mean that empirical quantitative research is impossible. For example, Sandra Resnick and colleagues used principal components analysis and confirmatory factor analysis to identify four domains of a recovery orientation in patients: empowerment, hope and optimism, knowledge, and life satisfaction[138]. This allows the prevalence of a recovery orientation among service users, and the impact of interventions on this orientation, to be investigated empirically.

We have presented clinical recovery and personal recovery as having fundamentally different meanings. Is this distinction valid?

Are clinical recovery and personal recovery incompatible?

Two overlapping but nonetheless different understandings of recovery have been proposed. Not all authors identify two meanings of recovery. For example, Ruth Ralph and Patrick Corrigan propose three definitions of recovery[117]:

1. Recovery is a naturally occurring phenomenon.

   Some people who meet diagnostic criteria for a serious mental illness are able to overcome their disabilities and fully enjoy a life in which their life goals are accomplished without any kind of treatment.

2. As with other medical illnesses, people can recover from mental illness with proper treatment.

   Others who do not enjoy spontaneous recovery from mental illness are able to achieve a similar state of goal attainment and life satisfaction as a result of participating in a variety of services.

3. Recovery reintroduces the idea of hope in understanding serious mental illness

   . . . It means that even though a person is diagnosed with schizophrenia or other serious psychiatric disorder, his or her life need not be limited to institutions.

(pp. 4–5)

They note that mental health professionals gravitate towards the second definition (clinical recovery), whereas consumers typically find more value in the first (spontaneous recovery) and third (personal recovery).

These three definitions are also used in the joint statement on recovery issued by the Care Service Improvement Partnership, the Royal College of Psychiatrists and the Social Care Institute for Excellence in the UK[139]. Each definition is valued: 'Many concerns about engaging with a recovery approach arise from thinking that these different conceptions are in competition with one another, whereas they are complementary and synergistic . . . Adopting a recovery approach harnesses the value of current treatments but is directed at living with and beyond these continuing limitations' (p. 2). This book takes a different position. It envisages a future in which the goal of mental health services is more explicitly the promotion and support of personal recovery. Clinical recovery has value, as one approach to supporting personal recovery. However, a primary focus on personal recovery would fundamentally change the values, goals and working practices of mental health services. Clinical recovery is subordinate to personal recovery.

Personal recovery encompasses the three types of recovery listed above. Spontaneous recovery occurs for some people, when the individual's biological, psychological, social and spiritual self-righting skills and supports combine to manage the mental illness. Personal recovery occurs for some people through receiving evidence-based treatments, so treatment is an important element of mental health services. But, crucially, personal recovery is underpinned for all people by hope, meaning, identity and personal responsibility.

A primary focus on clinical recovery is incompatible with a primary focus on personal recovery. This is a strong statement, so we will illustrate with examples of how the current focus on clinical recovery can hinder personal recovery in three domains: hope, meaning and symptoms.

Clinical recovery and hope

Hope is central to personal recovery. It leads to action based on approach rather than avoidance motivation[140] – having positive goals, rather than trying to avoid negative outcomes. It also sustains through the inevitable (but otherwise unbearable) setbacks and suffering: 'Having some hope is crucial to recovery; none of us would strive if we believed it a futile effort'[141] (p. 32); 'The thing that keeps me going is the knowledge that I'm going to get better. The one thing I do know about my illness, if history tells me anything, is that I bounce back. And when I bounce back the trick is to bounce back and stay well'[55] (p. 60).

Hope is a problem in mental health services. The rhetoric is clear: services should work in ways which foster hope and optimism[142]. However, the reality for many people who use mental health services is quite the opposite[143]: 'The belief held by hospital staff was that I would be powerless to influence the return of psychotic symptoms that could at any moment strike again. For me to escape this prophecy, it felt like wading through miles and miles of swamp. This was an incredibly lonely journey. I had no guides, no specialist support, no stories of success' (p. 307). This is not a new problem. In 1959, Menninger commented on mental health professional training that: 'I perceived vividly how hopelessness breeds hopelessness, how the non-expectant, hope-lacking or "unimaginative" teacher can bequeath to his students a sense of impotence and futility, utterly out of keeping with facts known to both of them'[144]. This leads to a situation where the possibility of a good future is rarely communicated by mental health professionals. It is therefore all too easy for people using services to develop the belief that they will never recover, and the self-fulfilling nature of such a belief is obvious. This is why people exposed to the idea of recovery often express surprise and disbelief[55]: 'About two years ago I realised that I really could recover. I find that quite an amazing fact, because over the years no one has actually said, "You can recover". I thought once you had mental health problems you were just going to be stuck with it' (p. 38).

Some consumers find that interactions with mental health professionals engender feelings of being disrespected, discouraged and hopeless. This phenomenon is labelled as 'spirit breaking' by Patricia Deegan[145]:

> The experience of spirit breaking occurs as a result of those cumulative experiences in which we are humiliated and made to feel less than human, in which our will to live is deeply shaken or broken, in which our hopes are shattered and in which 'giving up', apathy and indifference become a way of surviving and protecting the last vestiges of the wounded self.
>
> (p. 306)

This lack of hope has toxic consequences. The self-fulfilling nature of being told by an expert that you'll never be able to work, or live independently, or have children or be treatment-free is profoundly damaging. The reason that clinicians should never make these statements (either explicitly or – more commonly – implicitly) is not some vague notion of withholding damaging information. It is because these statements are often wrong. The evidence about recovery rates was reviewed earlier in this chapter. Work is a specifically important contributor to recovery, yet one study found that 44% of people with mental illness who had obtained employment had been previously told by a clinician that they would never work again[146]. A focus on clinical recovery, with its emphasis on engendering realistic (i.e. low) expectations, can destroy hope.

Clinical recovery and meaning

Finding meaning in life is a central challenge for anyone, with or without mental illness. It involves making sense of experience, and generating a story which fits for the person.

This gives a narrative of how they come to be where they are in life. Often there is a liberating aspect to the narrative, such as a discovery that we don't need to be a prisoner of our auto-biography or a slave to our genes. It also provides a context and purpose for the future – it is the spring-board for hope.

The importance attached to meaning has been downgraded in contemporary mental health services[83]. In Chapter 2 we identified how imposing a biomedical or biopsychosocial model on the person's experience can remove its meaning. For example, depicting delusions as 'empty speech acts, whose informational content refers to neither world nor self'[147] does not support individuals to meet the universal life challenge of finding how to understand and grow from experience.

How do people develop meaning? Alain Topor interviewed 16 people with severe mental illness who both self-defined and met professional criteria for recovery[148]. They identified experimenting with four types of explanatory model:

1. Life history (e.g. a difficult childhood)
2. Medical, often expressed with ambivalence, such as a view of medication as a 'necessary evil' (with recovery as present when medication had ceased to be an 'issue')
3. Spiritual, in line with other studies[107]
4. Social, especially constructing a self-narrative through telling one's story, and negotiating or compromising on the basis of the listener's response.

The implication of this diversity is that imposing any single explanatory model can be damaging. It is more productive to support the person in their quest for meaning through a stance of offering an understanding rather than imposing an explanation.

One response by mental health professionals to a call to emphasise the development of meaning is to invoke issues of insight: people with mental illness *by definition* cannot make sense of their experiences, because it is exactly that capacity for self-awareness which is impaired by the illness. The professional knows what is going on whereas the patient may or may not.

The embedded assumptions, that there is an absolute reality to know and that one party has privileged access to it, are challenged in Chapter 4. However, even within a clinical frame of reference, empirical studies do not support an automatic focus on promoting insight. Pat McGorry cautions against adding 'insight to injury', by ignoring the individual's readiness to accept an illness explanation[149]. Indeed, a shift in the first 6 months from integration to sealing over is associated with symptomatic improvement[150] and increased self-esteem[151]. Or, to put it in the language of lived experience, isolation and withdrawal from life and reality is 'a perpetual suspended animation that is better than never-ending pain' (p. 71). This is not to argue that what clinicians perceive as a lack of insight is desirable, but it may be necessary.

In a service focussed on personal recovery, disagreement with a clinical model simply does not matter – what is important is that the person finds their own meaning, which makes some sense of their experience and provides hope for the future. Why? Because suffering with meaning is bearable – meaningless suffering is what drives you mad. Finding meaning *is* moving on. By contrast, in a mental health service focussed on clinical recovery, lack of insight is always to be avoided, because it is a symptom of illness and symptoms are by definition undesirable. We turn now to symptoms.

Clinical recovery and symptoms

For clinical recovery, symptom abatement is necessary. For personal recovery, there is no universal stance about symptoms. This issue plays out in the realm of medication. Even if pharmacotherapy consistently reduced symptoms (which it does not – see Chapter 6), compliance with prescribed medication limits its effectiveness. If symptom reduction is a predefined goal of mental health services, then increasingly coercive approaches to ensuring medication compliance are justified. If, by contrast, empowerment, autonomy and self-determination are primary goals, then judgements about compulsion are more individual-ised. The issue does not reduce to a simplistic clinician versus patient power battle. For example, some consumers argue for a tiered approach to decision-making, with transfer of control gradually happening as the individual re-obtains capacity[152], whereas others argue that it is precisely at times of acute crisis when empowerment is most important[153].

There are at least two pragmatic reasons not to view symptom reduction as the primary goal of mental health services. First, it leads to this escalating cycle of increasing compul-sion. Second, a view of symptoms as always undesirable ignores the potential benefits. This is not intended in any way to romanticise the suffering commonly occurring in mental illness, but rather to note the reality that symptoms of mental illness are not always all bad. In Chapter 2 we described how mental illness can co-exist with high achievement, or contribute to a richness in life. Even more challengingly, some people report that the experience of symptoms can itself be therapeutic or cathartic[55]:

> I think sometimes there can be confusion between getting better and being symptom free. It is often during the times when I have had the most PTSD (Post Traumatic Stress Disorder) symptoms that I have achieved greater gains in recovery. For example, when new memories are surfacing my speech may be affected, but once I get through the difficult patches I am better than before.
>
> (p. 30)

Personal recovery is not always about symptoms, although it is almost always about the relationship with the symptoms[127]: 'I have taken ownership of my illness and I take responsibility for what I do and do not do. I don't let it control me. And it is an "it". It's not the whole of my life; It's part of my life now.'

Personal recovery and mental health services

We have argued that clinical recovery and personal recovery are different, and in some respects incompatible as primary goals for a mental health system. Specifically, the values, goals and working practices associated with clinical recovery are one of several approaches to promoting personal recovery. Clinical recovery is a sub-set of personal recovery. There-fore, prioritising clinical recovery is helpful for many people in supporting their personal recovery, but inadequate for others, and toxic for some.

Having made this distinction, we will now argue that mental health services should be focussed on the promotion of personal recovery, and not of clinical recovery. Five justifications for giving primacy to personal recovery over clinical recovery are presented in Section 2.

1. Epistemological – personal recovery places more value than clinical recovery on the knowledge of the individual
2. Ethical – acting in the professionally defined best interests of the patient should not be a primary value of mental health services
3. Effectiveness – the most common treatment (medication) does not cure, so the central promise of a clinical recovery approach is simply not fulfilled.
4. Empowerment – 'their' life has not been safe in our hands
5. Policy-based – national policy requires a focus on personal recovery.

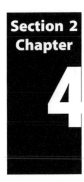

The primacy of personal recovery
Epistemological rationale

Summary of the epistemological rationale

Evidence-based medicine is based on Enlightenment principles, and downgrades the importance of subjective experience. Since mental illness is fundamentally subjective, constructivism would provide a better basis for mental health services, as it values both expertise-by-training and expertise-by-experience.

The epistemological basis of clinical research was developed during the Enlightenment. Shortcomings of this approach to knowledge will be outlined, and alternatives identified.

What is knowledge?

Epistemology is the branch of philosophy which deals with knowledge and belief, including the nature of knowledge itself, how it is obtained, what people know, and how knowledge relates to concepts such as truth and belief. A central assumption in the field of epistemology shifted during the Enlightenment.

Classical understanding of knowledge was influenced by the Greek philosophical worldview. Aristotle defined truth and falsehood: 'To say of something which is that it is not, or to say of something which is not that it is, is false. However, to say of something which is that it is, or of something which is not that it is not, is true'. Drawing on this assumption of objective truth, Plato identified knowledge as a subset of that which is both true and believed.

The existence of absolutes and the centrality of belief dominated thinking until the Age of Enlightenment in the seventeenth and eighteenth centuries. The period is sometimes called the Age of Reason, as it involved a move from belief to reason as the primary basis of authority. The transition is sometimes called *the mechanisation of the world-picture*[154], and followed from wider cultural assumptions, such as empiricism (basing cognition in experience common to all) and the democratisation of knowledge. The idea of an experiment – '*a question we put to nature*' through intervention and observation – was developed by Francis Bacon[155] and others during this period. Crucially, the central goal of science was to establish causal relationships and processes which allow predictions to be made about what will happen in the future. The goal is not understanding meaning or reasons.

Scientific principles emerging from the Enlightenment emphasise a particular type of knowledge, called nomothetic knowledge. The distinction between nomothetic and idiographic knowledge was introduced by Wilhelm Windelband. **Nomothetic knowledge** is based on what Kant described as a tendency to generalise, and involves the effort to derive laws that explain objective phenomena. It is derived from the study of groups which represent populations, normally using quantitative methodologies. **Idiographic knowledge**, by contrast, is based on the tendency to specify, and involves efforts to understand the meaning of contingent, accidental and often subjective phenomena. It is derived from the study of individuals and the properties which set them apart from other individuals, normally using qualitative methodologies.

Research focussed on the development of nomothetic knowledge seeks to develop generalisable explanations of the world derived from group-level experimentation. This involves **reductionism**: squeezing all the subjectivity or meaning or perspective out of a situation, so that truth can be revealed. Reductionism in the natural sciences is an asset – it indicates a robust theory, and allows reproducibility of a theory to be established through experimentation.

This world-view is the cultural and scientific context in which clinical research has developed, and accounts for why evidence from the randomised controlled trial has become dominant. The evidence-based medicine movement has developed the hierarchy of knowledge (which is in fact a hierarchy of method):

Highest (i.e. strongest) type of knowledge:

Systematic review and meta-analysis of randomised controlled trials

Followed in order by

Randomised controlled trials with definitive results

Randomised controlled trials with non-definitive results

Cohort studies

Case-control studies

Cross-sectional surveys

Lowest (i.e. least compelling) type of knowledge

Case reports

It goes without saying (because it has been said many times[156–158]) that this hierarchy brings benefits. The focus on randomised controlled trials (RCTs) as the gold standard of research methodology means that uncontrolled or poorly controlled studies are given less weight, more importance is attached to methodological issues, and more caution is exercised in evaluating outcome. As Derek Bolton puts it[159]: 'RCTs are here to stay. They are based on deep philosophical and cultural assumptions about nature and knowledge, assumptions that have well proved their effectiveness elsewhere.' How applicable to mental illness are scientific methods based on Enlightenment principles?

The development of a science of mental illness

We argued in Chapter 2 that mental illness is, before all else, a subjective experience. Therefore the object of mental illness research is the inner subjective world of experience. This gives rise to a basic problem: it is not possible to directly access subjective experience. It is only possible to investigate the observable world, either inside the body (e.g. biochemistry, neuroanatomy, self-reported cognitions) or outside (e.g. life events, social context, familial history). Clearly these inside and outside phenomena influence experience, and so research into the relationship between observable phenomena and subjective experience may be informative. But if the essence of mental illness is the inner subjective world, then only the person themselves can access this stratum.

The central challenge for any science of mental illness is to accommodate knowledge from both observation and subjective experience. This integration has been problematic. Two broad (and opposing) philosophies have dominated thinking.

On the one hand, **subjectivism** holds that the existence of every object depends on someone's subjective awareness of it – that perception is reality and that there is no underlying, true reality independent of perception. For example, Wittgenstein argued that 'the subject doesn't belong to the world, but it is a limit of the world'[160]. The problem with subjectivism is that this reduces clinical insight to intuition – if there is no objective reality, then clinical feel is as good a guide as any.

On the other hand, the end-point of an emphasis on observable reality is Ayn Rand's **objectivism**, which holds that there is a mind-independent reality, that contact with this reality is through sensory perception, and that objective knowledge is obtained from this perception by measurement[161].

A transition from subjectivism to objectivism in mental health services occurred with the development of descriptive taxonomies. Perhaps the most celebrated development in psychiatry is Emil Kraepelin's description of dementia præcox[162], the underpinning for what was re-christened by Eugen Bleuler as a 'group of schizophrenias'[163]. In Chapter 3 we noted the unhelpful assumptions of chronicity and deteriorating course which are embedded in these descriptions of dementia at a precocious age and of a splitting in the mind through loss of integration between mental functions. Nonetheless, this framework forms the basis for modern psychiatric practice. Arieti describes post-Kraepelin developments[164]:

> Once he defined this syndrome, Kraepelin tried his best to give an accurate description of it . . . one cannot help admiring the accurateness of his description; however, his description is remarkable for its extension and completeness, not for its depth. The patient appears as a collection of symptoms, not as a person; or if he appears as a person, he looks as if he belongs to a special species and thus should be differentiated from the rest of humanity and put into the insane asylum. The psychiatric hospital is a zoological garden with many different species.
>
> (pp. 11–12)

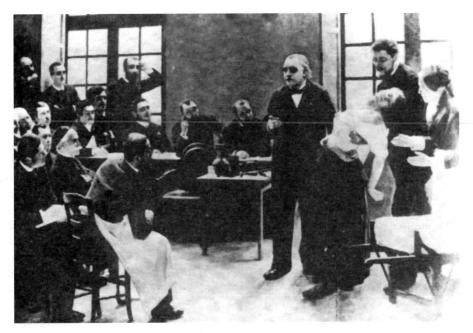

Figure 4.1 Charcot's presentation of a case of hysteria.

The problem with pure objectivism is that the patient becomes an object of enquiry. This is illustrated by Charcot's presentation of a case of hysteria at the Salpêtriére in 1887 (Figure 4.1).

Evidence-based medicine is vulnerable to this process of objectifying the person with mental illness. This may sound like an exaggeration, so we will explore it further.

Problems with evidence-based medicine

In the natural sciences there is a great emphasis on reproducibility – the ability to repeat an experiment and produce the same result. This does not translate directly into effectiveness research in the human sciences, because (as we noted in Chapter 2) causation is generative, not successionist. Unlike humans, a chemical cannot refuse consent, or be thinking of something else, or have a preference for treatment modality. The human sciences analogue of reproducibility is the use of inferential statistics – evaluating the likelihood of intervention X producing outcome Y. This likelihood is expressed as the Number Needed to Treat (NNT) statistic, meaning the number of persons who must be treated to either achieve a positive outcome or prevent a negative outcome for one extra person. The aim of effectiveness research is to identify optimal (i.e. lowest NNT) treatment strategies, which at least in theory (and sometimes in practice[165]) can be expressed as a deterministic flowchart.

The problem with using this model of reproducibility is twofold[166]. First, clinicians in general treat individuals not groups. Therefore the scientific question of interest is not what would a group of people benefit from, but rather what would this individual benefit from? This particular person may be in the group who don't benefit from the intervention with the lowest NNT. Second, the relationship between an intervention and its effect is mediated by a host of complex internal and external factors. Exploration of groups cannot directly illuminate individual processes. Idiographic knowledge is needed to predict the impact of an intervention on an individual. A generative notion of causality[46] involves a context (in this case, the patient in their environment) mediating the association between a mechanism (a treatment) and outcome. Asking group-level questions, trying to ignore the contextual issues by random allocation of confounders, and then applying the results to individuals is the wrong method. It is missing the necessary idiographic knowledge about the person receiving the treatment.

Evidence-based medicine defenders might counter that these are technical problems, simply pointing to the need to better understand the mediators of treatment effectiveness, through techniques such as process evaluation[167]. For example, pharmacogenomics investigates the influence of genetic variation in individuals on drug response, by correlating gene expression or DNA-sequence variations with a drug's efficacy. The aim is to optimise pharmacological treatments on the basis of the individual's unique genetic profile. Similarly, psychological therapies are more effective for some individuals than others. Psychological mindedness is the umbrella term for predictors of response to psychodynamic therapy, and includes belief in the benefit of discussing problems, ability to access feelings, interest in meaning, and openness to change[168]. Predictors of effectiveness can be empirically identified. For example, response to hypothetical contradiction – the ability to entertain the possibility of beliefs being wrong – is associated with a better response to cognitive behavioural therapy for psychosis[169].

Each of these developments is desirable. Any effort to identify for the individual patient whether a treatment will be helpful is to be welcomed. However, the reliance on nomothetic data means that these are necessarily broad-brush efforts. A swab test cannot capture expectancy based on past experiences, or personal preferences for treatment modality, or cultural beliefs, or a host of other predictors of treatment response. Similarly, nobody would suggest that people who don't exhibit adequate psychological mindedness or demonstrate the ability to respond to hypothetical contradiction be denied access to psychological therapies.

The current science of mental illness remains slanted towards the objectivist position. Clinical guidelines and research are focussed on diagnostic groups. Evidence-based practice uses nomothetic knowledge developed using randomised controlled trial methodology. Interventions are evaluated in order to identify generalisable rules expressed as NNT statistics.

The central problem is that nomothetic knowledge only provides half the story, because mental illness research is a human science, not a natural science. Humans differ in important ways from the objects of study of the natural sciences: we have attitudes, we are active agents in our world, we have consciousness, we can make decisions and change our minds. These attributes mean that Enlightenment principles which work so well in the natural sciences do not work as well in clinical settings.

In the human sciences, reductionism is a problem, not an asset. It objectifies the person by squeezing all the meaning out of their experiences. $2C_2H_5OH+CO_2$ may always be champagne. Is labelling a person as 295.3 (DSM-IV code for paranoid schizophrenia) really the same type of activity? By ignoring all that makes the person human, what is left is an undifferentiated shadow of humanity. It may be possible to describe this shadow in detail, and the shadow is related to the human, but it remains a shadow. The loss of meaning arising from biomedical and biopsychosocial models was explored in Chapter 2. Why then have these models been so embraced in mental health services? We suggest there is a higher-level, societal explanation.

The distinction between nomothetic and idiographic knowledge parallels a deeper dichotomy. In Greek mythology, Apollo and Dionysius were the sons of Zeus. Apollo was the god of the sun, lightness, music and poetry. Dionysius was the god of wine, ecstasy and intoxication. These two gods have come to be associated with two world-views.

The Apollonian view of the world is characterised by a focus on truth, logic and order. For the Apollonian, the best society is one which emphasises order and predictability. The guiding ethical principle is utilitarianism, expressed in Jeremy Bentham's rule of utility: the good is whatever brings the greatest happiness to the greatest number of people[170]. An Apollonian society emphasises uniformity and group norms, and meeting obligations such as work and relationships. Dissent is actively discouraged.

By contrast, the Dionysian view emphasises spontaneity, intuition and rebellion. The ethical framework is focussed on personal fulfilment and hedonism. A Dionysian society emphasises freedom, liberation from previous constraints, and the central importance of creativity and subversion of existing power structures.

To flesh out this distinction, Table 4.1 shows other words identified by Michael Thro as associated with each perspective[171].

Societies oscillate between the two ends of this spectrum over time. For example, in England the most prominent recent Dionysian eras were the 1920s (the Roaring Twenties) and the 1960s (the Swinging Sixties). The last swing toward the Apollonian end was in the 1940s and 1950s (World War II and the austerity years). At present, society is also leaning towards an Apollonian phase, shown by the development of league tables in education and health services, restrictions on human rights in the context of the 'War on Terror', an escalating series of policy and legislative initiatives in every area of government, and so forth.

Table 4.1 Poles of the Apollonian–Dionysian continuum

Apollo	Dionysus
Sun	Earth
Ego	Id
Psyche	Eros
Stoic	Epicurean
Mind	Heart
Reason	Emotion
Thinking	Feeling
Order	Chaos
Restraint	Excess
Male	Female
Hierarchy	Equality
Science	Art
System	Spontaneity
Compulsiveness	Impulsiveness
City	Country
Classicism	Romanticism
Civilisation	Nature

What is the relevance of this dichotomy to mental health services? An Apollonian society provides a context in which the values of traditional evidence-based medicine are more likely to dominate. An emphasis on the needs of the group over the perspective of the individual means that nomothetic knowledge fits the zeitgeist better than idiographic knowledge. The desire for order and uniformity leads to an increasing emphasis on evidence-based treatments, i.e. with the lowest Number Needed to Treat score and hence the most likelihood of benefiting the group, irrespective of their impact on individual patients. Clinical judgement is seen as a potential source of bias to be reduced through increasingly prescriptive clinical guidelines, rather than a creative resource in the mental health workforce.

This Apollonian–Dionysian spectrum underpins the changing definition of recovery. The 'get back to normal' everyday meaning is Apollonian – concerned with re-establishing social order, valuing being normal (i.e. lacking in any individuality) and conforming to social norms. Personal recovery is Dionysian – concerned with individual well-being, valuing idiosyncrasy, and liberating from stigma and discrimination.

The dominance of nomothetic knowledge

The mental health system values nomothetic knowledge more than idiographic knowledge, for at least three reasons.

First, the evidence-based medicine movement has successfully equated 'evidence' with nomothetic knowledge. Since it is prima facie undesirable to work other than on the basis of evidence (e.g. on the basis of clinical anecdote, historical precedent or personal whim) then the acquisition and application of nomothetic knowledge becomes an ethical imperative for clinicians.

Second, clinical guidelines are based on the hierarchy of evidence shown earlier, which gives primacy to nomothetic knowledge. Clinical guidelines are becoming increasingly influential in informing resource allocation decisions, such as mental health team composition. Since personal concerns such as being employed and having a reasonable degree of status loom large for most professionals, this development is likely to shape research and clinical discourse. Psychoanalytic psychotherapists, for example, have traditionally been negatively disposed towards randomised controlled trials, but are now issuing urgent calls to develop a credible (i.e. nomothetic, clinical trial-based) evidence base[172].

Third, it fits the perceived role requirement. If the clinician's job is to make authoritative pronouncements in highly emotional situations, then the ability to make decisions quickly and with confidence is needed. Using nomothetic knowledge meets this need. Assessment primarily involves allocating the individual to the right group, and since action is based on predefined priorities and behavioural templates it leads to more apparent certainty than idiographic knowledge.

However, downgrading the importance of idiographic knowledge creates blind spots for clinicians, including an over-emphasis on current treatment vogues (e.g. medication – see Chapter 6), difficulty in using multiple models of understanding experience to offer genuine choice, and a belief that a diagnosis is true rather than a hypothesis.

The epistemological tension

There is a fundamental epistemological tension between nomothetic and idiographic know-ledge. We will illustrate this tension in relation to professions, science and service users.

Emphasising nomothetic knowledge leads to the job of a professional being understood in terms of 'technical rationality'[173]:

> Technical rationality holds that practitioners are instrumental problem solvers.
> Who select technical means best suited to particular purposes. Rigorous professional
> practitioners solve well-formed instrumental problems by applying theory and
> technique derived from systematic preferably scientific knowledge.
>
> (pp. 3–4)

But technical rationality is an inadequate approach for addressing human problems[174]:

> If the model of Technical Rationality is incomplete, in that it fails to account for
> practical competence in 'divergent' situations, so much the worse for the model. Let us
> search instead for an epistemology of practice implicit in the artistic, intuitive
> processes which some practitioners do bring to situations of uncertainty, instability,
> uniqueness, and value conflict.
>
> (p. 49)

Eraut notes the 'ideological exclusivity of a paradigm in which only knowledge supported by rigorous empirical research is accorded any validity'[175] (p. 10). In relation to education, Grimmett refers to[176]: 'the unmindful aping of natural science paradigms in the social sciences (sometimes referred to as scientism) that seems so pervasive in the professional schools of universities' (p. 25).

Giving primacy to nomothetic knowledge also impoverishes scientific discourse. For example, sociological research is almost totally absent from mental health literature[177], due to the 'troubled relationship between sociology and psychiatry'[178]. This makes some contentious issues – such as compliance[179], patient aggression[180], schizophrenia[181] and being a patient[182] – less visible.

To illustrate, Galbraith's work on countervailing powers involves the proposal that powers are dynamically related to each other, so increasing power in one group is linked with the possibility of resistance and reassertion of power by another[183]. Bridget Hamilton argues that the construct of insight requires a notion of identity in the patient (who expresses a view as to whether they have a mental illness or not) which is stable and located in the mind, whereas the post-modern notion of subjectivity highlights the socially con-structed and constantly changing subjective experience of self[177]. The assumption of insight as an objective reality therefore ignores the power relationships which it supports[184]. A discourse in which the position of the professional expert is given primacy over the 'lay' patient is an exercise of power. Therefore disagreement about the explanatory model of illness and the consequent need for treatment is an act of resistance by the patient to this dominant discourse. Framing this resistance as a lack of insight can then be seen as a means of reversing this power exchange. It is noteworthy that guidance for DSM-IV-TR recognises the importance of listening to the patient in the psychiatric assessment because this gives the opportunity to 'correct any distortions'[185] (p. 29).

Sociological research challenges the belief that scientific development involves the dispassionate and disinterested aggregation of knowledge over time, with each new level of understanding building on the strong foundations of established fact. Only by stepping outside the clinical frame of reference do the contradictions caused by this tension become evident. For example, assumptions about what matters become apparent when service users lead research. User-focussed monitoring is a consumer-led research method which has been used to find out from service users what they want from mental health services[186]:

- acceptance
- shared experience and shared identity (i.e. meeting others who have had the same experiences)
- emotional support
- a reason for living
- finding meaning and purpose in their lives
- peace of mind, relaxation
- taking control and having choices
- security and safety
- pleasure

Two points emerge from this list. First, they are very different to clinical preoccupations around symptom reduction, risk management and crisis containment. Second, they are all positive and forward-looking – not at all about getting rid of things like symptoms or social disability. In psychological terminology, they relate to approach motivation rather than avoidance motivation. They point to a completely different way of constructing the job of a mental health professional.

Individual service users give primacy to idiographic knowledge. There are several reasons for this. Individuals hold detailed self-knowledge about what makes them the person they are. Emphasising group membership (e.g. a diagnostic category) over individual difference does not value this self-knowledge. There is also a fear that nomothetic knowledge will be used to justify actions which lead to damage for the individual. For example, if the clinician believes that evidence shows that medication works, and this person refuses their medication, so they need to be compulsorily medicated, then the end-point is the individual experiencing coercion. The evidence-based medicine movement does not give primacy to individual choice. Finally, there is a close association between nomothetic knowledge and clinical practice. Some consumers experience services as aversive and unhelpful, and so by extension reject the evidence base underpinning the service.

On the other side of the epistemological tension, no one would argue for the abandonment of nomothetic knowledge in favour of *vulgar situatedness*[187]. An exclusive focus on idiographic knowledge leads to a number of blind spots, including a difficulty in separating what is helpful for the individual from what is helpful for others, instinctive mistrust of professionals who operate on the basis of nomothetic evidence – 'they don't listen to us', 'they don't give us genuine choices' – and an oppositional discourse, highlighting short-comings in the mental health system and implicitly or explicitly blaming mental health professionals for problems.

We can and must do better than simply relying on clinical anecdote (in which care depends on the intuition of the clinician), historical precedent (since, as we will discuss in Chapter 7, this has not been an auspicious success), or even consumer demand – the person is seeking help precisely because they are stuck and don't know the way forward. So how can this tension be resolved?

Epistemology and personal recovery

And so we come (at last!) to the central implication. A focus on personal recovery addresses the epistemological challenges outlined above. It places value on observable and nomothetic data – nobody wants treatment provided on the whim of the clinician who happens to see them. It also places value on idiographic knowledge – which is solely accessible by the patient. The practical implication for mental health services is that the application of evidence-based treatments is an important, but not exclusive, element of mental health services. As Rob Whitley put it in relation to the idiographic endeavour of cultural competence[188]: 'Cultural competence can ensure that evidence-based practices do not transmogrify into one-size-fits-all mindless technical application. Similarly, evidence-based medicine can ensure that cultural competence does not dissolve into anarchic reinvention of treatment for every individual' (p. 1589).

A good life involves a balance of the Apollonian and Dionysian – doing what you must and doing what you want. The absence of either element leads to an impoverished existence. This is a perennial truth – in 2400 BC the Egyptian Ptahhoptep wrote 'One that reckoneth accounts all the day passeth not a happy moment. One that gladdeneth his heart all the day provideth not for his house. The bowman hitteth the mark, as the steersman reacheth land, by diversity of aim'[189]. Or, as Maria Edgeworth put it in more modern parlance, 'All work and no play makes Jack a dull boy – All play and no work makes Jack a mere toy'[190].

A central proposition of this book is that both nomothetic and idiographic knowledge are necessary types of evidence. Both are authentic: they each tell us something meaningful and valid about the world. Both types are also necessary to provide a full and balanced picture of the world. This integrative stance mirrors modern resolutions of other dualisms. Donald Hebb responded to a journalist's question about whether nature or nurture contributed more to personality by asking whether the length or width of a rectangle contributes more to its area[191]. Similarly, Peter Chadwick commented on the mind–body dualism that *psychology without brain is like biology without mind*[67].

As noted in Chapter 1, this book is written to illustrate the blending of both types of knowledge. It combines insights from many individuals with arguments based on nomothetic studies. My interest in personal recovery in part emerged from noticing discordance between, on the one hand, the dissatisfaction I heard in conversations with patients and when reading first-hand accounts of recovered individuals (idiographic knowledge), and on the other hand the much more positive picture of increasingly effective psychological and pharmacological interventions emerging as nomothetic knowledge in the last 20 years in the academic literature.

Neither nomothetic nor idiographic knowledge in isolation are a sufficient underpinning for clinical practice. Some commentators draw nihilistic conclusions[22]: 'My solution – to the problem of mental illness – is that there is and can be no general solution. There is no general theory that can inform our decisions . . . [Unlike general medicine] In psychiatry there are no such basic principles . . . The ultimate criteria in deciding what to do in a psychiatric emergency are ethical, not scientific' (p. 73).

I agree that foundational or universal theories are suspect, but disagree with the pessimistic implications. A suspicion about the universality of theory simply places in the foreground the importance of values – as Bracken and Thomas put it, ethics before technology[26]. Theories differ in their implicit values, and the choice of theory is not value-free. Therefore, debate about theory *is* debate about values. We propose key values relating to personal recovery in Chapter 15. For now, we identify an alternative epistemological basis.

Constructivism – a more helpful epistemological basis

A balance point between subjectivism and objectivism can be found in the epistemology of constructivism. This holds that all knowledge is constructed, and does not necessarily reflect external reality, but rather depends on convention, individual perception and social experience. It specifically criticises the notion of ontological reality (i.e. reality as it is in itself) as incoherent, since one must already know what reality consists of in order to confirm it.

This perspective is not new. Gautama Buddha (560–477 BC) wrote 'We are what we think. All that we are arises with our thoughts. With our thoughts we make the world'. Heraclitus (540–475 BC) said that 'one cannot step into the same river twice . . . all is flux; all is becoming' (i.e. neither the person nor the river is ever the same). More recently, Immanuel Kant (1724–1804) described the mind as an active organ 'which transforms the chaotic multiplicity of experience into the orderly unit of thought'. The Swiss philosopher and psychologist Jean Piaget is credited with the development of formal constructivist epistemology[192].

Mahoney identifies five basic themes in constructivism: activity; order; identity; social-symbolic processes; and dynamic, dialectical development[193]:

> Constructivism views the living system as a proactive agent that participates in its own life dynamics. This portrayal is in contrast to traditional physical science renditions, in which the living system is a passive conduit of energies, forces and masses that are moved or modified only by being impacted by other external entities. In constructivism, complex systems – and certainly those we call 'living systems' – are organic processes expressing self-movement and ongoing self-organization.
>
> (p. 747)

A key theme in constructivism is the role of disorder, as a trigger for dialectical development (i.e. change generated by contrasts). Disorder, the opposite of order, is necessary for the development of complex systems, so processes of disorder are not pathologised as opponents of health. This observation underpins the discussion of risk in Chapter 20. New life patterns emerge from the chaos and dysfunction that occur when previous patterns are no longer viable[194]. The accounts of people with a diagnosis of schizophrenia contain many examples of this type of personal growth[195]:

> Before when I was a kid and not having any really bad symptoms, if I saw somebody who really looked [odd], stood out, I might giggle like the rest of the kids. Now, I would have compassion for the person.
>
> It [having schizophrenia] made me more human . . . it made me really have compassion and empathy.
>
> I still had to struggle with was I ever going to get a Bachelor's degree and . . . ever have kids and I've come to terms with those two things – no and no . . . Strangely

enough, it doesn't bother me. I just felt a release of negative energy when I gave up those aspirations.

Well, it, my illness, actually got me writing poetry. For which I've been published. I got some recognition.

This does not of course mean the experience of mental illness should be romanticised, or that the personal growth opportunities are readily apparent or proximal. It does, however, suggest caution in viewing mental illness as a wholly negative experience. This is consistent with consumer narratives reviewed in Chapter 3, which indicated that the experience of mental illness can bring both burden and benefit.

From a constructivist perspective, identity is not a single stable entity, or a collection of enduring personality traits. Rather, it is an embodied and emerging process, combining both consistency and diversity. Furthermore, this process is embedded in a social and symbolic context, in which the development of personal identity occurs within human and other relationships. A prime focus in supporting recovery is therefore on relationships, covered in Chapters 10 to 13.

In common with other knowledge bodies (e.g. cultural studies, ecological ethics, linguistics, human rights movements), a key assumption in constructivism is that everything and everyone is connected. This emphasis on intrapsychic and interpersonal process and the dynamic, changing nature of development provides a more helpful model of self when applied in mental illness. It opens up the possibility of adaptation, re-orientation, integration, and other responses to the experience by the individual. It also recognises the dynamic nature of social role negotiation – if everyone treats the person as being mentally ill, then this inexorably influences the self-image of the person, just as the behaviour of the person influences how others respond to them. In particular, the *way* that mental health staff work with people in the 'patient' role may be as important as *what* they do. The role of identity and social roles underpins the Personal Recovery Framework developed in Chapter 9.

A key advantage of constructivism is that it encourages a scientific and professional self-awareness and tentativeness. A constructivist perspective is mindful of being an ideology rather than 'how things are' – unlike the evidence-based health care (EBHC) lack of awareness[196]:

> EBHC is an ideology . . . but one that violates its own ideology. Indeed, one of the basic tenets is that only what has been scientifically proven in RCTs is credible, and it is a matter of faith that only what has been proven in such research is safe to be used in health care to improve health . . . Evidence-based medicine is for believers . . . EBHC adepts will be in the belief state forever.
>
> (p. 1374)

Constructivism is also pro-scientific in the wider sense of the term, whilst recognising the limitations of any universal or foundational theory. As Foucault put it[197]:

> The intellectual's role is no longer to place himself 'somewhat ahead and to the side' in order to express the stifled truth of the collectivity; rather, it is to struggle against the forms of power that transform him into its object and instrument in the sphere of 'knowledge', 'truth', 'consciousness' and 'discourse'.
>
> (pp. 207–208)

Constructivism offers the opportunity to integrate the knowledge underpinning clinical models with the uniqueness of the individual.

Box 4.1 Principles for a mental health service based on a constructivist epistemology

Principle 1:	Clinicians are not dispassionate scientists – our values, beliefs and actions influence the sense we make of the patient
Principle 2:	A clinical model produces a hypothesis – it is not reality, and so may need amending or discounting
Principle 3:	A clinical model is valuable when the hypothesis it generates is useful to the patient
Principle 4:	Clinical work is inherently a collaborative endeavour, involving the patient and the clinician working to re-construct new and more helpful understandings about the person and their world

Mental health services need to work in ways which value both professional (nomothetic) and personal (idiographic) knowledge. We have proposed constructivism as a more helpful epistemological basis, which integrates these two approaches. A constructivist perspective would lead to four principles for mental health services, shown in Box 4.1.

These principles are highly supportive of personal recovery. They emphasise the importance of both professional knowledge and the self-knowledge of the consumer. The clinician's job is more than a technical role implementing treatments defined in clinical guidelines. It is to be an active and influential person working in partnership with the consumer, bringing nomothetic expertise-by-training to complement the person's idiographic expertise-by-experience. A key tool in the clinician's armoury is the ability to apply well-developed clinical models as one means of making sense of the person's experience. The crucial advantage offered by a constructivist perspective is that the focus is on utility – does the clinical model help the person? If not, change the model, rather than trying to change the person.

Epistemology is, as we have noted, intimately entangled with values. We therefore turn now to the issue of ethics – the values prioritised by mental health services and systems.

5 Ethical rationale

Summary of the ethical rationale

The consumer is in general better placed than the mental health professional to identify what is in their best interests. Therefore care should normally be provided on the basis of the consumer's goals and preferences. The two ethical justifications for compulsion are the interests of society and the best interests of the patient. Best interests are better defined by the patient or their nominated proxy decision-maker than by mental health professionals.

The aim of this chapter is not to provide an overarching ethical framework or describe the legal justification for compulsion, since that is a task better left to experts[198;199]. Rather it is to make the point that an orientation towards doing things to a person on the basis of professional views about their best interests does not promote personal recovery. A better guiding principle is to orient action by clinicians as far as possible around the consumer's goals, rather than professional goals. We then consider the exceptions to this principle.

Working with the consumer

We start with a guiding ethical principle: that mental health services should as far as possible be oriented towards supporting the individual to achieve personally valued goals, rather than towards the goals professionals might have for them. This sounds like an orientation to which every mental health professional would sign up, and yet the emergent properties of the system are not always consistent with this principle. For example, care plans typically focussed on amelioration of deficits, resolution of symptoms, avoidance of hospitalisation and relapse, and restoration of social functioning are based on clinical goals rather than life goals. These aspects may be necessary stepping stones, but these are not in themselves life goals. Practical approaches to identifying the individual's life goals will be described in Chapter 17.

An orientation towards giving primacy to consumer-defined goals means the primary job of mental health services is to support the person to progress towards their own life goals, not to provide treatment to meet clinical goals. Treatment is one important resource available from mental health professionals, but it should be a means to an end of the individual's life goals, not an end in itself. Clinical skills remain central. For example the clinician may observe consistent links between a particular behaviour of a patient (e.g. self-neglecting, becoming euphoric, reporting an increase in preoccupation with voices, stopping medication, having arguments with neighbours) and an undesirable outcome. This is important information, which the professional should actively highlight in their work with the patient, and support the person to engage in processing. But the difference is that this professional expertise is a resource to be offered to the consumer, as we discuss in Chapter 18.

This principle is the ethical justification for a focus on personal recovery. However, there are obligations conferred on mental health professionals which require some things to be done which are not based on the individual's life goals, and with which the individual may not agree[200]. Until there is a change in political stance about concepts such as responsibility, mental health professionals need to meet this obligation. The remainder of this chapter explores when compulsion is acceptable. This underpins the approach described in Section 3, where recovery-focussed approaches to medication (Chapter 19), risk (Chapter 20) and crisis (Chapter 21) are outlined.

We suggest that there are two justifications for doing things to people against their will.

Compulsion justification 1: benefit to society

Societies have values. The extent to which deviance is valued or tolerated, the balance between individual and community good, the role of the state in the protection of minors, the importance of public safety and the acceptability of suicide are all examples of societal values. They reflect the relative importance attached at a given point in time to individual freedom and group freedom: the Apollonian–Dionysian spectrum described in Chapter 4. Societal values change over time, but at any one time they are invariant. Societal values are expressed as mandated behavioural constraints. Most commonly in relation to mental health these constraints are that no one will be left to die (whether wilfully through suicide or unintentionally through self-neglect) or allowed to harm others. These behavioural constraints are non-negotiable.

One obligation placed on mental health professionals is to constrain behaviour in order to uphold these societal values. This obligation is conferred either directly through mental health legislation or indirectly through codes of conduct and mental health policy. It is an obligation which cannot and should not be ignored in a recovery-focussed mental health system. These societally imposed, non-negotiable constraints on behaviour provide one ethical justification for compulsion.

Distinguishing between intervening to benefit society and intervening to benefit the patient is helpful. It is honest, and places responsibility for this decision where it belongs – with society, rather than the individual professional. Professional judgement about whether the person has crossed over the societally mandated line remains central, but the line itself is not a professional judgement. It also makes clear that compulsion is not necessarily in the patient's best interests. For example, the responses of people who have experienced compulsory detention are highly variable, ranging from extremely positive ('It saved my life') to extremely negative ('It traumatised me')[201]. As another example, for people showing a pattern of disengagement, relapse and compulsory admissions, the professional response of taking responsibility may well ultimately be damaging for some patients, if it gets in the way of the individual taking personal responsibility for their own well-being. Since we cannot predict with certainty whether a specific patient will benefit from a compulsory intervention, we cannot know if it is in the patient's best interest. The justification for intervening is to uphold societal rules (which we can know), rather than for the benefit of the patient (which we cannot know).

Compulsion justification 2: best interests

Over and above societally mandated boundaries of behaviour, there is an ethical justification to intervene in situations where there is a risk of damage to the person's life, health and well-being. There is no law that says someone cannot give away all their money or ruin their marriage through promiscuous behaviour when manic, or isolate themselves when depressed, or blot out voices with alcohol, or any of the other dilemmas with which mental health professionals routinely become involved. Yet the right to autonomy is reasonably over-ridden for some people at some points in their life by considerations of best interests. This is recognised in mental health legislation. For example, in England the legal justification for compulsion is risk to self or others (i.e. the societal rules justification) or risk to health (i.e. the best interests justification). A recovery orientation does not mean standing back, on the grounds that the person refuses help, whilst their life thins out and slips away.

This ethical justification for compulsion is paternalism: a clinician is acting paternalistically towards a patient when: his action benefits the patient; his action involves violating a moral rule with regard to the patient; his action does not have the patient's past, present or immediately forthcoming consent; and the clinician believes they can make their own decision[202]. Some clinicians might reject the label of paternalism, viewing their work as client-centred and not involving compulsion. The argument which we will present is as applicable to the more acceptable ethical principle of beneficence: doing things to a person on the basis of professional beliefs about what is in their best interests.

The idea of doing things to the patient in their best interest has been a consistent theme in the evolution of the mental health system, as we discuss in Chapter 7. The marker of a service in which ethical imperatives such as paternalism or beneficence are given primacy is a discourse in which actions are justified on the basis of duty (e.g. 'I'm a Doctor, so I treat people'), with professional (rather than the individual's) perceptions about their best interests driving care. This approach arises from a world-view that treatments are effective, and the privileged access of health professionals to these effective interventions places an ethical requirement on those practitioners to provide treatment. This has led to an often unchallenged assumption that best interests are necessarily defined by professionals. There are four challenges to this assumption.

First, this ethical imperative is increasingly out of step with wider societal values, which instead emphasise personal responsibility, informed choice and the right to self-determination. In other areas of life there is a recognition that the goals, aspirations and values of the individual should (in a moral sense) take primacy over those of the professional. This is eloquently expressed by consumer-activist Judi Chamberlin[203]:

> The ethical system . . . that drives the involuntary treatment system is paternalism, the idea that one group (the one in power, not oddly) knows what is best for another group (which lacks power). The history of civilisation is, in part, the struggle against paternalism and for self-determination. People in power are always saying that they know what is best for those they rule over, even if those poor unfortunate individuals think they know best what they want . . . The struggle for freedom has always been seen by the powerful as a denial of the obvious truth of the superiority of the rulers.
>
> (p. 406)

It is also recognised by professionals[26]:

> Until now, most psychiatrists wanted to hold on to an identity centred on the idea that they were delivering science-based technologies to patients suffering from certain identified illnesses . . . As such, psychiatry is very much a modernist venture. Its primary discourse is scientific, mainly around biology and positivistic versions of psychology. Issues such as meaning, values and assumptions are not dismissed but they are relatively unimportant, secondary concerns.
>
> (p. 5)

Second, health professionals no longer have sole access to information about treatments. Many patients have easy access through the internet to diverse sources of information about their mental illness. More deeply, in the previous chapter we identified changes in the world-view occurring during the Enlightenment. An implicit dichotomy that developed was between knowledge which is held by professionals and belief which is held by lay (i.e. non-professional) people. The implication of this dichotomy is that professional knowledge is more highly valued than lay beliefs. This distinction is challenged in a constructivist epistemology (outlined in the previous chapter), in which all forms of knowing are positioned as belief, and there is no true, unchanging knowledge.

The third challenge to the professional judging what is in the best interests of the individual arises from an awareness that the interests of people with mental illness have not been well served when responsibility for their well-being is assumed by others. This aspect will be elaborated in Chapter 7. Clinicians recognise the issue[198]:

> Ethical concerns about the psychiatrist's role and functions have dogged the
> profession for at least three centuries . . . Moral harms have emerged from the misuse
> of the asylum as a custodial 'warehouse', misunderstanding of the transference
> relationship, the gruesome effects of physical treatments such as leucotomy and
> insulin coma (to name but two), the misuse of psychiatry for political purposes (as
> occurred in the former Soviet Union) and systems of healthcare that jeopardise the
> needs of the individual, purportedly to benefit the many.
>
> (p. 7)

The final challenge to giving primacy to a professional perspective on best interests is that it is inconsistent with modern capacity-based legislation. For example, in England and Wales the Mental Capacity Act[204] defines best interests as what the patient would have chosen for themselves in the situation if they had capacity. This necessarily requires attention to the person's goals, values and preferences.

So we argue that: (a) best interests are a justification for compulsion; AND (b) in a recovery-focussed system, the closer to the individual's view of their own best interests the compulsion is, the more it can be ethically justified. How can the person's views of what is in their best interest be identified? The best approach is for the person themselves to state in advance what they wish to happen when in crisis. Where this is not possible, a proxy decision-maker is the next best alternative. Since family or friends will often know the person better than the clinician, professional judgement is not in general the best approach to identifying what the person themselves would have chosen. If neither the individual's preference nor a nominated proxy decision-maker is available, then a clinical perspective on best interests may be the best remaining approach. In Chapter 21 we explore what this means in practice.

We have argued that the two justifications for compulsion are non-negotiable behavioural constraints mandated by society and the best interests of the patient, and that best interests are better defined by the patient or their nominated proxy decision-maker than the clinician. This points to a need for professional certainty and tentativeness: certainty about the non-negotiable behavioural constraints, and tentativeness about what is in the best interests of the patient.

Balancing ethical imperatives

Acting to uphold societal rules or in the person's best interests can conflict with other values[198]. For example, the post-Enlightenment focus on 'self' as a primary unit of analysis leads to a view that distress is internal, individual, unhealthy and unnatural. This understanding of rationality emerges from, and has the embedded assumptions of, a White, male, Western perspective. The existence of other perspectives raises important questions[26]:

> If psychiatry is the product of a culture which was preoccupied with rationality and the individual self, what sort of mental health care is appropriate in the postmodern, multicultural world in which many of these preoccupations are losing their dominance? . . . Should we not attempt to develop a discourse about distress that incorporates insights from more than 30 years of feminist and postcolonial thinking and writing in this realm? Is Western psychiatry appropriate to cultural groups which do not share Enlightenment preoccupations, but instead value a spiritual ordering of the world and an ethical emphasis on the importance of family and community?
>
> (p. 12)

Clinical judgement is a central approach to balancing conflicting values. In a recovery-focussed service this is even more true, because developing decision-making approaches in which the consumer is more empowered will create new ethical dilemmas, especially in relation to professional accountability where what the person wants is incompatible with the clinical perspective[205].

If values need to be balanced, how is this done? One approach is values-based practice, which we discuss in Chapter 15. Another approach is to draw from biomedical ethics. Beauchamp and Childress propose four guiding principles[206]:

1. Respect for autonomy: the importance of personal choice and self-determination is emphasised
2. Non-maleficence: there is an active focus on avoiding hopelessness and dependency
3. Beneficence: there is an equally active focus on providing effective treatments and interventions
4. Justice: there is support to exercise citizenship rights.

In their framework, actions justified on the basis of beneficence are balanced by the need to promote autonomy and support citizenship.

A third approach is to use different values. We explore this in Chapter 15. For example, a modern version of the Hippocratic Oath, written by Louis Lasagna in 1964, puts this well:

> I will respect the hard-won scientific gains of those physicians in whose steps I walk . . . I will apply, for the benefit of the sick, all measures [that] are required, avoiding those twin traps of overtreatment and therapeutic nihilism . . . I will remember that there is art to medicine as well as science, and that warmth, sympathy, and understanding may outweigh the surgeon's knife or the chemist's drug . . . I will not be ashamed to say 'I know not,' nor will I fail to call in my colleagues when the skills of another are needed for a patient's recovery . . . I will remember that I do not treat a fever chart, a cancerous growth, but a sick human being, whose illness may affect the person's family and economic stability. My responsibility includes these related problems, if I am to care adequately for the sick.

Incorporating these values into mental health services would change basic assumptions. At present it is difficult to identify any use of the concept of 'overtreatment'. The result is that many patients receive unnecessary and (for some) harmful treatments. Similarly, few clinicians admit 'I know not', even when patients present with the most intractable of life difficulties. The rationale is the importance of maintaining therapeutic optimism, but the stance is underpinned by Enlightenment principles: the triumph of rationality and the dominance of evidence-based medicine. Admitting ignorance would destroy the illusion that the clinician will be responsible for the patient, but would also give back responsibility to the patient for finding their own way forward. We explore the implications for clinician–consumer relationships in Chapter 13.

Many of the case studies in this book illustrate what a greater emphasis on values looks like in practice. As a precursor, the Soteria Project[207] focussed on the values expected of workers[26]:

- *Do no harm*
- *Do unto others as you would have done unto yourself*
- *Be flexible and responsive*
- *In general the user knows best*
- *Valuing choice, self-determination, the right to refuse and informed consent*
- *Anger, dependency, sexuality and personal growth are acceptable and expected*
- *Where possible, legitimate needs should be met*
- *Take risks*
- *Make power relationships explicit* (pp. 265–266)

An emphasis on values positions the application of scientific knowledge as a means, not an end. Debates about method become recognised as debates about values and ethics. This change is happening in other areas of society, such as a questioning by the organic food movement of the primacy given to efficiency. In mental health services, a focus on values challenges the predefined goal of transforming the abnormal human into a normal human. Rather, the goals (and resulting methods) of mental health services become truly patient-centred: based on what individuals themselves aspire to in their life.

Chapter 6

Effectiveness rationale

Summary of the effectiveness rationale

The effectiveness of medication for mental illness has been exaggerated, the indications widened, and the potential disadvantages under-stated. Having a balanced and evidence-based approach to medication, rather than predefining it as a necessity, will focus services on personal rather than clinical recovery priorities.

Medication is the dominant treatment offered for mental illness. Across all users of specialist mental health services, 92% have taken medication for their mental illness in the previous year[208], rising to 98–100% for people admitted to in-patient units[209]. More widely, there has been a huge increase in prescription of medication for common mental disorders in primary care. For example, primary care prescriptions for antidepressants in England have tripled, from 9.9 million in 1992 to 27.7 million in 2003[210]. Primary care physicians are well aware of clinical guidelines that medication should not be a first-line treatment for mild to moderate depression[211], but prescribe antidepressants because of the lack of available alternatives. In the past three years, 78% of primary care physicians prescribed where they thought an alternative approach would have been more appropriate, including 66% because the alternative was not available and 62% because of the waiting list for the suitable alternative[212]. Similarly, for severe mental illnesses such as psychosis, treatment almost always involves medication, with a much lower level of provision of psychological and social interventions[213].

The intention in this book is not to be anti-medication but pro-choice, and in Chapter 19 we discuss the contribution of medication to recovery. However, in this chapter we argue that the dominance of medication as a treatment strategy is empirically unjustified. We make this case by critically outlining the stages by which medication comes to be seen as a necessity.

Creating markets

Before a drug can be tested, it needs a condition (or, from the perspective of pharmaceutical companies, a market). One means of opening up a new market is to identify a new condition. However, if done overtly the profit motive would be transparent and invoke suspicion. Pharmaceutical companies therefore use covert strategies to develop new markets. One method is to get the sufferers to raise awareness – a particularly powerful approach, since who can criticise the patient voice? Many user or consumer or patient groups receive funding from drug companies. For example, Andrew Herxheimer[214] notes that the Global Alliance of Mental Illness Advocacy (GAMIAN Europe) was founded by Bristol-Myers-Squibb, and in the USA the National Alliance for the Mentally Ill 'between 1996 and 1998 received almost $12m from 18 drug companies, led by Eli Lilly. The organisation promotes the nationwide expansion of PACT (Program of Assertive Community

Treatment), which includes home deliveries of psychiatric drugs backed by court order' (p. 1209).

Eloquent explorations of disease mongering – widening the boundaries of medicine to grow markets for those who sell and deliver treatments[215] – are becoming available, and should be required reading for professionals who view a diagnosis (such as bipolar disorder[216], attention deficit hyperactivity disorder[217], social phobia[218] or post-traumatic stress disorder[219]) as revealed truth rather than social construction.

Once the existence of the condition is established, whether through lobbying by sufferers or other forms of disease awareness campaigns[53], it is then more acceptable for pharmaceutical companies to propose their product as the solution. This is done under the guise of providing information – again, who could deny that people have a right to information?

The problem is that the information is biased. This is shown by experiences from the USA and New Zealand, the only countries so far to allow direct to consumer advertising (DTCA) by pharmaceutical companies. For example, after legalising DTCA in 1997 with regulation by the Food and Drug Administration (FDA), spending on advertisements in USA went from $266m in 1994 to $2.5bn in 2000[220]. A review concluded[221]: 'DTCA is also often inaccurate . . . From 1997 to 2001, the FDA issued 94 notices of violations, mostly because benefits of the drug were hyped up and risk minimised' (p. 1709).

The 'science' of commercially funded drug trials

What about the science? Drug research is not independent. Pharmaceutical companies directly fund between 70%[222] and 90%[223] of all drug trials. Even where the funding is from non-industry sources, between one quarter[224] and one third[225] of investigators have industry affiliations. Increasingly in the USA, drug trials are performed by commercial organisations called contract research organizations who compete with each other for business. This means that there is a financial incentive to design and perform trials in ways which produce advantage for the customer – the drug company[26].

Research funded by a pharmaceutical company is more likely to show benefit for their product, due to selection of an inappropriate comparator or publication bias[226]. Biased scientific designs include exposing the control group to a washout period (i.e. creating a withdrawal effect)[26] or using older drugs with worse side-effect profiles as the comparator[227], or even dropping 'under-performing' sites altogether[228].

This bias in scientific quality is then amplified by bias in reporting of results. Publication bias is strongly present in reporting of drug-company funded research. One strategy is multiple publication of results favouring their product[229], disguised through author rotation and substitution[230]. For example, the 1999 Cochrane review of the effectiveness of one popular atypical antipsychotic (olanzapine) found the same study cited in 83 separate publications[230]. The 2005 update concluded[231]:

> A great deal of global effect / mental state data are missing from the studies supplied by Eli Lilly . . . We find it surprising that a compound worth $3.69bn per year is so successful even though there is a lack of important data for people with schizophrenia, their families and professional carers . . . We have found no evidence of an attempt to conceal the fact that the hundreds of presentations relate to a limited number of studies but inclusion of the unique company trial codes in each presentation would have helped piece together the few sausages from the very thinly sliced salami.

This is in no way a company-specific issue. Publication bias has also been shown for another popular anti-psychotic – clozapine[232].

A second strategy is selective reporting and publishing of mixed results[233]. For example, a review investigated the association between FDA-registered antidepressant studies (with FDA ratings of efficacy) and resulting publications[234]. They considered 74 studies, involving 12 antidepressants and 12 564 patients. Of 38 studies rated by the FDA as positive for the sponsoring drug company, 37 were published. Of the 36 studies rated either negative ($n=24$) or questionable ($n=12$), 22 were not published, 11 were published as positive, and 3 were published as not positive. This publishing bias inflates the apparent effect size of each individual drug (ranging from 11% to 69% inflation), and the FDA-rated overall mean weighted effect size of 0.31 was inflated to an apparent effect size of 0.41. A similar picture emerges in Sweden[229]. (Disconcertingly, immediately after writing this paragraph I looked at the online BBC news to find the lead article titled 'Anti-depressants "of little use"', about a new study indicating drug–placebo differences only occurring in very severe depression[235] – media interest may change practice more than scientific findings.)

Presumably mindful of potential litigation, surprisingly few commentators label these practices as fraud for profit. If industry-funded studies are to be viewed as research (which they apparently are, given their publication in academic journals), then these practices are unethical. If (as they perhaps should be) they are treated as marketing material, then their status is a matter of commercial ethics, but they should not be accorded the status of academic research.

There are numerous other areas of concern, including:

- Pharmaceutical industry links with political leaders[236]
- Industry funding of regulatory bodies in Europe[237] and the USA[238]
- Citing 'data on file' and 'educational information' (i.e. not peer-reviewed) in marketing material given to professionals[228]
- Use of popular internet sites to propagate a financially advantageous biomedical model of schizophrenia[239]
- Industry influence on clinical guideline development[240].

The depth of the problem is becoming apparent in increasingly common reviews in medical journals[234;235;241;242]. A former editor of the New England Journal of Medicine, Marcia Angell, commented on the pharmaceutical companies that[243]: 'This is an industry that in some ways is like the Wizard of Oz – still full of bluster but now being exposed as something far different from its image. Instead of being an engine of innovation, it is a vast marketing machine' (p. 20). It is not clear why this particular journal seems to so galvanise its editors about the issue, but another former editor, Arnold Relman, goes further (cited by Moynihan [244]): 'The medical profession is being bought by the pharmaceutical industry, not only in terms of the practice of medicine, but also in terms of teaching and research' (p. 1190).

The actual effectiveness of pharmacotherapy

Can we get an unbiased view about the effectiveness of psychotropic medication? Two approaches have been used.

First, analysis of results from studies registered in the Food and Drug Administration (FDA) database: this addresses several sources of bias – it includes full disclosure of all data from world-wide testing of a drug (so selective or multiple reporting and dropping of sites is minimised), and has robust quality standards (so poor comparators and methodology are minimised). For antipsychotics ($n=10\,118$), annual rates of suicide and attempted suicide were 1.8% and 3.3% for placebo, 0.9% and 5.7% for typical antipsychotic, and 0.7% and

5.0% for atypical antipsychotic[245]. Symptom reduction was experienced by 1.1% of participants for placebo (n=462), 17.3% for typical antipsychotic (n=261) and 16.6% for atypical antipsychotic (n=1203). For antidepressants (n=19 639), annual rates of suicide and attempted suicide were 0.4% and 2.7% with placebo, 0.7% and 3.4% with active comparators (i.e. control group antidepressants), and 0.8% and 2.8% with investigational antidepressants[246]. Symptom reduction was experienced by 30.9% with placebo (n=2805), 41.7% with active comparators (n=1416), and 40.7% with investigational antidepressants (n=4510). These data suggest nil or marginal benefit from psychotropic medication – certainly not the uniform substantial benefit that would justify current prescription levels.

A second approach has been used in the UK and USA, where non-industry funded pragmatic trials of first-generation (typical) versus second-generation (atypical) antipsychotics have been completed. The US Clinical Antipsychotic Trials of Intervention Effectiveness (CATIE) Study (n=1493) and the UK Cost Utility of the Latest Antipsychotic Drugs in Schizophrenia Studies (CUtLASS) (n=363) had consistent findings[247]: 'Our conclusion must be that first-generation drugs, if carefully prescribed, are as good as most second-generation drugs in many if not most patients with established schizophrenia' (p. 163).

The conclusion drawn by the principal investigators of the two studies is interesting[247]:

> It is worth reflecting on how crudely we often use antipsychotic drugs. Polypharmacy, the prescribing of two or more antipsychotics in parallel, is widespread despite the lack of evidence to support it and the knowledge that it doubles cost and multiplies safety risk. Off-label prescribing is common. It is perhaps not surprising that, in the context of a severe, chronic illness, clinicians are tempted to resort to untested measures. It is the same sense of frustration that allowed us to be 'beguiled' . . . by the promise of a new class of drugs. These trials emphasise again the urgent need for discovering new, safe, effective medications, as well as knowing how to best use our effective treatments.
>
> (p. 163)

My conclusion is different. CUtLASS, CATIE and studies reviewed earlier in the chapter all indicate that the benefits of each generation of medication have been systematically exaggerated, both in absolute terms and relative to previous generations. The winners from this arrangement are pharmaceutical companies, who make more money, and those who prescribe, whose status is enhanced. The losers are patients.

The close ties with pharmaceutical companies and the support for a model locating mental illness as a biochemical disturbance may come to be seen as the central failure of the profession of psychiatry in the late twentieth century. In the words of the President of the American Psychiatric Association[248]: 'as a profession, we have allowed the biopsychosocial model to become the bio-bio-bio model . . . Drug company representatives bearing gifts are frequent visitors to psychiatrists' offices and consulting rooms. We should have the wisdom and distance to call these gifts what they are – kickbacks and bribes' (p. 3).

An empirically supported view of medication

Clinical guidelines[142] emphasise the value of maintenance medication, with the results that psychotropic medication prescription is near universal in mental health services[213]. This needs to change.

Overall, a balanced appraisal of the effectiveness of medication would be that medication has some benefits, generally modest, for some people some of the time. The development of better medications is of course welcome, and pharmacological treatment should be available to all. But prescription of medication should be a genuine choice for patients. This has important implications.

Because medication will have a neutral or harmful impact on some patients, the professional orientation towards prescribing when in doubt is damaging. For example, polypharmacy becomes the norm, and difficult to address through quality improvement approaches[249]. I have yet to meet a prescriber who states that they prescribe when in doubt, and yet the level of prescribing especially in specialist mental health services suggests that this belief exists and influences practice. David Whitwell – a practising psychiatrist – asks an important question[22]: 'If only 50% derive benefit from the drugs, why are 100% still being encouraged to take them? The 50% who do not benefit may be positively disadvantaged by the unwanted effects of the drug. Efforts to raise the amount that patients actually take of the prescribed drugs fail to address well-founded patient scepticism' (p. 21).

Almost all clinical trial evidence in favour of antipsychotic medication involves short-term (i.e. less than two years) follow-up[250]. Even accounting for the bias in presentation of medication trials reviewed earlier, consistent benefits at the group level are shown for symptom reduction during acute relapse. What is less clear is the need for long-term maintenance medication as a prophylactic against relapse. The Vermont longitudinal study[113] found different approaches to medication among the recovered patients:

- 20% were prescribed no psychotropic medication
- 30% were prescribed but did not take any medication (i.e. non-compliance)
- 25% were prescribed and made targeted use (i.e. partial compliance)
- 25% were prescribed and 'religiously' took their medication (i.e. full compliance).

The view that prophylactic medication should in all cases be prescribed long-term (the euphemism meaning for life, unless the patient complains) is neither empirically supported nor promoting of personal recovery. Literature on this subject inadvertently highlights the values embedded in prescribing[250]: 'Although we should understand and respect our patients' decision to opt for a trial off medication, in the majority of cases it would be most responsible to recommend maintenance of antipsychotic medication on an indefinite basis' (pp. 286 and 290). A recovery-promoting approach would involve the availability of medication long-term, for the individual patient to use (in an active sense) if *in their judgement* the benefits outweigh the costs.

The view that there is something irrational (linked to lack of capacity) in not taking psychotropic medication as prescribed is common, but also not empirically supported. Rates of compliance in physical and mental illness are broadly similar. One review found 58% of prescribed antipsychotic medication was taken, 65% of antidepressant medication and 76% of medication for physical illness[251]. Other studies find no difference between compliance rates[252].

Reasons for not taking prescribed psychotropic medication are varied. For example, a study investigating the predictors of medication compliance in 228 people admitted to acute units in England and Wales found that coercion during admission, an unhelpful relationship with the prescribing clinician, low involvement in treatment decisions, prominent side-effects, poor 'insight' and negative attitude to treatment all predicted poorer compliance[253]. More generally, a key emerging determinant is the match between the explanatory model of the patient and the prescriber[254]. Unsurprisingly, therefore, collaborative decision-making is associated with improved adherence[255]. Finally, there is now preliminary evidence that use of neuroleptic medication on first presentation may not be necessary[256], and that discontinuation can in itself be harmful[257]. Non-compliance may be a highly rational response for some patients.

If decision-making is based on realistic concerns, why does medication seem to be the focus for so much of mental health services? Again, Whitwell's analysis is clear[22]: 'There is an expectation in psychiatric hospitals that people will be given medication . . . If none is prescribed it will lead to the question being asked of whether the person is really ill and really needs to be in hospital . . . there are no serious psychiatric illnesses for which no drugs are indicated' (p. 32).

We need to move away from professional imperatives to prescribe, and towards genuinely patient-led approaches which place the individual at the heart of decision-making. Some patients will take medication as suggested by the prescriber. Some will negotiate the dose, type or duration of prescription. Some will choose non-pharmacological approaches to self-management. All choices are valid, because making choices promotes self-determination and personal responsibility. Can we estimate the proportions in each group? The Soteria Project is an approach developed by the late Loren Mosher to provide care for people experiencing acute psychosis, which emphasised the role of the environment and relationships ('interpersonal phenomenology') rather than medication[207]. The approach was not anti-medication but pro-choice. At two-year follow-up, 58% of people had received neuroleptic medication at any time and 19% continuously during the two-year period[258]. The overall approach was associated with improved outcomes[258] and reduced costs[259] compared with admission to standard acute units. In Chapter 19 we will explore what a recovery-supporting approach to medication looks like in practice.

This will not be a simple shift. What is the compassionate clinician to do when confronted with someone experiencing severe and disabling symptoms? How can the experienced professional respond when the person seems intent on following a path of action which looks certain to repeat previous damaging cycles? These real-life clinical dilemmas will be addressed in Section 3. We now turn to the fourth rationale for focussing on personal recovery.

Empowerment rationale

Summary of the empowerment rationale

The interests of people with mental illness have consistently been subordinated to the interests of other dominant groups in society. 'Their' life has not been safe in our hands. Consumers should have primacy in decision-making about their own lives.

In this chapter we provide some illustrations of the ways in which the emergent properties of the mental health system have subordinated the interests of people with mental illness to the interests of other dominant groups in society.

For convenience the presentation is chronological, but the chapter is not intended to be a history of the mental health system. Nor is it intended to be balanced. The point of this chapter is to note some of the many examples when the lives of people with mental illness have not been safe in the hands of the mental health system. It is about emergent system properties, not about individual practitioners or specific professional groups. It is a description not a criticism – although there are lessons to be learned, which are suggested at the end of the chapter.

The changing treatment of mental illness

The idea that mental illness was a legitimate focus of medicine emerged after the European Enlightenment[26]. The historian Roy Porter summarises this development[260]:

> The enterprise of the age of reason, gaining authority from the mid-seventeenth century onward, was to criticise, condemn and crush whatever its protagonists considered to be foolish or unreasonable . . . And all that was so labelled could be deemed inimical to society or the state – indeed could be regarded as a menace to the proper workings of an orderly, efficient, progressive, rational society.
>
> (p. 14)

The primary purpose in creating asylums was to socially exclude these unreasonable people. There were of course other purposes: asylums were (initially) humane places, often with uplifting architecture, open spaces and compassionate attention to human needs. As with much to come in this chapter, the intention is not to judge past actions through current values. The aim is to highlight examples of things being done to people with mental illness.

1750–1900: madness as illness

Medical involvement was initially to treat physical illness and offer moral guidance[26], but changed into a process of systematically ordering and classifying the inmates after a battle between the medical profession and the legal profession for control of the asylum[261]. Madness came to be seen as illness, with a consequent focus on treatment and charity.

Since madness was an illness, the pre-Enlightenment focus on expunging the evil from the individual was replaced by a twin focus on protecting the vulnerable and segregating the ill – further contributing to the rise of asylums. A range of treatment regimes were employed, included bleeding patients, spinning them, dunking in cold water, holding underwater until unconscious, and tranquiliser chairs. How were these treatments justified? In line with Enlightenment values, the emphasis on rationality underpinned a view that those who had lost their ability to reason were de facto not fully human, and therefore any approach to restore rationality was defensible.

Alongside these developments, England and France saw the growth of moral treatment. For example, the Retreat in York was opened by William Tuke in 1796, and later run by Samuel Tuke[262]. Aversive medical treatments for insanity were de-emphasised in favour of creating a relaxed and therapeutic environment focussed on nursing care. Simultaneously Philippe Pinel was appointed by the revolutionary government in France to run the Parisian institutes of the Salpêtrière for women and the Bicêtre for men. Pinel focussed on management of the mind, involving talking and listening to the patient rather than medically treating them. Both these early clinical models emphasised the twin virtues of kindness and empathy: kindness towards the individual with their illness, and empathy implying for the first time there may be meaning in the experiences. These two values were associated with a challenge to treatments that worked by breaking the patient. The first shoots of an expansion in this approach, such as the opening of an asylum in Philadelphia modelled on York[26], soon dwindled as the focus of mental health care shifted back to technological responses to madness.

1900–1950: madness as 'other'

The early twentieth century saw the rise of the eugenics movement, a *soi-disant* science which viewed madness as a spreading genetic disorder. The short step to viewing people with mental illness themselves as a threat to civilised society was soon made, leading to forcible incarceration in asylums to protect the vulnerable (it was never entirely clear if this meant people with mental illness or the public). Compulsory sterilisation was introduced as a progressive health measure. Asylum budgets, and the results on inmates, were bare-bones – consistent with a socially devalued role for people with mental illness.

Changes to the public view of insanity were accompanied by new clinical developments. Novel treatments included gastrointestinal surgery, water therapies (keeping patients in water for several days), induction of fever, and refrigeration therapy (cooling patients until they lost consciousness). The most widely used physical treatments were insulin coma therapy, metrazole convulsive therapy and electro-convulsive therapy – all intended to work by changing the brain[227]. For example, insulin coma therapy was proposed as a scientific treatment, after its discovery in 1927 by Manfred Sakel, a neuropsychiatrist from Berlin. After publication in 1933, it became a widely used treatment for schizophrenia in Europe and the USA. Scientific text-books on the treatment highlight the embedded Enlightenment assumptions about what matters and, consequently, what doesn't. For example[263]:

> Careful investigations have shown that in patients with a prolonged series of deep comas there is sometimes a mild degree of intellectual impairment . . . The degree of impairment has been of practical importance in only a handful of patients reported in the literature, and is in any case not comparable with the disability caused by the disease itself.

Insulin coma therapy was abandoned in the 1960s, partly because controlled trials showed it to be ineffective[264], and partly due to the advent of neuroleptics.

The ultimate expression of the cure-at-all-costs approach was brain surgery, which was publicised as a miracle therapy for madness[227]. Prefrontal lobotomies were widespread in the 1930s and 1940s, and were seen as a safe treatment – indeed, the Portugese neurosurgeon Egas Moniz received the Nobel Prize for Medicine in 1949. Over 40 000 lobotomies were performed in the USA, about 17 000 in the UK, and 9300 across Norway, Sweden and Denmark. Now widely (though not totally) abandoned, the reason for their enthusiastic introduction is clear[265]:

> Lobotomy . . . exemplified a common characteristic of medical practice, in which doctors and patients have often felt the need to 'do something' in the face of seemingly hopeless situations . . . Sometimes, the interventions are the first step toward a successful remedy; in other instances, they prove worthless.
>
> (p. 120)

It is reasonable to want to do something to alleviate suffering. It is reasonable to try new approaches, although the non-use of randomised controlled trial approaches when developing these treatments was indefensible given that these were established methods – the first randomised controlled trial was published in 1753[266]. But any treatment should be both scientifically justified and ethically defensible. The evidence-based medicine movement has created a framework for a scientific justification for new treatments. This is to be welcomed. The remaining challenge is ethical – to both listen to and act on what people receiving treatments and interventions say is of importance to them: which brings us to the present day.

1950 onwards: madness as neurotransmitter disturbance

The 1950s saw the chemical revolution. The first antipsychotic medication – chlorpromazine – became available, rapidly followed by several others. The early marketing as a chemical lobotomy or as a means of producing symptoms of encephalitis lethargic virus changed by the 1960s to describing chlorpromazine and other neuroleptics as a safe, antischizophrenic medication[227]. The message communicated to the public was that antipsychotics: (i) are effective; (ii) normalise the overactive dopamine systems in the brains of people with schizophrenia; and (iii) are safe. However, none of these assertions is true. We addressed the effectiveness question in Chapter 6. We now consider the second and third claims.

Neuroleptics do not restore disturbed homeostasis. They work by antagonising (blocking) dopamine D2 binding. In other words, they have affinity but no efficacy (biological response) for dopamine receptors. This difference from homeostasis is important, because it produces several problems on discontinuation: cholinergic rebound, supersensitivity psychosis (also known as rebound psychosis), withdrawal dyskinesias and activation syndrome[267]. Furthermore, the dopamine hypothesis of supersensitive dopamine receptors is an argument equivalent to observing that aspirin relieves pain, and concluding that pain is caused by an absence of aspirin[268]. Of course, it is now possible to contextualise neurotransmitter changes with greater clarity: as a final common pathway, as related to D2, also involving serotonin (5-HT1, 5-HT2, 5-HT3), as a component of a neurodevelopmental hypothesis, etc. However, these are descriptions rather than explanations of overactivity. The question of *why* is not asked. Writing about schizophrenia 30 years ago, Anthony Clare suggested that[269]: 'For all the advances, in understanding and treatment, the condition remains a baffling and enigmatic one, a harrowing experience for the individual sufferer, and a challenge to the ingenuity and skill of those intent on unlocking its secrets' (pp. 214–215). Major investment has not brought major advances in genetic[270;271] or psychophar-macological[245;247] research. There is much description, but not much explanation, for schizophrenia. This suggests the need for modesty rather than certainty in working with people with mental illness, especially when considering doing things to them.

Antipsychotics are also not safe. Neuroleptics have many side-effects (i.e. directly cause many health problems), including dystonia, akathisia, parkinsonism, tardive dyskinesia, tachycardia, hypotension, impotence, lethargy, seizures, hyperprolactinaemia, weight gain, diabetes mellitus, agranulocytosis and neuroleptic malignant syndrome. Alongside these direct health effects, they are also stigmatising. The characteristic shuffling gait associated with the parkinsonian symptoms marked out people as from the local asylum. When I entered mental health work, patients with these features were colloquially referred to as doing the modecate shuffle or the haloperidol hop. In the 1990s a new form of atypical antipsychotic medications was brought to market. These were hailed as safer and more effective than the previous generation of typical antipsychotics. The exaggerated claims about their effectiveness were discussed in Chapter 6. In relation to safety, these atypicals have a different side-effect profile (i.e. cause a different set of health problems), such as diabetes and agranulocytosis. Whether this is safer than health problems caused by typical antipsychotics is clearly an individual judgement which can only be made by the person taking the medication.

The empowerment rationale for personal recovery

Of course, there have been many desirable developments in mental health services: the closure of the total institution[71] in which patients with a mental illness lived, died and were buried in graves identified by numbers, not names[272]; an awareness of the importance of environment, such as Dutch social psychiatrist Arie Querido's development of community-based mental health services for people in acute distress[273]; the application of anti-discrimination legislation to people with mental illness, creating a legal framework to challenge social exclusion; the development and evaluation of specific health care structures, which foster specialisation for different patient groups; availability of a broader range of interventions (e.g. vocational rehabilitation, cognitive behaviour therapy), which creates the possibility of choice; and so forth.

However, the selective presentation in this chapter emphasises the negative to make three points.

First, to raise the issue of whether an apology is justified. This question arises in any situation where the dominant group has inflicted harm on the subordinate group over a sustained period. It is not an issue of mental health or even health services, but a general socio-political concern about how best to respond to past wrongs. Recent examples include the Truth and Reconciliation Commission in the post-apartheid era in South Africa, and the apologies for Nazi atrocities by German Chancellor Konrad Adenhauer and for the associated role of the Roman Catholic church by Pope Benedict. Politicians face calls for this. In the UK, Tony Blair expressed deep sorrow in 2006 for the role of England in the slave trade. In Australia, John Howard refused to apologise for the treatment of indigenous Australian people, but this was the first act by Kevin Rudd following a change of Government in 2008. In the same year, Stephen Harper apologised for Canada having forced 150 000 aboriginal children to attend state-funded Christian boarding schools aimed at assimilating them. Real reconciliation and partnership may only be possible once a line has been drawn through the symbolism of an apology, which explicitly recognises the need for a new trajectory in the future[274]. Public acknowledgements of harm from the mental health system have been made, such as to the 185 former psychiatric patients of the Lake Alice Hospital child and adolescent unit in New Zealand for 'sexual abuse, being locked up with adult service users, and being punished using unmodified electro-convulsive therapy and paraldehyde'[91] (p. 35). A few other examples of local apologies exist[272], but no general apology for maltreatment (however well-intentioned) of people with mental illnesses has ever been made by a government or a mental health professional body. The Confidential Forum for Psychiatric In-Patients of Psychiatric Hospitals sought to understand the experiences of former in-patients in New Zealand. It was held between 2005 and 2007, and after hearing the accounts of many former in-patients concluded[275]: 'Many expressed a hope for a public acknowledgement by the Government that their experiences in psychiatric institutions had been humiliating and demeaning and had often taken a lifelong toll' (p. 3). There has been no formal response.

Second, to underscore the message of Chapter 5 about caution in pronouncing on what is in the person's best interests. Mental health professionals are with very few exceptions good people, wanting to help and make life better for the people they are working with. However, doing things to patients on the basis of professional perspectives about their best interests or because something needs to be done has inadvertently inflicted harm on many people. It would surely be arrogant to assume things are different now.

Finally, to raise awareness for people entering the mental health professions, who do not understand why there is such an oppositional discourse from some consumer perspectives. There is a clear pattern of the citizenship rights of individuals being consistently subjugated to the needs of other, more powerful groups in society. Whether the subjugation was of women through moral insanity justifying incarceration for adultery[276], or of homosexual people whose deviance was treated with aversion therapy (i.e. electrocution)[277], or of political dissidents previously in the Soviet Union[278] and currently in relation to the Falun Gong sect in China[279;280], or simply of the everyday people who experienced the systematic stripping away of their identity[71], the implication is the same. The mental health system internationally has, at times, been a means of oppression.

How can oppression be addressed? The only sustainable approach is to not have the power to oppress. The primary agenda of the mental health system in the nineteenth century was protection, and in the twentieth century was treatment. In the next chapter we suggest that the policy direction indicates the primary agenda for the twenty-first century will be about recovery. Without engagement in discussions of power, there is a real danger that this agenda simply becomes the next thing to do to people with mental illness.

If personal recovery is about anything, it is about empowerment. A focus on personal recovery will involve giving primacy to the preferences, wishes and values of the individual. This will require social and political debate about responsibility, difference and risk, but it may be the only effective way to ensure people with mental illness are not harmed by the mental health system.

8. Policy rationale

Summary of the policy rationale

Public sector mental health professionals have been told to develop a focus on personal recovery in mental health services.

The final rationale is that there is an emerging policy consensus that the primary goal of mental health services is to promote personal recovery. Quite simply, mental health services should be focussed on supporting personal recovery because that is what, at a policy level, has been identified as the goal of mental health services[281].

This will be illustrated by reviewing mental health policy from five countries.

Policy in the United States of America

In 2003, the President's New Freedom Commission on Mental Health concluded that[282]:

> the system is not oriented to the single most important goal of the people it
> serves – the hope of recovery . . . Most individuals could recover from even the most
> serious mental illnesses if they had access in their communities to treatment and
> supports that are tailored to their needs.
>
> (p. 3)

The Commission explicitly identified recovery as the goal of a transformed system. It defined recovery:

> *Recovery* refers to the process in which people are able to live, work, learn and
> participate fully in their communities. For some individuals, recovery is the ability to
> live a fulfilling and productive life despite a disability. For others, recovery implies the
> reduction or complete remission of symptoms. Science has shown that having hope
> plays an integral role in an individual's recovery.
>
> (p. 5)

Two principles for system transformation were identified:

> **First, services and treatments must be consumer and family centered**, geared to give
> consumers real and meaningful choices about treatment options and providers –
> not oriented to the requirements of bureaucracies
>   **Second, care must focus on increasing consumers' ability to successfully cope
> with life's challenges, on facilitating recovery, and on building resilience**, not just on
> managing symptoms.
>
> (p. 5)

The profession of psychiatry in the USA has signed up to this orientation[283]. Individual States differ in their progress. Those with more advanced implementation of a recovery orientation include California (www.dmh.ca.gov), Connecticut (www.ct.gov/dmhas),

Georgia (mhddad.dhr.georgia.gov), Massachusetts (www.mass.gov/dmh), New York (www.omh.state.ny.us) and Philadelphia (www.phila.gov/dbhmrs).

Policy in Australia

The approach to developing mental health policy in Australia has since 1992 involved a consecutive series of five-year National Mental Health Plans. The latest plan states[284]:

> These [mental health] services should provide continuity of care, adopt a recovery orientation and promote wellness.
>
> (p. 4)

The plan defines what a recovery orientation involves:

> A recovery orientation emphasises the development of new meaning and purpose for consumers and the ability to pursue personal goals.
>
> (p. 11)

This federal plan is then interpreted at State level. For example, the plan for Queensland identifies five common elements necessary to support individuals during their recovery journey: Hope, Active sense of self, Personal responsibility, Discovery and Connectedness[285]. In South Australia, the emergent emphasis from local consultation was that 'the prevailing organisational culture of the mental health system should be an orientation to recovery'[286]. Pro-recovery State-level guidance has also been issued by Australian Capital Territories[287], Tasmania[288], Victoria[289] and Western Australia[290].

Policy in New Zealand

In New Zealand, the development of mental health services is led by the Mental Health Commission, a body established by the government in 1996. The vision statement of the Commission is[91]:

> To ensure that people with mental illness live in an environment which respects their rights, provides fair and equal opportunities, and have access to a fully developed range of mental health services which is provided by the right combination of people responding appropriately to people's needs in order to achieve the best possible outcomes and recovery.

In 1998 the Mental Health Commission published the Blueprint[291], setting out the guiding principles for mental health services. The Mental Health Commission (www.mhc.govt.nz) has been highly active in producing recovery-oriented research and practice guidance[107;124–126;292–297], which are described in Case Study 22.

Policy in Scotland

In Scotland, a national mental health plan was launched in 2006, called *Delivering for mental health*[298]. The vision stated:

> We must ensure that we deliver on our commitments in respect of equality, social inclusion, recovery and rights. Doing this is central to our vision and to the success of the plan.
>
> (p. vi)

A number of initiatives have been supported by the Scottish Executive in order to deliver on this plan, including an anti-stigma programme (www.seemescotland.org), making information about recovery more visible (www.scottishrecovery.net), training for staff working with children and young people (www.headsupscotland.com), and a telephone listening service for people experiencing low mood, targeted at men (www.breathingspacescotland.co.uk).

The vision was underpinned by a number of commitments. For example, Commitment 1 states 'We will develop a tool to assess the degree to which organisations and programmes meet our expectations in respect of equality, social inclusion, recovery and rights'. The Scottish Recovery Indicator has been developed and is now being piloted[299]. Commitment 2 states 'We will have in place a training programme for peer support workers by 2008 with peer support workers being employed in three board areas later that year'. This work was informed by a briefing paper from the Scottish Recovery Network in 2005[300], and the development process is described in Case Study 4.

Policy in England and Wales

In 2001 the Department of Health issued a policy statement in relation to recovery[301]:

> We need to create an optimistic, positive approach to all people who use mental health services. The vast majority have real prospects of recovery – if they are supported by appropriate services, driven by the right values and attitudes.
>
> The mental health system must support people in settings of their own choosing, enable access to community resources including housing, education, work, friendships – or whatever they think is critical to their own recovery.

This direction of travel has been reinforced by a series of policy initiatives in relation to the Expert Patient[302], self-management[303], social inclusion[304] and choice[305]. The recovery approach has been signed up to by all main mental health professions, including psychiatry[139], clinical psychology[268] and occupational therapy[306]. For example, a new strategic direction for mental health nursing was set following a national review by the Chief Nursing Officer[307]: 'The key principles and values of the Recovery Approach will inform mental health nursing practice in all areas'.

Implementation toolkits have been developed[308], including a values-based workbook[309]. Skills in Promoting Recovery are identified as one of the ten Essential Shared Capabilities needed across the mental health workforce[310], and a training programme has been developed[311]. An innovative policy development has been a consultation around guidance for how people's mental health problems should be understood[312]. Another specific focus has been on modernising day services[313], which identified 'opportunities for people with mental health problems to run their own services' as one of the four key functions because 'Many people particularly value help from others who are, or have been, in similar situations'.

Summary of the policy rationale

This brief review has outlined the policy support for a focus on personal recovery in the USA, Australia, New Zealand, Scotland and England. In other countries including Ireland[314;315], Canada[316] and the German-speaking world[317], there is an emerging focus on recovery reflected in policy and practice.

This is not of course to ignore two challenging realities. First, policy is often inconsistent. An emphasis on recovery can and does simultaneously co-occur with policy encouraging a focus on risk, deficit and segregation. Second, policy is not practice. This chapter is not about implementation, but rather is focussed on the policy context in which practice occurs.

There is a consensus at a policy level, especially in the Anglophone world, about the centrality of personal recovery. Section 3 addresses the translation of this rhetoric into reality.

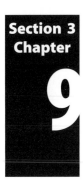

Section 3
Chapter

9

Recovery-focussed mental health services
The Personal Recovery Framework

In this chapter we develop an overarching Personal Recovery Framework, describing the processes involved in personal recovery.

The framework is intended to be theoretically based, empirically informed and widely applicable. It is underpinned by a constructivist epistemology (described in Chapter 4), which points to the changing and negotiated nature of experience. Therefore this framework is not intended to be prescriptive about what recovery is, since there can be no invariant generalisable theory or model. Rather, the aim is to provide a trans-theoretical framework to guide mental health professionals in supporting personal recovery. One aim is to identify how clinical models can help, and hinder, recovery. Another aim, consistent with the issues identified in Chapter 2, is to focus attention on the person rather than the illness, and on the person in their social context rather than decontextualising the individual.

Empirical foundations

The framework will be based on empirical research into the domains and stages of personal recovery.

The domains of personal recovery

Several writers identify key domains relevant to personal recovery. Leroy Spaniol and colleagues identify four negative impacts following from being diagnosed with a mental illness[87]:

- Loss of a sense of self, as it is replaced by an identity as a mental patient
- Loss of power, including agency, choice and personal values
- Loss of meaning, such as through loss of valued social roles
- Loss of hope, leading to giving up and withdrawal.

Ruth Ralph extracted four processes from a review of personal accounts[131]:

- Internal factors, such as awakening, insight and determination
- Self-managed care, including coping with difficulties
- External factors, especially connection with others who express hope for the person
- Empowerment, combining internal strength and interconnectedness with others.

Larry Davidson and colleagues reviewed published qualitative accounts of recovery, and identified common themes of redefining self, being supported by others, renewing a sense of hope and commitment, accepting illness, being involved in meaningful activities and expanded social roles, managing symptoms, resuming control over and responsibility for one's life, overcoming stigma, and exercising one's citizenship[128].

Lapsley and colleagues organised the findings from their narrative research with 40 New Zealand people in recovery into the HEART acronym[107]:

- Hope
- Esteem (self-esteem)
- Agency
- Relationship
- Transitions in identity, comprising
  - Personal Identity
  - Māori identity
  - Cultural identity (other than Māori)
  - Achieving lesbian or gay identities
  - Leaving behind illness identities

A particularly relevant framework was developed by Retta Andresen and colleagues on the basis of a review of consumer accounts of recovery. They extracted four emergent themes[123]:

- Hope as a frequent self-reported component of recovery
- Self-identity, including current and future self-image
- Meaning in life, including life purpose and goals
- Responsibility – the ability to take personal responsibility for one's own recovery.

Synthesising these and other accounts[318], four key domains involved in personal recovery are proposed in Table 9.1.

Table 9.1 The four key domains of personal recovery

Domain	Definition	The central question	Importance in mental illness
1. Hope	A primarily future-oriented expectation of attaining personally valued goals, relationships or spirituality which lead to meaning and are subjectively considered possible[135]	*What will happen to me?*	Mental illness and its devaluing consequences can take away hope for a good future
2. Identity	Those persistent characteristics which make us unique and by which we are connected to the rest of the world	*Who am I?*	Mental illness undermines personal and social identity
3. Meaning			
Direct meaning	An understanding which makes adequate personal sense of the 'mental illness' experience	*What has happened?*	Mental illness is a profound experience, which requires a personally satisfactory explanation
Indirect meaning	An integration of the direct meaning into personal and social identity	*What does this mean for me?*	Mental illness leads to re-evaluation of values and personally meaningful life goals
4. Personal responsibility	A constellation of values, cognitions, emotions and behaviours which lead to full engagement in life	*What can I do?*	The mental illness itself and responses from the person, mental health services and wider society can all undermine the ability to be responsible for one's own life

The stages of personal recovery

Several studies have mapped the stages through which people recovering from mental illness typically pass. Davidson and Strauss interviewed 66 people with mental illness over a 3-year period, to investigate the processes involved in reconstructing a sense of self in recovery[121]. They identified four stages:

1. Discovering the possibility of experiencing agency
2. Taking stock of one's strengths and limitations
3. Putting aspects of the self into action
4. Using this enhanced sense of self as a resource in recovery.

Baxter and Diehl interviewed 40 people about their recovery experiences, and identified three psychological events[319]:

1. Crisis, followed by a stage of recuperation, accompanied by denial, confusion and despair
2. Decision to get going, followed by rebuilding the ability to resume normal life roles, suffering setbacks and developing a more integrated sense of self
3. Awakening to restructured personhood, followed by the stage of recovery and rebuilding healthy interdependence – a stage characterised by future goals, meaningful work, advocacy and fun.

Young and Ensing synthesised the views of 18 people with mental illness who were living independently, to identify three phases[320]:

1. Initiating recovery, involving accepting the illness, finding hope, and the desire to change
2. Regaining what was lost and moving forward, including taking responsibility, self-redefinition, and a return to basic functioning
3. Improving quality of life, involving an overall sense of well-being and striving for new potentials.

Pettie and Triolo developed a detailed understanding of recovery in two people, leading them to suggest two phases[321]:

1. 'Why me?' followed by the search for the meaning to the illness
2. 'What now?' followed by the task of developing a new identity and positive sense of self.

Spaniol and colleagues undertook a longitudinal qualitative investigation of the recovery experiences of 12 people, and identified four phases[130]:

1. Overwhelmed by the disability, feeling confused, out of control of life, lacking self-confidence and connection with others
2. Struggling with the disability, involving finding an explanation for the illness, learning to cope, fear of failure and building strengths
3. Living with the disability – managing it, developing a stronger sense of self, more meaningful roles and a satisfying life within the limits of the disability
4. Living beyond the disability – living a contributing life, unlimited by the disability, with a sense of meaning and purpose to life.

In an effort to synthesise these studies, Retta Andresen and colleagues proposed five stages[123], shown in Box 9.1.

An alternative formulation is provided by the National Institute of Mental Health for England (NIMHE)[318], derived from earlier work in Ohio[322]. They identify four levels, shown in Box 9.2.

Box 9.1 Andresen's five-stage model of recovery

1. **Moratorium** – characterised by denial, confusion, hopelessness, identity confusion and self-protective withdrawal.
2. **Awareness** – the first glimmer of hope for a better life, and that recovery is possible. This can emerge from within or be triggered by a significant other, a role model or a clinician. It involves a developing awareness of a possible self other than that of mental patient.
3. **Preparation** – the person resolves to start working on recovery, e.g. by taking stock of personal resources, values and limitations, by learning about mental illness and available services, becoming involved in groups and connecting with others who are in recovery.
4. **Rebuilding** – the hard work stage, involving forging a more positive identity, setting and striving towards personally valued goals, reassessing old values, taking responsibility for managing illness and for control of life, and showing tenacity by takings risks and suffering setbacks.
5. **Growth** – [may also be considered the outcome of the previous recovery processes] whether or not symptom-free, the person knows how to manage their illness and stay well. Associated characteristics are resilience, self-confidence and optimism about the future. The sense of self is positive, and there is a belief that the experience has made them a better person.

Box 9.2 NIMHE four-stage model of recovery

Stage 1: Dependent / Unaware
Stage 2: Dependent / Aware
Stage 3: Independent / Aware
Stage 4: Interdependent / Aware

A stage model was also developed by a group of consumers across the USA[137]. The Recovery Advisory Group Recovery Model proposed non-linear development through six stages:

1. Anguish – described as *bottoming out*
2. Awakening – a *turning point*
3. Insight – the *beginning of hope*
4. Action plan – *finding a way*
5. Determined commitment – *to be well*
6. Well-being, empowerment, recovery.

Any stage model necessarily suffers from at least two shortcomings. First, it imposes an order on human growth and development which may not fit some people's experiences. In other words, its external validity is limited. An image of a spiral rather than linear stages may be a more helpful metaphor. Second, it can easily become seen as a model for what *should* happen, with consequent feelings of failure incurred for people who do not seem to be recovering. The response to these concerns is to distinguish between a map and a route. Providing a map of the terrain does not prescribe the best way through it. Similarly, providing a synthesis of the kinds of domains and processes involved in the recovery journey of others has value in a general way, but does not provide an individualised list of instructions to follow. Each person needs to find their own way forward.

Stage models of recovery have several important clinical advantages:

1. They contribute to therapeutic optimism. The very fact of established pathways to recovery becoming more visible combats the clinician's illusion that no-one recovers (supported by the evidence that clinicians only see people when in crisis and not when well[323]), and has the potential to impact on the (often implicit) prognostic communications embedded in clinical discourse.

2. They provide a way of making sense both of progress and of lack of discernible progress in a non-stigmatising and non-pathologising way.

3. They help clinicians to become more sophisticated in providing support matched to the person's stage of recovery, with different sorts of action needed to support people at different stages of recovery. For example, encouraging someone who lacks hope to take personal responsibility may simply accentuate the feelings of failure and despair.

So on the basis of the lived experience of people with mental illness, it has been possible to identify common domains and stages involved in a journey of personal recovery. Building on this theoretical basis, we now develop a framework for personal recovery.

The ultimate goal of personal recovery is healing – a taboo word in mental health services. This involves reclaiming or regaining or restoring or discovering oneself and one's world. It is a much deeper process than treating mental illness. The starting point is to consider who or what is in need of healing, which involves the concept of identity.

Identity

What does identity mean? A comprehensive analysis of the concept has been provided elsewhere[324]. Broadly, the term is used differently by psychologists and sociologists.

Psychologists use identity as a term to describe *personal identity* – the things that make a person unique. Being unique is the different, idiosyncratic, interesting, damaged, impassioned part of us. Components of a personal identity include a mental model (or self-image) of oneself, self-esteem (a valued personal identity) and individuation (the process of differentiated components becoming a more indivisible whole), along with a capacity for self-reflection and awareness of self. Personal identity involves that which sets us apart – having our own aspirations, dreams and preferences which make us a person. This individuality is the reason why there cannot be one model of recovery which fits all people, why professionals should be cautious about saying (or thinking) 'we do recovery', and why the individual's views on what matters to them have to be given primacy.

Sociologists more commonly use the term as meaning *social identity* – the collection of group memberships that define the individual. Components of this understanding include role-behaviour, discrimination towards outsiders by members of the in-group, and identity negotiation in which the person negotiates with society about the meaning and value of their identity. Social identity encompasses that which joins us. It involves the development of a contextual richness to identity, which gives a sense of being like others and provides a buffer against identity challenges. This contextual richness comes through having layers of identity. The most intimate or proximal layers are those that define our views of who we most deeply are, and whose loss would fracture our self-image. More distally, there are the range of other identities and social roles which prop up and reinforce our overall sense of self.

Both these definitions are underpinned by the philosophical definition of identity. Philosophers use the term as meaning persistence – the existence of a persisting entity particular to a given person. Components of this understanding include change, time and sameness. Identity is that which is preserved from the previous version in time when it was modified, or it is the recognisable individual characteristics by which a person is known.

Combining these schools of thought allows a definition of identity to be proposed:

Identity comprises those persistent characteristics which make us unique and by which we are connected to the rest of the world.

This definition encompasses those things which differentiate and those which integrate us. It does not capture all forms of identity. For example, the identity of indigenous Australian people is interwoven with the physical world[325]. Spiritual identity is shared with the land, a description of reality which clearly incorporates a concept of identity quite different from the psychological, sociological and philosophical definitions presented above. Similarly, Native American conceptions of health involve a relational or cyclical world-view, balancing context, mind, body and spirit[326]. Māori and Pacific Islanders in New Zealand also have a cultural identity influenced by Whānau Ora – the diverse families embedded in the culture.

Having noted its limitations, the above definition of identity will be used. Emergent identity in this definition can be weighted more towards either personal identity or social identity. It therefore encompasses both a Western view of the world in which the person is the unit of identity, and a more familial or cultural definition of personhood in which the person-in-context is the unit of identity. Indeed, it recognises that personal and social identity will often overlap. I am a clinical psychologist, partly because my own professional training encourages that self-definition (personal identity), and partly because this role shapes the interactions I have with others (social identity).

This approach to identity is deliberately trans-theoretical. It can be described in cognitive models as core schema, in psychoanalytic models as object-relations, in behavioural models as learned behaviours, in genetic terms as phenotypic expression, in personal construct counselling as self-constructs, and so on. The intention is to construct a framework for personal recovery which is not specific to one therapeutic orientation or professional group, since no single clinical model or profession has a monopoly on knowledge.

To illustrate the richness of the concept, Box 9.3 lists some types of identity.

Box 9.3 illustrates a few of the many dimensions in which people create and maintain their sense of self. It is noteworthy that few of these identities are rooted in biological or biochemical or anatomical modalities. This is one reason why physical means of understanding (and consequently treating) are not concordant with the dimensions used by most people to form and shape their identity[63]. Given this discordance, it is easy to see how mental health professionals and consumers can sometimes be speaking different languages.

Applying the definition of identity to mental illness, there are three component elements of an identity as someone with a mental illness:

(a) I see myself as a person with mental illness (personal identity)

(b) Others relate to me, and I relate to others, as a person with mental illness (social identity)

(c) Both (a) and (b) are ongoing (permanence).

In general, people with mental illness do not struggle to feel different – the associated social and clinical messages reinforce this personal identity. Indeed, the engulfing role of mental patient leads to what Erving Goffman called a spoiled identity[327], or what Glynis Breakwell calls a threatened identity[328]. After an ethnographic study involving living for 9 months as a client of an assertive community treatment team, Sue Estroff came to a view of schizophrenia as a disease of the self[329]: 'Schizophrenia is an "I am" illness, one which may take over and redefine the identity of the person'. This fits with the accounts of people experiencing

Box 9.3 Some of the many dimensions and types of identity		
Individual dimension	**Social dimension**	**Cultural dimension**
I am an optimist/realist/pessimist	I am a citizen	I am an Eritrean
I am important/unimportant	I am a campaigner	I am a European
I can/cannot cope	I am a volunteer worker	I come/do not come from one culture
I am fat/thin	I am a neighbour	I live/do not live within my culture
I am tall/short	I am employed/unemployed	I am defined by my culture
I am a moral/immoral person	I am popular	I am proud of/shamed by my culture
Interpersonal dimension	**Spiritual dimension**	**Sexual dimension**
I am a wife/husband	I am a Muslim	I am a lover
I am a carer	I am a Christian	I am straight/gay/bisexual
I am a good/bad friend	I am a humanist	I am attractive/repulsive
I am a loner	I am an agnostic/atheist	I am faithful
I am a father/mother	I am in touch with God	I am asexual

psychosis, who use terms such as phantom, demon, machine, robot, a 'nobody nowhere' and a 'nothing' to describe this feeling of being something other than, or less than, fully human[330]. The challenge is most often feeling connected to and like others. This can involve connecting in a new way with yourself (personal identity) or with the world (social identity).

Engaging with this complexity, rather than fixating on an impoverished deficit-focussed view of the self, is a vital step on the road to recovery. Recovery begins when you find somewhere to connect to. Or as Elizabeth Baxter, a psychiatrist who experienced a severe psychosis, notes[331]: 'One crucial reason people with serious mental illnesses recover is because they find someone who believes in them and their recovery'.

If promotion of personal recovery is the goal, then it is important to establish the tasks involved in personal recovery.

The four tasks of recovery

Four recovery tasks can be identified: developing a positive identity, framing the mental illness, self-managing the mental illness, and developing socially valued roles. Each will now be considered.

Recovery task 1: developing a positive identity

The first task of recovery is developing a positive identity outside of being a person with a mental illness. This process involves establishing the conditions in which it is possible to experience life as a person not an illness. This can be described as the *me–it* difference. Over-developing the *it* – the identity as one who has a chronic illness – is one iatrogenic impact of current mental health services. Developing a positive identity involves finding the *me* who has the *it* – the mental illness. This ability to differentiate self (me) from the diagnosis and illness experience (it) is associated with a positive long-term outcome in schizophrenia[121].

A positive identity gives the possibility of a personally valued future. This is why the recovery literature emphasises so strongly the importance of hope. Identity elements which are vitally important to one person may be far less significant to another, which underlines that only the person can decide what constitutes a personally valued future *for them*.

Overall, the goal for people with mental illness is to move from an either-or stance to a both-and stance – I am a person in my own right *and* I have a mental illness (or whatever other frame of meaning is helpful). This involves two elements: amplifying the sense of self, and diminishing the identity as a person with mental illness. This push-pull strategy may involve approaches for both promoting well-being and treating illness.

This is not making a case for denial. The argument being made is not that mental illness and its impact should be ignored and then all will be well. Even if the mental illness were removed (or cured) totally, an imprint on identity would remain. Rather, the point is that the direction of the spot-light dictates what you see – if the sole focus of the person, other significant people in their life and mental health professionals is on the mental illness part, then this is all that will be seen, which sets the context for the mental illness to become an engulfing role. To extend the metaphor, the brighter the spotlight the deeper the shadow – an exclusive focus on illness both enhances its apparent importance and also makes it harder to develop or maintain a sense of self separate from the illness.

However, forming a new or altered identity is a slow and potentially painful process, involving changes to core beliefs and giving up previously cherished self-images. Although it is necessary to operationalise recovery as an outcome to allow scientific study, it is in essence an ongoing process, a journey, an attitude, a readiness to embrace the challenges of life. It is not an end-point, a result (e.g. of treatment), or a state. It takes a long time.

How does recovery happen? Relationships lie at the heart of identity. A positive identity is developed by establishing or re-establishing identity-enhancing relationships. Each relationship may be a relationship with aspects of the self (a positive personal identity), or a relationship with things outside the person (a positive social identity), including but not limited to other people, social role, higher beings, and social or cultural or political identities.

The process of developing a positive identity can involve establishing new or different relationships, or re-establishing previous relationships. This is because people start from different places. The NIMHE framework described in Box 9.2 differentiates six meanings of recovery[318]:

1. A return to a state of wellness
2. Achievement of a personally acceptable quality of life
3. A process or period of recovering
4. A process of gaining or restoring something
5. An act of obtaining usable resources from apparently unusable sources
6. Recovering an optimum quality of life in disconnected circumstances.

For some people, developing a positive identity will mean re-connecting with their previous sense of self. This is the closest meaning to the everyday sense of the term recovery as synonymous with cure. For others, it will involve replacing their previous sense of self with a new and more constructive identity achieved through personal growth[121]. For others, it involves finding a sense of who they are now[332]: 'We can never go back to our "premorbid" selves. The experience of disability and stigma attached to it, changes us forever' (p. 87). In all cases, the essence of this recovery task is moving from an identity focussed on illness and difference to one which contains the possibility of a better future. This, of course, requires hope.

Recovery task 2: framing the 'mental illness'

The second recovery task involves developing a personally satisfactory meaning to frame the experience which professionals would understand as mental illness. This involves making sense of the experience so that it can be put in a box: framed as a part of the person but not as the whole person. This meaning might be expressed as a diagnosis, or as a formulation, or it may have nothing to do with clinical models – a spiritual or cultural or existential crisis (hence the quotes in the task title). The actual meaning does not matter, since (consistent with a constructivist perspective) there is no one way to interpret reality. What matters is that the meaning both provides a constraining frame for the experience, and can serve as a springboard to a better future.

This task is important because it is difficult, perhaps impossible, to recover when mental illness is the wallpaper of your world. Unframed mental illness experience creates an enveloping role which diminishes agency:

I can't do that because . . .

> *. . . I have an illness*
> *. . . I need to go to a day centre*
> *. . . I might have a relapse*
> *. . . I am an illness – no-one expects anything else of me*
> *. . . Others know more about me than I do*
> *. . . I'll have to ask the doctor first*

Which over time leads to:

I can't do that because . . . I am different

Framing involves making sense of the experience. To re-iterate, this may or may not be as a mental illness. What matters is finding a way of framing the experience which makes the experience comprehensible and allows for a positive future. People get stuck at the '*Why me?*' point, and need to find a personal meaning before they can move on. This might involve understanding the cause, but this is only helpful if it provides a springboard to meaning. The understood cause might simply be fate – '*It just happened to me . . . there's no reason . . . I was just unlucky*'. The aim of this process is to move from the '*Why me?*' point to the '*Yes . . . but*' point:

> Yes, I have a mental illness, but at least I can now get treatment
> Yes, I will always be a schizophrenic, but at least I now understand what is happening to me
> Yes, I have had these devastating bouts of depression, but now I know that the bouts don't last forever
> Yes, I have been the battleground for satanic forces, but now I know what's going on is nothing to do with me
> Yes, I have offended my ancestors, but now I realise that I can make amends

Framing also requires a level of acceptance or integration of the mental illness experience into broader identity – what we called in Table 9.1 the indirect meaning of the mental illness. It avoids either extreme – total denial of any problem leading to maladaptive strategies focussed on maintaining this denial, and total loss of self in the engulfing role as a person with a mental illness. This does not mean accepting any one particular conceptual or clinical model of illness. Rather, framing one's illness involves redefining how a person understands this particular life challenge in the context of a broader sense of self[128]. As Onken and colleagues put it[333]: 'Recovery involves replacing a view of the self as centered on psychiatric disability to that of one who is a whole person facing challenges, thus broadening the telling of one's life story through transformation of suffering into a significant life experience' (p. 13).

Recovery task 3: self-managing the mental illness

Framing the mental illness experience provides a context in which it becomes one of life's challenges, allowing the ability to self-manage to develop. The goal of self-management might involve (for different people):

- Cure – getting rid of it
- Adaptation – learning ways of living with it
- Positive re-framing – finding value in it
- Minimising – downgrading its impact on identity
- Displacing – getting on with more important things

Self-managing mental illness is not easy, but then who said life would be easy? Finding a way of living with or journeying beyond the experience of mental illness is a challenge requiring strength, resilience, hope, support, etc. In other words, just the same qualities as everyone else needs to meet their challenges. But the emerging stories of successful individuals show that personal recovery is possible.

The key transition is from being clinically managed to taking personal responsibility through self-management. The term self-management does not mean doing everything on your own. It means being responsible for your own well-being, including seeking help and support from others when necessary –the Aware / Interdependent phase in Box 9.2. An eloquent description is provided by Patricia Deegan[334]:

> To me, recovery means I try to stay in the driver's seat of my life. I don't let my illness run me. Over the years I have worked hard to become an expert in my own self-care. For me, being in recovery means I don't just take medications. Just taking medications is a passive stance. Rather I use medications as part of my recovery process. In the same way, I don't just go into hospital. Just 'going into hospital' is a passive stance. Rather, I use hospital when I need to.

Why are framing and self-managing not the first tasks? Because a person who is focussed on personal recovery gives primacy to well-being over illness. Passively receiving treatment with the intention of subsequently re-establishing a positive identity once better runs the very real risk of becoming stuck in the mental illness role. This pattern is commonly observed in mental health services. People using mental health services receive an increasingly aggressive (in both the medical and lay senses) programme of interventions and treatments, as they journey from acute care through rehabilitation to continuing care, with the initial therapeutic optimism gradually being replaced by labels such as treatment-resistant, non-compliant and, ultimately, heart-sink patient.

Developing a positive identity is closely connected with framing and self-managing the mental illness. The positive identity creates a push on the mental illness part, and framing and self-managing create a pull. The positive identity is then supported by the final recovery task, of creating and maintaining an embedding network of valued social roles.

Recovery task 4: developing valued social roles

The final recovery task involves the acquisition of previous, modified or new valued social roles. This normally involves social roles which have nothing to do with mental illness. The exception to this is the consumer activist, who uses their own experiences of mental illness as a springboard to working in mental health services (see Chapter 12) or to social activism (see Chapter 23). Valued social roles provide scaffolding for the emerging identity of recovering person.

This process overlaps with the development of a positive identity, but differs in two ways:

1. It is about who I am to others and in the world, rather than who I am to me. The focus is on identities which are created and maintained in the world – which will tend to be social rather than personal identities

2. It is about the development of scaffolding that supports the positive identity, by providing a rich and layered identity in which no one element (such as '*I am mentally well*') is the only element that really matters. It also creates fall-back positions to deal with identity challenge – '*Well, if I'm not in work, at least I can do more painting*'.

What is a *valued* social role? Like identity, it comprises two parts – personal and social value. A person may feel good about themselves (personal value) for having shown the determination to create a role as an independent thinker, even if others do not seem to value this role. Alternatively, someone may enjoy the social status of their job (social value), even if they do not personally see the job as very important. Social roles which are valued by both the person and their environment are the easiest to maintain, as they are reinforced both individually and socially.

Identity and relationships

All four recovery tasks involve relationships, because identity involves relationships – either with ourselves (personal identity) or with the world and other people in it (social identity). This is consistent with the emphasis put on relationships in the accounts of people who have experienced recovery from mental illness. Why are relationships so vital?

The earlier description of identity was informed by Erik Erikson's theory of psychosocial development[335] and George Kelly's personal construct theory[77]. Both theories emphasise the importance of social interaction in negotiating and defining a sense of identity[336]. Current identity research suggests that identity formation and maintenance is a more active process than Erikson envisaged, involving continuous creation, challenge and re-creation[337]. Identity is not a fixed construct, but consists of a configuration of *possible selves*[338] or self-constructs. Key possible selves are the feared self (the self we are afraid of becoming) and the ideal self (the self we would like to become)[339]. Two relevant findings emerge from identity research.

First, the primacy and influence of these various past, present and future selves is influenced by social interactions. For example, highly valorised previous identities can influence the social identity of the person for the rest of their life, including both positively valorised identities (e.g. astronaut, popular politician, Olympic gold medal winner) and negatively valorised identities (e.g. murderer, paedophile). But so can present identity over-ride even highly valorised previous identities: Ronald Reagan is not primarily remembered as an actor. So identities can change, and are influenced by the social environment.

Second, the ideal or hoped-for self is a key motivator for action and change. For example, Dunkel and Anthis[340] examined the relationship between hoped-for or feared-for selves and *identity commitment*[341] – level of personal commitment to achieving and maintaining the identity. They found a positive relationship between identity commitment and consistency of hoped-for positive selves, such as happiness, healthiness and job satisfaction. This relationship was not present between identity commitment and feared selves, such as loneliness, poverty and terminal illness. The hoped-for self is consistent with the ideal self in intentional change theory[339], and can act as goals for the individual. Feared-for selves create negative emotions, reduce motivation and limit the ability to identify and work towards an ideal self. The practical implication is that focussing on strengths and hoped-for selves is more likely to foster positive affect, future orientation and change than focussing on deficits and feared-for selves (e.g. by discourse centred on symptoms and prevention of relapse and hospitalisation)[342].

Relationships are therefore central to identity development, for two reasons: they provide the context in which different possible selves emerge and are reinforced or constrained, and they provide a means of fostering change through focussing on hoped-for rather than feared-for identities.

The emphasis in academic theory on the link between relationships and identity is concordant with the reports of people who have recovered from mental illness. Developing a positive identity involves the relationship with self:

> In the early stages I thought that the answers to my personal recovery lay outside of me. But now I see recovery more as a personal journey of discovery and I am much better at trusting my own instincts and paying attention to feelings instead of suppressing or trying to contain them.[55]
>
> (p. 32)

> One of the elements that makes recovery possible is the regaining of one's belief in oneself.[343]
>
> (p. 9)

Framing and self-managing the 'mental illness' involves the relationship with the illness:

> Me. That's what's changed! Me! It was a control thing. For 20 years there was an unconscious release of control on my part . . . I let the symptoms of my illness become the centre of my universe, and I realise now that the symptoms of my illness are not the centre of my universe.[55]
>
> (p. 6)

> In the early 1980s I was diagnosed as schizophrenic . . . In 1993 I gave up being schizophrenic and decided to be Ron Coleman. Giving up being a schizophrenic is not an easy thing to do, for it means taking back responsibility for yourself, it means that you can no longer blame your illness for your actions . . . but more important, it means that you stop being a victim of your experience and start being the owner of your experience.[116]

Developing valued social roles involves the relationship with the world and those in it. External relationships which are vitally important to one person may be far less significant to another, so it is not possible to create a universally applicable list. However, four types of relationships often feature in stories of recovery:

1. Relationship with a higher being (e.g. spirituality) or connection with others (e.g. culture, society)

> My wife was sitting in the car with me. And I asked her to pray for me and I was just kind of out of control and I was very intense. And, um, so she just laid hands on me and started to pray and I just had a sense that this, yeah, this anxiety went through the top of my head . . . and it, uh, just kind of went to nothing.[107]
>
> (p. 52)

I admitted I was wrong and that was the key to my changing. I was wrong. When I thought about it, this repentance I talked about, I collapsed in the shower. I said . . . 'I'm sorry' to God, 'My life is not what you intended. It could not have been'. So things changed from then on.[107]

(p. 53)

One of the major things for me since my recovery started was feeling integrated and part of the wider community, society, or whatever you want to call it . . . Recovery for me is a discovery of self, or an ongoing spiritual journey to find who you really are.[55]

(pp. 50–51)

2. Close relationships (with partner, spouse, family, friends, neighbours, pets)

I couldn't do what I do every day if it wasn't for my partner . . . She knows that I can do it. Nobody had ever done that for me before, they always wanted to change me or change something, but she likes me the way I am.[55]

(p. 11)

They [my family] were giving me the space but they expected me to come back . . . It was like a grieving time, it really was, you've had your time to grieve, you have responsibilities that require you to see to them, come back and do it![107]

(p. 51)

The hospital was very close to my home and that was very helpful. I couldn't be in my flat on my own to begin with, but I have a cat I wanted to take care of. Pretty soon I had to go there twice a day, morning and evening, whether I liked it or not. So looking after my cat was a major factor in my making my first steps towards recovery.[55]

(p. 44)

3. Relationship with other mental health service users

A person does not have to be 'fully recovered' to serve as a role model. Very often a person who is only a few 'steps' ahead of another person can be more effective than one whose achievements seem overly impressive and distanced.[119]

I realised, sitting there in the acute ward . . . amongst all the other loonies in there, I actually felt safe and comfortable, first time in my life that I could remember.[107]

(p. 54)

4. Relationship with a specific mental health professional

The turning point in my life was . . . where I started to get hope that I could actually make the leap from being sick to being well . . . Dr Charles believed I could. And Rev. Goodwin believed that I could . . . Certain people believed that I could make the leap. And held that belief even when I didn't believe it myself.[344]

. . . it may have been because [my nurse] really seemed to pay a lot of particular attention to me . . . she knew I had potential and talent and all this and that I could get better, and I knew it too.[121]

My relationship over this time with my social worker has been the key thing for me. I began to realise that there were people who believed that there was more to me than my mental health.[55]

(p. 26)

The Personal Recovery Framework

Four recovery tasks have been identified: developing a positive identity, framing the 'mental illness', self-managing the mental illness and developing valued social roles. These recovery tasks and the central importance of relationships inform a framework for personal recovery.

The framework is consistent with the four key domains of personal recovery outlined in Box 9.2. Hope arises when the possibility of a more positive identity is felt. Identity involves reclaiming a sense of personhood outside of being a person with a mental illness, by developing a positive personal identity and valued social roles. Meaning involves framing the mental illness – finding a way of making sense of it (direct meaning) and its implications for the person (indirect meaning). Personal responsibility involves the development of the ability to self-manage the mental illness and other life challenges.

These processes are based on the insights derived from stage models that there are characteristic transitions experienced by people in recovery. The four tasks of recovery are thus loosely ordered, to suggest a general but not universal ordering from belief to action and from personal to social.

This Personal Recovery Framework is summarised in Figure 9.1.

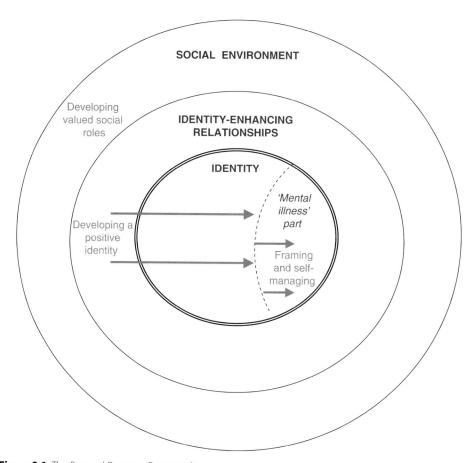

Figure 9.1 The Personal Recovery Framework.

The social environment comprises the world and others in it. Identity-enhancing relationships can be with the self, the mental illness or with the social environment. Figuratively, the process of recovery involves reclaiming a positive identity in two ways (shown as arrows in Figure 9.1): by identity-enhancing relationships and promotion of well-being which push the mental illness into being a smaller component of identity, and by framing and self-managing which pull the mental illness part. These processes take place in a social context which provides scaffolding for the development of an identity as a person in recovery.

Consistency with other frameworks

This framework is consistent with other approaches. For example, in seeking to implement a recovery strategy in New Zealand, the Mental Health Commission published a recovery framework based on the narratives of 40 people who have recovered from mental illness[107]. Their framework has the acronym RECOVER, and is shown in Box 9.4.

The RECOVER framework is consistent with the Personal Recovery Framework – it emphasises self-management, growth through the sustained development of a positive personal and social identity, and the importance of supportive relationships.

An alternative framework is provided by David Whitwell, who identifies seven naturalistic factors which impact on recovery: Time; Relationships; Life events; Employment; Shock (something which jolts the person out of the mindset of identity as a person with a mental illness); Development of new interests; and Access to money and housing[22]. This is

---

Box 9.4 The RECOVER framework

Reading, researching and learning from others about mental health

Learning to recognise the signs of ill health

Emotional growth

Change of circumstances

Change of residence, Making a new commitment to employment or further education, New family responsibilities

Others: experiencing social support

Family/Whānau assisting recovery, Faith, Active support, Challenge in the context of support, Partners, Friends, Mental health workers, Health providers as counsellors, Quality of relationship, Health providers as teachers, Health providers creating an appropriate cultural setting, Support groups, Miscellaneous supportive others (boss, work colleague, pet)

Virtues – practising them

Good general health practices, Avoiding known triggers and stressors, Recognising warning signs of impending mental health problems and taking preventive action, Using medication thoughtfully, Emotional release, Psychological/cognitive techniques to overcome thoughts and behaviour symptomatic of ill health, Spiritual practices, Pushing at limitations

Etcetera

Individual strategies, e.g. money

Repeat strategies that work and realise that recovery takes time

compatible with the Personal Recovery Framework. It emphasises that recovery happens in stages, arises from an interplay between the person and their environment, and that relationships and the ability to access normal social resources are crucial.

What does the Personal Recovery Framework imply for the job of mental health professionals?

The job of mental health professionals

A personal recovery-focussed mental health service would be organised to support individuals to undertake the four recovery tasks, and underpinned by an emphasis on relationships. Since personal recovery is something the individual experiences, the job of the mental health professional is to support the person in their journey towards recovery. Drawing on the synthesis of the four key domains of recovery shown in Table 9.1, four groups of support task can be identified.

The task of supporting hope

Mental health professionals can support the development of hope by fostering relationships. We explore this in Chapters 10 to 13. Additionally, because hope dies without opportunity,

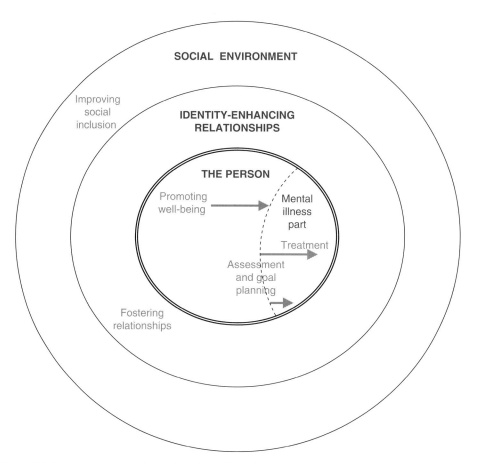

Figure 9.2 The recovery support tasks of mental health professionals.

an important job of a recovery-focussed mental health professional is to improve social inclusion, as discussed in Chapter 23.

The task of supporting identity

Mental health professionals can support the development of a positive identity by promoting well-being (discussed in Chapter 14) and goal-planning (Chapter 17) which encourages personal growth and development.

The task of supporting meaning

Mental health professionals can use the assessment process to support the person to find their own meaning in their experiences, discussed in Chapter 16.

The task of supporting personal responsibility

Treatment matters, and offering evidence-based interventions which foster self-management is often a vital contribution to recovery, as discussed in Chapter 18.

In Figure 9.2 these support tasks are positioned in the Personal Recovery Framework.

We begin at the beginning, with relationships. In Chapter 10 we consider relationships with a higher being, and in Chapter 11 close relationships with others. Chapter 12 identifies the central importance of relationship with other people who have experienced mental illness. In Chapter 13 we consider the relationship between the mental health professional and the consumer.

10 Fostering relationships with a higher being

What truly heals? This chapter unpicks some aspects of healing.

Healing

People need to recover not only from the mental illness itself, but from its emotional, physical, intellectual, social and, most importantly for some, spiritual consequences. Healing may not be supported by mental health services until they attend to these broader and deeper impacts[333]:

> The healing process not only incorporates a new way of living with and controlling symptoms, but also an increasing adeptness of navigating social realms to overcome stigmatizing and discriminatory social-structural beliefs and practices. Re-authoring hinges on reclaiming a positive self-concept.
>
> (p. 14)

Healing is a complex activity, which can be understood in spiritual terms[345]:

> Spirituality is an extraordinary part of the ordinary lives of people. From birth to death, spirituality is manifest in life's turning points, revealing mystery and depth during these pivotal moments in time . . . In crisis and catastrophe, spirituality is often intertwined in the struggle to comprehend the seemingly incomprehensible and to manage the seemingly unmanageable.
>
> (p. 3)

Many clinicians find spirituality problematic. When supervising cognitive-behavioural work with clients whose delusional content is religious, I have observed that the therapist often experiences a conflict of values. On the one hand, the standard cognitive therapy approach to delusions involves empirical reality testing. On the other, the social value of not directly challenging another's religious beliefs is difficult to violate, and the expectation that religious beliefs should accord with the same standards of proof we would expect of other unusual beliefs (e.g. that the neighbours are plotting against us) feels wrong.

More generally, clinical staff often feel under-skilled in relation to spirituality, anxious about causing offence, and uncertain of the link between the clinical and the spiritual. Perhaps this is a legacy of Freudian views of religion as regressive and pathological. Perhaps it is because professionals have (statistically) abnormal spiritual views – 90% of the US population believe in a personal God, compared with 24% of clinical or counselling psychologists[345]. Whatever the reason, the resulting behaviour does not foster spiritual development. Sometimes people are even discouraged from spiritual exploration, in case it exacerbates religiose delusions. More commonly, terms such as healing, God and soul are rarely uttered by clinicians, let alone discussed or supported as a primary focus of work. This silence sends a powerful message about what matters, which actively impedes the journey of many people towards recovery. The reality is that many people in recovery identify that having some form of faith is an important source of love, support and a sense of belonging when they feel abandoned by others[107;346].

Spirituality

How could this change? First, some conceptual clarity. In relation to mental health services, it is helpful to separate spirituality from religion. Pargament defines religion as a broad individual and institutional domain that serves a variety of purposes, secular as well as sacred, whereas spirituality represents the unique function of religion[347]. Spirituality can then be defined as *a search for the sacred*. The *search* can involve: traditional religious institutions (e.g. church, mosque, temple) or non-traditional organisations (e.g. Twelve Steps, meditation centres); belief systems from early organised religions (e.g. Jewish, Buddhist, Christian) or from newer spiritual movements (e.g. feminist, goddess, ecological spiritualities); and conventional religious practices (e.g. scripture reading, prayer, rites of passage) or other human expressions that have as their goal the search for the sacred (e.g. yoga, art, music, social action).

Sacred has been defined as including[348]:

> concepts of God, the divine, and the transcendent. However, other objects can become sacred or take on extraordinary power by virtue of their association with, or representation of, divinity[347]. Sacred objects include time and space (the Sabbath, churches); events and transitions (birth, death); materials (wine, crucifix); cultural products (music, literature); people (saints, cult leaders); psychological attributes (self, meaning); social attributes (compassion, community); and roles (marriage, parenting, work).
>
> (p. 647)

Separating religion from spirituality makes discussion of spirituality more possible in a mental health context. A search for the sacred, or trying to find a connection with a higher meaning or purpose in life, is a unifying human endeavour. Religion, whatever else one may say about it, does not unify humanity. In a conversation about spirituality, the focus is not on what religious group the clinician does or might belong to. Rather, the topic is how the consumer can develop as a spiritual being. There is less concern about an implicit agenda of conversion. The personal beliefs of the clinician then become less relevant, which paradoxically liberates the clinician (if consistent with their therapeutic orientation) to refer to their own spiritual experiences where helpful.

A second rationale for focussing on spirituality is that it makes visible commonalities across different traditions. For example, spiritual methods of coping with adversity include marking boundaries, spiritual purification and spiritual reframing[349]. Averill suggests that important elements of spiritual experience can be understood in either secular or spiritual terms[350], shown in Table 10.1.

The need to feel alive, to have uplifting experiences and to be part of something larger than oneself is central to the recovery narratives of many people. The consistent theme is a recognition that we cannot always help ourselves by personal effort, and that connection with a higher being is enriching.

Mental health services can support spiritual development

How can the person be supported by mental health professionals in their spiritual development? A straightforward strategy is simply to ask the person about meaning and purpose in

Table 10.1 Elements of a spiritual experience

	Description	Secular perspective	Spiritual perspective
Vitality	A powerful force, a creative attitude, being 'free-spirited', adventurous, open to new experiences, or growing through inner exploration or meditation	Health Energy Enthusiasm	Soul Grace Sanctity
Meaningfulness	Spiritual experiences are deeply felt, sometimes life-changing. Meaning may take time to emerge. This can be associated with a sense of mystery and awe	Art Science Literature	Faith Scriptures Revelation
Connectedness	A feeling of union or harmony with another being or thing. This may involve connection with a living, dead or imagined person, a cultural or ethnic group, humanity or nature. The common theme is self-transcendence – an identification with something beyond the self.	Family Lovers Nature	God Fellowship Church

their life. This will be stepping outside the clinician's sphere of expertise, but may also be stepping into the patient's sphere of need. What has the experience of mental illness taught the person? How has the person's sense of what life is about changed over time? When does the person feel most alive, or most connected with something or someone else?

Whitwell notes that spirituality – inner life, meaning and purpose, the 'ground' in which the person is the figure – can all be demolished (either temporarily or permanently) by the experience of profound mental distress[22]. The path to recovery can then involve reconnecting with previous sources of comfort and sustenance, which is a much more active and transformative process than going back to how you were. Or it can involve developing new sources of support, new meanings in life, and even new realisations about the self which lead to the positive aspects of mental illness described in Chapter 2. The task of the mental health professional is to set a context in which these powerful processes can happen.

Resources to help clinicians to support spiritual development are becoming available (e.g. www.spiritualcrisisnetwork.org.uk, www.spiritualcompetency.com). Although spiritual development is not easily amenable to action planning, mental health professionals can encourage this process by supporting the person:

- to nurture a positive view of the self, by demonstrating compassion in how the professional responds to the consumer when they report difficulties and setbacks
- to have spiritual experiences, such as reading scripture, prayer, attending places of worship, accessing on-line religious resources
- to have uplifting secular experiences, through exposure to art, literature, poetry, dance, music, science, nature
- to access opportunities for self-discovery, such as through personal therapy, keeping a diary, writing a poem or a song, developing a narrative about oneself
- to give back to others, e.g. voluntary work, having a pet, having responsibility for something or someone
- to develop a different relationship with their thoughts, e.g. by learning how to meditate, or through CBT
- to develop social capital, e.g. by experiencing citizenship, becoming politically active (including as a consumer activist)
- to develop cultural identity, e.g. by accessing culture-specific groups and through healing and purifying cultural ceremonies

- to access self-help and mutual support groups
- to undertake recovery planning activities, such as the Personal Recovery Plan developed by Ron Coleman[116], or the Wellness Recovery Action Planning developed by Mary Ellen Copeland[351]
- to have time to think, including a quiet place to go, and prompts which aid contemplation
- to take action: engaging in life rather than disengaging from life; making connections with the world, and other human and non-human beings in it; acting on the basis of approach rather than avoidance motivations.

This involves working in a very different way. Our first case study illustrates one approach to supporting this experience of connection.

Case study 1: Peace Ranch

Peace Ranch is set in 25 acres of countryside in Caledon Hills, north of Toronto. It was established in 1990, and provides opportunities for people with mental illness to experience agriculture, animal husbandry and country life. It is a working farm, with goats, sheep, hens, peacocks, cats, donkeys, horses and a frighteningly large pot-bellied pig. Staff have a range of training, including therapeutic riding, horticultural therapy, social recreation and farming. The emphasis is on supporting individuals: 'through doing things for themselves, our residents learn the value of managing their own lives'. Ten residents live in the farmhouse, and 100 people attend the day programme.

Residents start the day with barn chores: feeding and cleaning for animals. Moving into a role where you are caring for someone 'moves the person to being a champion' – it encourages empathy and caring for others. The sense of responsibility and accomplishment is something worth getting up for. Daytime activities include therapeutic garden design, animal care, horseback riding, apple cider pressing, farmhouse cooking, hiking, maple syrup production and country crafts (e.g. pumpkin-carving). Many activities are community-focussed. Produce is grown both for sale at markets and for entering into local competitions. Peace Ranch-on-wheels involves visiting seniors in their home and supporting them to plant, maintain and use herbs and other produce. Preparing the baby animals to appear in a petting zoo involves spending time holding and caring for them, because loved animals give love back. Going on to work in the petting zoo at local events gives an experience of mastery when children ask about the animals, and is a way of being a contributing member of the community.

Even a brief exposure can be transformative. The 'day in the country' programme offers a 'penetrative, rejuvenating silence' away from the pace of life in cities. The experience at Peace Ranch is all about discovering things outside yourself: conversation is focussed on the person's farm jobs and on nature rather than on illness. One resident identified the benefit that plants and animals don't judge: caring for them is 'one way you don't have to rely on other's perceptions'. This experience of authentic connection to nature, growth and food is new for many attenders. For example, gardening requires a focus on here-and-now activity. This grounding experience of living in the moment fosters peace of mind and a sense of being connected to the cycles of life. Growing something from a seed, nurturing the seedling and feeling pride at the result can invoke a sense of awe: something magical is happening. The doubt about whether the seed will make it is also a metaphor for the need for hope in life.

The economic impact of Peace Ranch is positive – after accounting for operating costs, over US$500 000 is saved per year through reduced hospitalisation rates. The personal impact is also clear, with some people experiencing their time in the programme as a punctuation point

Case study 1: (*cont.*)

in their life. One ex-resident described coming for a day's taster, then a 6-month trial, followed by two years living on the farm. He reported that working with animals relaxed him – his mind stayed calm because he felt a bond with the animals. Sitting out at night under the stars in a non-light-polluted setting was also experienced as a powerful process – 'it touches the soul'. The routine of farm life provided him with a basis to address drug issues, and the consequent stability allowed him to move into independent accommodation. He is now working in the market gardening and petting zoo projects.

Further information: www.peaceranch.com

The overall challenge is to develop an orientation towards fostering spiritual development. Emerging approaches such as supported spirituality[352] are one contribution, which seek to harness its healing potential. This encompasses many aspects: sustaining through difficult times in life; providing a way of making sense of the struggle for meaning, providing coping mechanisms; a means of accessing natural social support; a context for wellness and rules of behaviour (GOD as Good Orderly Direction in life); a valuing of acceptance of the need for help and of dependence; and a means of finding absolution for feelings of guilt and shame. Some relevant resources are available at ssw.asu.edu/portal/ research/spirituality.

Spiritual development has the potential to generate hope. As we will discuss in Chapter 21, any crisis (e.g. a mental health crisis) requires a resilient response if the person is to move from succumbing to surviving and even thriving. In the language of positive psychology (described in Chapter 14), flourishing is possible even in the midst of adversity. What gets in the way is pessimism, negative thinking, wishful thinking, self-blame, unhelpful avoidance – things that sap a person's ability to engage with, and ultimately grow from, the crisis. The antidote to these negative influences is hope. The development of hope reconnects the person with their innate, self-righting capacity, and can be a deeply spiritual experience.

We turn now to more proximal relationships, with close friends and family in the person's social world.

Chapter 11

Fostering close relationships

Close relationships are the important relationships between the person with mental illness and others (e.g. family, friends, neighbours, pets) with whom they are in meaningful contact. People with mental illness often have reduced social networks[4], so remaining relationships are vital. If the primary goal of mental health professionals in fostering close relationships is to support the person's recovery, then what does this mean in practice?

To illustrate, consider a mother who expresses concern to a clinician about her son John, a voice-hearer, who is sleeping late in bed every day, and regularly smoking cannabis. One response would be:

> I can see why you're concerned. We know that people who isolate themselves are more vulnerable to an increase in auditory hallucinations, losing motivation and becoming depressed. There is also good evidence that cannabis makes a psychotic relapse more likely. So you need to find some way to get him into a normal pattern of getting up, but without criticising him or treating him like a child. He has to make his own choices, you see – otherwise if you take over he's again more likely to relapse. I'll also encourage him to get out of bed earlier the next time I see him.

The explicit communication is empirically supported – self-monitoring deficits are increased in the absence of external stimuli[353], cannabis is associated with increased likelihood of relapse[354], and emotional over-involvement and critical comments do contribute to increased relapse rates[355]. However, the implicit communication has a number of anti-recovery components:

1. The clinician is the expert, shown by discourse markers ('We [i.e. I] know that ...', 'There is also good evidence that ...') and use of jargon
2. The assumed job of the clinician is to provide advice to fix the problem
3. The advice is focussed on avoiding bad things happening to John, such as symptoms or relapse
4. The focus on symptoms and difficulties communicates that positive change is unlikely
5. The advice puts the mother in a double bind – damned if she does try to badger John out of his bed, damned if she doesn't
6. Improvement in John will happen on the basis of action by the clinician or by John's mother.

Consider this alternative response:

> I can see why you're concerned. John is isolating himself, which means his voices may get worse, and it's also hard for him to get much enjoyment, so there's a risk his mood will drop. And you'll know that cannabis can make John's voices get worse. So we need to understand what stops John from being a bit more active. Now, you know him better than I do. What good things does John have to get up for? ... If there's nothing,

then I have a check-list of things some people find enjoyable. Can you ask him to fill it in – do go through it with him if he wants – and then try to discuss with John how to develop some opportunities? Could you also ask him to bring it along the next time he sees me, as I'd be interested to see what he puts?

The explicit communication is the same. However, the implicit communication has a number of more helpful contributions to promoting personal recovery:

1. The clinician has relevant expertise, but does not position themselves as the expert – shown by discourse markers ('you know him better than I do'), expectations of knowledge being shared rather than exclusive ('You'll know that . . .'), and lack of jargon

2. The job of the clinician is to work with the mother to support John in developing his own solution

3. The clinician's response is focussed on increasing the chance of good things happening to John, such as finding something he enjoys

4. The response is positive but realistic – change is actively expected, but the concerns are real and the goal is to be 'a bit more active'

5. The mother has a concrete task to do, but one which is collaborative rather than prescriptive. The concern about Expressed Emotion therefore doesn't need to be voiced.

6. John has the answers, although he may need very active support from his mother and the clinician to find a way forward.

Of course, it is possible that John simply wants an alternative lifestyle. For example, I supervised work with a service user who wanted to be a musician, and whose ideal day was rising mid-afternoon, playing a gig in a local pub then jamming with friends until going to bed at sunrise. This person did not lack motivation for his own goals, but he did for the service goal of a normal sleep pattern. Returning to John, it would probably be unhelpful to invalidate the mother's concerns by exploring this issue with her. In individual work with John, the clinician may explore his lifestyle choices. What kind of person does he want to be? Who does he aspire to be like? What would his ideal day look like? If it emerged that John wanted a more nocturnal life, then of course that should be accepted, valued and supported.

The general principle is that close relationships are vital: they shape identity, and contribute to or hinder well-being. Supporting close relationships can be a powerful means of promoting hope. The clinical challenge is to balance this goal with the recognition that not all close relationships are beneficial. This involves the normal clinical skill of balancing inter-dependence on others with the promotion of personal autonomy. Frameworks are now becoming available to inform decision-making in this area[356], which highlight that clinical judgement remains centrally important. Ceding power to the consumer does not remove the expectations on clinicians to apply their professional expertise and wisdom in their work. Many clinical dilemmas are complex, with no simple, or even right, solution[198]. The challenge is to develop a values base such that the clinical bias is towards actions that promote, rather than hinder, personal recovery.

One approach to harnessing the recovery-promoting potential of family members is to involve carers in mental health services. This approach is used in the next case study.

What about intimate relationships, such as marriage and lesbian, gay and straight partnerships? International comparisons highlight marked differences in relationship rates. A recent authoritative study found that nearly three-quarters of Indian people with a diagnosis of schizophrenia were married at follow-up, compared with about one-third from the developed world[114]. So the likelihood of an intimate relationship is influenced by cultural factors.

Case study 2: family peer support workers

The ORYGEN Youth Health service employs trained family peer support workers, who are parents of people who have previously developed mental health issues. Their role is to act as 'carer consultants', providing a service to other parents and family of people referred to ORYGEN. Family peer workers actively seek to engage with families, including phone and face-to-face contact, through liaison with other ORYGEN services, particularly out-patient case-managers and through visiting the in-patient unit. They have also set up a family resource room which families can access when they bring their young person along to the main ORYGEN site.

A key feature is that their role is to be a paid non-professional with lived experience, whilst they actively work alongside the mental health clinicians at ORYGEN. A central value is to integrate this programme with the clinical services, not to create parallel systems. Some case managers initially expressed concern about working at cross-purposes with the family peer workers, for example in relation to what advice they would offer. This has been addressed by providing the family peer support workers with regular supervision from an experienced clinician and having clear guidelines about the role of family peer support workers. Case managers are also invited to family peer supervision meetings, where they can discuss referrals and management plans. Information that will assist family peer support workers with supporting the family is helpful. Some of the family peer support worker duties include:

- acting as a positive link between the service and the carer
- understanding and giving *emotional* support as another family member who has been through a similar situation
- encouraging the family member to feel empowered and to discuss specific questions with the case manager, and offering to be a go-between where helpful.

Further information: info@orygen.org.au

The challenge for mental health professionals is then to avoid communicating impoverished expectations to patients about the possibility of their experiencing a rich and fulfilling intimate relationship. It goes without saying that any discussion about this should take account of the individual's sexuality, so staff need to demonstrate sensitivity to the different patterns and compositions of intimate relationships. However, the deeper problem is one of silence – sexuality and intimate relationships are routinely not discussed with patients, other than when screening for problems during the Sexual History element of a Mental State Examination. For example, the Camberwell Assessment of Need is a standardised assessment of 22 domains of health and social needs for people with severe mental illness[357], and Sexual Expression is the domain most frequently rated as 'Not known' by staff[358]. This is worrying not only because of the clinical importance of asking about a domain of life commonly impacted on by side-effects of neuroleptic medication, but also because it may reflect unstated staff beliefs that a fulfilling sex life is not available to people with mental illness.

This absence of enquiry may also be linked to the treatment-focussed training of professionals – a belief that if they identify an unmet need then it's their job to do something about it, and what can they do in this domain? One aspect of personal recovery that is liberating for staff is that responsibility for improving the person's situation shifts from them to the consumer. It becomes more possible to have open discussions about a life challenge, without the clinician feeling obliged to fix it. This links with the discussion in Chapter 5 about acknowledging 'I know not' in the face of complex life difficulties, rather than adopting an expert 'Do what I say and all will be well' stance.

The roles of coach or mentor are more helpful (and enjoyable) for staff in relation to complex social issues such as an unfulfilled sex life, because they open up new possibilities of action. In Chapter 23 we will show that the best employment approach is to experience real-life work, rather than training the person until they are ready for work. Similarly (though without the empirical evidence base), the best response to someone who wants an intimate relationship might involve supporting them to do things which give access to a pool of potential partners, such as joining a social or sports club, doing voluntary work, using an internet dating service, or going on a speed dating event. These proactive approaches are stretching, in different ways, for the individual and the clinician. The individual may need support to take on these challenges, and it may be more helpful to frame them as learning opportunities rather than expecting initial success. Ongoing involvement and debriefing may well be required as the person learns to cope with the ups-and-downs these experiences will involve. Similarly, the clinician may need support through supervision to move beyond constraining clinical beliefs, such as the importance of being better before doing normal things like dating. Of course, some of these actions will be premature for people in the early stages of recovery, but the principle is to ensure that impoverished expectations and stigmatising beliefs do not preclude normal, mainstream ways of addressing common (in both senses) human problems.

We now turn to the relationship between people with mental illness and others who may be further along their road to recovery from mental illness.

12 Peer relationships

There is a growing recognition that peers – people with their own experience of mental illness – can directly contribute to the recovery of others[300;359;360]. Meaningful peer involvement is universally associated with innovative recovery-focussed services internationally.

A recommendation for engendering hope is cited by Kirkpatrick and colleages[361]: 'My suggestion is to get as many success stories as possible from those who have schizophrenia to give a sense of hope to those just beginning their journey'. How can this be done? Three levels of peer support for recovery can be differentiated: mutual self-help groups, peer support specialists and consumer-operated services.

Mutual self-help groups

Mental health systems traditionally give primacy to expert knowledge gained through professional training and education. A direct consequence, from the service user's perspective, can be that the mental health system is structured to give professionals control over the service and people using the service[362]. As a consequence, self-help or mutual support groups have in general developed outside mental health services. They give primacy to lived experience, leading to structures based on the assumption that all participants have something to contribute. Organisational structures tend to be more egalitarian and less hierarchical, with a wide range of role and participation opportunities[363]. They also promote political and social activity[333]: 'Connections among peers allow a nonpathologizing community discourse that is less susceptible to judgment and fosters expressions of power and collective social action ... These actions serve to counteract the stigma imposed by society and internalized by individuals while instilling meaning in life pursuits' (p. 16).

Mutual self-help groups vary in their level of connection with traditional mental health service values and beliefs. For example, the Hearing Voices Network (www.hearing-voices.org) runs groups which offer a safe haven in which voice-hearing people can feel secure and comfortable whilst working towards regaining some power over their lives. It emerged from the work of Marius Romme[42], and emphasises accepting and living with voices. Schizophrenics Anonymous (www.sanonymous.org), by contrast, is a self-help organisation for people with a diagnosis of schizophrenia which aligns with a biomedical model of mental disorder[195], yet the guiding principles of Schizophrenics Anonymous are clearly pro-personal recovery:

1. I surrender ... I admit I need help; I can't do it alone
2. I choose ... I choose to be well. I take full responsibility for my choices and realise that the choices I make directly influence the quality of my days
3. I believe ... I now come to believe that I have great inner resources and I will try to use these resources to help myself and others

4. I forgive . . . I forgive myself for all the mistakes I have made. I also forgive and release everyone who has injured or harmed me in any way

5. I understand . . . I now realise that erroneous, self-defeating thinking contributes to my problems, unhappiness, failures and fears. I am ready to have my belief system altered so my life can be transformed

6. I decide . . . I make a decision to turn my life over to the care of God, as I understand Him, surrendering my will and false beliefs. I ask to be changed in depth.

Katie Randall and Deborah Salem identify four key elements of mutual self-help groups[195]:

1. *Personal stories and community narratives*

   Personal stories are told, often repeatedly, within settings which shape self-understanding and identity. These normative narrative communities[364] promote recovery by helping participants make sense of their experiences in less stigmatising ways. Telling one's story is cathartic, promotes reflection, is reciprocal, and for some people may only be possible peer-to-peer.

2. *Role models*

   Leaders within the self-help group are visible role models. Hearing the experiences of others struggling with similar issues is normalising (i.e. the opposite of stigmatising), and can be inspiring and promote hope.

3. *Opportunity role structures*

   The core belief about all participants having value and something to offer translates into an assumption that all members can both give and receive help.

4. *Social support, sense of belonging, and connection*

   Self-help groups stress both the importance of taking personal responsibility and the need for support. Consequently they emphasise social support, belonging, connection and community.

Supporting access to an external mutual self-help group can be an important recovery support by a clinician for an individual consumer. However, the external positioning of mutual self-help groups reduces their direct impact on the mental health system. Since it can be challenging for clinicians to work in a recovery-focussed way – their instinctive responses are conditioned more by professional socialisation toward clinical rather than personal recovery – involving consumers as employees in the mental health system can have a transformative effect.

Peer support specialists

Terms such as peer support specialist[360], peer worker[365], consumer employee[366] and prosumer (professional consumer)[367] all describe roles in the mental health system for which personal experience of mental illness is required. The term peer support specialist (or simply peer) will be used here to describe this role.

Creating peer support specialist roles brings four types of benefit.

1. For the peer support specialist, it is a job with all the benefits that follow from this. Their own lived experience is valued, which can be a transformative reframing of an illness experience. They give to others, which is an important component of healing. Self-management and work-related skills are consolidated.

2. For other staff, their presence leads to increased awareness of personal values. Since very few mental health workers disclose a history of mental illness to their co-workers, there

is no challenge to the them-and-us beliefs about fundamental otherness held by many mental health professionals[70]. Interacting with peer colleagues challenges these beliefs in a natural rather than forced way. It is a common experience of staff to initially feel they can't talk freely when a peer joins the team, but over time this raised self-awareness becomes a means of identifying and addressing unhelpful values and beliefs.

3. For other consumers, exposure to peer support specialists provides visible role models of recovery – a powerful creator of hope. This type of benefit is increasingly being recognised in other areas of medicine, such as the importance of patient contact with survivors of cancer (www.acscsn.org, www.cancercenter.com). There may also be less social distance than with professionals, leading to more willingness to engage with services. For example, clients of an assertive outreach team who were allocated to receive input from a peer support specialist in addition to standard case management had greater levels of engagement and fewer needs[366]. Peers tend to focus on practical support needs, which can be vital. They are less constrained by social constructions of a professional relationship, so can offer friendship.

4. For the mental health system, peer support specialists can be carriers of culture. There is often less need to train and maintain a pro-recovery orientation in recovered consumers, because of their own lived experience. They promote these values in their interactions with other workers and with the system as a whole.

The peer support specialist role has policy support in many countries. For example, in England[301]: 'All mental health services will be expected to recruit and train service users as part of the workforce' (p. 21).

What skills are needed to work as a peer? Just as professionals need training, there is a need to train individuals who have experienced mental illness for working as a peer support specialist. The Intentional Peer Support approach of Shery Mead[360] identifies four cornerstones/tasks: Connection (engaging with others), Worldview (self-awareness about their own values), Mutuality and mutual responsibility (relationships in which both people have value and reciprocity is possible) and Moving Towards (harnessing approach motivation). In the USA there are now established training programmes, e.g. in Georgia[368], Arizona (see Case study 24) and Boston (see Case study 17). In other countries the infrastructure is developing, e.g. Scotland (see Case study 4). Even where no established training programme exists, it is still possible to prepare individuals for aspects of the role. For example, a necessary skill for working as a peer is the ability to tell one's own story. Many consumers are unaware that they have a story to tell which could be of benefit to themselves and others. The next case study is an initiative in Philadelphia which aims to develop this skill.

Case study 3: Sharing Your Recovery Story

The *Sharing Your Recovery Story* training helps people in recovery from mental illness to discover their story in a new way and begin to develop a simple structure for their story. The training focuses on helping people identify the 'recovery' portion of their story: what they did to get from the hard time to the place they are in now.

The training uses techniques drawn from the storytelling world of story listening and appreciations as a way to help people begin to develop their story in new ways. It is based on the belief that we are all born storytellers; we just lose touch with our story along the way. People express appreciation at the end of the training, and often make new peer-to-peer connections, providing extra avenues of support.

The training has been delivered in Philadelphia and surrounding counties, and has served as an entry point for people in recovery to connect to the system in new roles. People have moved on from this training to participate as trainers in other trainings, to share their story in public venues designed to increase awareness of recovery transformation and to decrease stigma, to become certified peer specialists and to assume other leadership roles within the mental health system.

The original storytelling training has been supplemented with several additional approaches:

- Family member storytelling training: focusses on the family experience when a loved one has a mental illness. Training has included parents of young and adult children, siblings, spouses and extended family members. Again, reviews have been overwhelmingly positive and this training is providing impetus to the family inclusion initiative in Philadelphia.
- Youth Storytelling Training: for adolescents who have received services in the system.
- Storytelling Training for staff: while staff are invited to participate in the original storytelling training this was developed to provide staff with additional skills to run storytelling groups at the programmes in which they work.

Further information: Joan Kenerson King (jking@netreach.net)

Many challenges arise from creating peer support specialist posts, and are worth considering in advance. A clear and distinct job description for the peer support specialist is important, or the role is vulnerable to being co-opted. It is tempting for service managers and administrators to consider reducing staffing costs by replacing expensive professionals with cheaper staff, but using peer support specialists to achieve a cheaper workforce doing the same tasks will neutralise their contribution.

Two concerns that are sometimes expressed relate to confidentiality and safety. The confidentiality concern is that peer specialists will have access to confidential clinical records. However, the same rules of confidentiality govern peer support specialists as any other type of employee. Employees breaching confidentiality policies should face disciplinary action. The safety concern is that some peer specialists may be damaging to those with whom they work. Whilst there certainly are people with experience of mental illness who should not work as peers, this risk is exaggerated due to stigmatising beliefs linking mental illness and violence (as we discuss in Chapter 20). The actual level of risk should be dealt with as per any other applicant – there should be a formal recruitment and selection process, and policies in place to deal with unacceptable behaviour.

Since not everyone with their own experience of mental illness will make a good peer, several issues should be explored during the recruitment process. Does the person show humility about their own experience, or will they attempt to impose their solution on others? Can the person talk about their own experiences, as a source of suffering from which they can draw, but with sufficient distance that they can use their experiences as a resource for others? Does the person accept their own limitations, show good self-management skills and a readiness to seek support from others? Does the person show passion, enjoyment in their own life, a sense of playfulness – or other evidence that they have transcended a role defined by mental illness and connected with the stress-buffering effects of play and pleasure[330]?

Working as a peer is not always easy. Common issues include uncertainty from clinical services about their value, credential barriers for potential peers with no formal qualifications, cultural tensions where services do not engage well with specific peers, a lack of training opportunities, lack of support to manage their own mental illness and meet the emotional and physical demands of paid work (especially if they are coming from unpaid, voluntary or no work), poor career development opportunities, the impact on welfare benefits, the lack of a living wage, and maintaining a (partial) identity as a consumer rather than a mini-professional. This last challenge arises because many peers report feeling an impostor – neither a proper consumer nor a qualified professional. Balancing these role tensions is not easy. A qualitative study of the experience of five peers identified six types of role strain[369]:

1. Super cool – they could not express a normal range of emotions in their work-place, e.g. anger, elation, being 'down in the dumps'
2. Super normal – they felt they needed to be conservative in appearance and behaviour
3. Super person – they felt they were expected to be experts in every area of mental health
4. Unskilled – they felt they were seen as unskilled, with colleagues assuming they had no other education and skills than what was inherent in being a consumer
5. Voyeurism – staff wanted to know details of illness and admission experiences without wanting to hear the lessons that could be learnt from them
6. Remuneration – the absence of pay scales created problems in getting a wage that reflected the work they did.

Participants identified approaches to dealing with these strains:

- Consumer humour (used with other consumers, parodying their consumer background and the 'normality' of non-consumer colleagues)
- Debriefing with other consumer colleagues, being open without the fear of being pathologised
- A thick skin to deal with the everyday ignorance and discrimination they experienced
- Perspective about the big picture – reminding themselves that they are there to change the culture, and having reminders (e.g. sitting in a ward)
- Supervision to deal with the stresses of employment.

Key organisational approaches to supporting the role were identified as policies and procedures, positive senior management support, a liaison person, a clear job description and expectations, having more than one peer in post, flexible working hours and acceptance that disability may require time off work. Good supervision, as for any other mental health worker, is vital. Challenging prejudicial beliefs about ability is also important. For example, a study in Connecticut showed that former consumers are as able to work as case managers as anyone else[370]. Our next case study describes how one country is developing a cohort of peer support specialists.

Case study 4: developing a peer support specialist infrastructure

International collaboration has underpinned Scotland's efforts to introduce peer workers as part of their mental health service system. In December 2005 a number of leading exponents of peer working from the USA were invited to speak at a conference organised by the Scottish Recovery Network (SRN), about the role and potential development of peer working in Scotland. Speakers included Larry Fricks, then of Georgia Certified Peer Specialist Project, and Gene Johnson and Lori Ashcraft from Arizona-based Meta Services (now known as Recovery Innovations).

This event generated huge interest in peer working in Scotland and eventually led to a Government commitment to support this new role where people with lived experience of mental health issues and recovery are trained and employed as specialist recovery workers.

Case study 4: (*cont.*)

The first peer support service in Scotland is called Plan2Change. Based in Edinburgh, it was developed initially as a partnership between NHS Lothian, Penumbra and the Scottish Recovery Network. This project was funded via Social Inclusion and aimed to work with people experiencing considerable life difficulties but not necessarily in receipt of secondary mental health services. Training for the peer workers, who link closely with local primary care and other service providers, was provided by Recovery Innovations in late 2006.

This intensive two-week course was then repeated in 2007, meaning that in total over 40 people had now been trained across Scotland as peer specialists. Some of these people have now gone on to take up roles as employed peer workers in a number of Health Board areas as part of an evaluated pilot project, linked to the Scottish Government's commitment, as described in Delivering for Mental Health[298].

Peer workers in these pilots are fulfilling roles within community and inpatient services. The majority are employed by NHS Boards but some are employed by a service-user-led organisation and placed within statutory services.

Further information: www.scottishrecovery.net

The development of peer support specialist roles also creates new ethical dilemmas. For example, there is professional consensus that it is never appropriate to have sex with a consumer. This invariant rule works well where there is a clear distinction between consumer and employee, but how does it apply when peers are employed in the workforce? Does becoming a peer support specialist mean that an existing sexual relationship with another consumer needs to be severed? What about where a new sexual relationship is likely to develop?

How do peer support specialists work? A key difference is in the way of relating to consumers: peers create partnership and real relationships rather than detached relationships – terms we elaborate in the next chapter. They exemplify the recovery coach – a term developed in the addictions field[371]:

The role of a recovery coach is a:

- *motivator and cheerleader (exhibits bold faith in individual/family capacity for change; encourages and celebrates achievement)*
- *ally and confidant (genuinely cares, listens, and can be trusted with confidences)*
- *truth-teller (provides a consistent source of honest feedback regarding self-destructive patterns of thinking, feeling and acting)*
- *role model and mentor (offers his/her life as living proof of transformative power of recovery; provides stage-appropriate recovery education and advice)*
- *problem solver (identifies and helps resolve personal and environmental obstacles to recovery)*
- *resource broker (links individuals/families to formal and indigenous sources of sober housing, recovery-conducive employment, health and social service, and recovery support)*
- *advocate (helps individuals and families navigate the service system, ensuring service access, service responsiveness and protection of rights)*
- *community organiser (helps develop and expand available recovery support resources)*
- *lifestyle consultant (assists individuals/families to develop sobriety-based rituals of daily living) and*
- *a friend (provides companionship)*

This list provides an outline of how peer support specialists work. A key focus is on enhancing recovery capital – the internal and external assets required for successful recovery initiation and maintenance[372]. The basic orientation of a peer support specialist is towards amplifying and supplementing natural recovery supports, rather than replacing these assets. This is no different to what we will argue (in the next chapter) a partnership relationship between a clinician and a consumer needs to look like if it is to support recovery. However, the two advantages of peers is that they have a personal experience of recovery to draw on, and they have not in general experienced the socialisation of professional training which can encourage a doing-to (i.e. replacing natural supports) mentality.

This means that the instinctive responses of peers can be highly supportive of recovery. They offer a counterpoint to the tendency of mental health professionals to unwittingly avoid certain topics, such as the experience of being compulsorily detained or being forcibly medicated. Peers also easily recognise the value of having time off from the illness experience, through activities such as gardening, travel, socialising and film-watching. These kinds of activities promote the experience we will discuss in Chapter 14 of being in flow, with all the consequent benefits for a meaningful life. They easily value the meaning found in the experience of contributing or giving back: 'I'm part of the world, I'm a human being, and human beings usually kind of do things together to help each other out'[373] (p. 288). This experience can take many forms: sending birthday cards; looking after a pet; taking part in research; becoming a peer worker. The common theme is that giving back contributes to the move from being someone who 'didn't feel like I deserved to have a halfway decent life' to coming to 'not be afraid to take things from people in return'[330] (p. 156).

Peer support specialists do not have to be people with substantial life experience – the main criterion is that they are further along the recovery road. At the ORYGEN Youth Health service in Melbourne, past programmers (i.e. people who have been through the programme) are employed as peers.

Case study 5: youth peer support workers

The ORYGEN Youth Health service employs peer support workers. Peers are recruited by interview into voluntary posts, and provided with monthly supervision from experienced clinicians about issues arising in their work. Though the position is considered voluntary, the young people are reimbursed for their time and travel.

The peer worker role is developing. For example, peer workers visit (in pairs) the acute in-patient mental health unit twice a week. Their goals during the visits are:
- to engage residents on the unit in meaningful activities and conversation
- to provide peer support
- to provide information about the ORYGEN service
- to provide the opportunity to mix with other young people who are further down their pathway to recovery
- to address the stigma associated with attending the ORYGEN programmes, and encourage involvement in the group programme
- to provide advocacy, e.g. signposting to complaints procedures.

Peer support workers also run a 'drop-in' room for several hours a week at the outpatient clinic. The drop-in room provides an opportunity for young people to meet together informally in a supportive, youth-friendly environment and to find out information from peers about ORYGEN services and other services available.

The peer support programme is embedded in a larger consumer-participation programme called The Platform Team, whose roles include contributing to service development,

involvement in interviewing panels, representing young people on committees, and providing a consumer advocacy service, including receiving media training before appearing on TV to discuss youth mental health.
Further information: info@orygen.org.au

If the involvement of peer support specialists in mental health services brings so many benefits, then the natural extension is to consider peer-run services and programmes.

Peer-run programmes

A peer-run programme, or consumer-operated service provider, is more than simply an organisation staffed by peers[359]. It is a service whose purpose is to promote personal recovery through its values and operating practices. This is shown by the Fidelity Assessment Common Ingredients Tool (FACIT)[374], which is a 46-item fidelity scale whose components are shown in Box 12.1.

Box 12.1 Components of the FACIT Scale

1. Programme structure
   - Consumer-operated (board participation; consumer staff; hiring decisions; budget control; volunteer opportunities)
   - Participant responsiveness (planning input; satisfaction/grievance response)
   - Linkage to other supports (traditional mental health services; other consumer-operated service providers; other service agencies)
2. Environment
   - Accessibility (local proximity; access; hours; cost; reasonable accommodation)
   - Safety (lack of coerciveness; programme rules)
   - Informal setting (physical and social environment; sense of community)
   - Reasonable accommodation
3. Belief systems
   - Peer principle
   - Helper's principle
   - Empowerment (personal empowerment, personal accountability, group empowerment)
   - Choice
   - Recovery
   - Acceptance and respect for dignity
   - Spiritual growth
4. Peer support
   - Peer support
   - Telling our stories: artistic expression
   - Consciousness-raising
   - Crisis prevention
   - Peer mentoring and teaching
5. Education
   - Self-management/problem-solving strategies
   - Education
6. Advocacy
   - Self advocacy, peer advocacy

There is an empirical evidence base underpinning peer-run programmes[359]. Reviews of their effectiveness have been undertaken by research groups in the USA[375-377], New Zealand[293] and England[378;379]. The findings are consistently positive[380]:

> Overall, these studies suggested that self-help and peer support programs can promote empowerment and recovery[381;382] ... preliminary evidence suggests that these programs decrease the need for acute mental health services and mental health hospitalizations[381;383;384]; increase social support, functioning, and activities[383;385;386]; decrease substance abuse[381;383]; and may benefit perceived quality of life[377;387].
>
> (p. 786)

A systematic review of six randomised controlled trials, seven comparative studies and 13 descriptive studies concluded[293]:

> Overall, research on consumer services reports very positive outcomes for clients. This review of effectiveness found some studies that reported high levels of satisfaction with services, general wellbeing and quality of life while others reported no significant differences ... No studies reported evidence of harm to service users or that consumer services were less effective than the equivalent services offered within a traditional setting.
>
> (p. 4)

For example, an eight-site randomised controlled trial across the USA investigated the impact of participation in consumer-operated service programmes[380]. The study found that participants experienced increased empowerment in services which implemented the active ingredients, and that a dose–effect relationship was present at the participant level.

The development of peer-led services is one of the most effective approaches to promoting personal recovery. For example, stigmatising beliefs are difficult or impossible to maintain when a majority of employees are peers. Peer-led services have a very different feel to traditional mental health services. They communicate the message that the experience of mental illness shows the strength to have come through adversity, rather than being a sign of weakness. The central goal of peer-led services is to support people to re-engage in determining their own future. Our next case study is an example of a peer-run telephone support service.

Case study 6: Warmline

Warmline (Waea Mahana in Māori) is a free peer support telephone helpline staffed by peer volunteers (i.e. people who self-identify as users or ex-users of mental health services). It is run by the Non-Governmental Organisation Wellink (Te Hononga Ora) in Wellington, and is the first peer support phone service in New Zealand. It aims to help callers to work out their own solutions to their problems over time.

The Warmline service features include:
- Confidential peer self-help
- Someone to talk to when feeling sad, lonely, anxious or frightened
- It involves open sharing of feelings
- It gives time to talk to someone who has been there
- It promotes awareness of ways to help yourself
- It gives a chance to discuss a decision.

It is not a crisis line or clinical service, but referral on to another service is possible. Confidentiality issues are addressed explicitly, with advertising material containing the

Case study 6: (*cont.*)

statement 'Anything you discuss with a Warmline volunteer is confidential within Warmline except in exceptional circumstances. Warmline would only contact other services if they had your implied consent'.

The service has about 30 volunteers, and new people are recruited through adverts in local papers, encouraging people with experience of using mental health services to apply. Applicants can be people who have had no contact with mental health services for several years, or people for whom Warmline provides a supportive work-experience opportunity, as a stepping-stone back towards paid work, especially in the mental health sector.

Further information: www.wellink.org.nz

Peer-led services create opportunities for meaningful involvement, shown in our next case study.

Case study 7: Rethink garden project

This project started as an activity offered by the local day centre. A centre worker who was keen on gardening negotiated with the local council to work a disused allotment, one plot among about 50 on the site. Service users attending the day centre could opt to do gardening, and they and the mental health professional worked the allotment together. Following the closure of the day centre the charity Rethink took over the gardening project and around that time a discussion resulted in the garden becoming totally user-led and -run.

The quarter-acre plot houses a polytunnel, fruit cage and raised and flat beds within which grow an impressive variety of delicious herbs, fruit and vegetables, from rhubarb, melons and plump strawberries to aubergines, some splendid-looking asparagus and large vibrantly coloured peppers. The raised beds have been built for easy wheelchair access and for those who struggle to bend down. All woodwork including the raised beds, fruit cage and sign on the front gate has been made by members, everyone tending to work to their talents and expertise although ready to muck in with the less appealing jobs, such as weeding, as and when required. Members are motivated to spend time maintaining and caring for the garden partly because its survival depends upon their input, and in turn this sense of responsibility and achievement develops self-esteem and purpose. Caring for the garden is a positive responsibility because it is 'a self-imposed discipline rather than imposed by a doctor' or mental health team; 'there is no coercion' to be involved. The members' efforts are also rewarded materially; the fresh produce divided between them provides a welcome addition to the cooking pot.

There is a core group of four people and a larger peripheral group. Nowadays people are not 'sent' to garden from any of the local services but the users who work the garden hold barbeques and rely on word-of-mouth to recruit new members. The garden is entirely user-led, bestowing agency and control. Members come and go as they want, generally putting in a couple of 3–4-hour sessions per week. Decisions about planting are made together during a meeting held in the winter, but planning isn't exact and the garden evolves: members describe 'learning as we go along'.

The garden is considered by members as providing an activity, a 'focus' and a 'structure to the week', and not necessarily thought of as a therapy: 'it gives you something to do and you get something back from it'. Satisfaction is derived from thinking about and planning what can be achieved in the garden even at times away from the garden: 'I think about it before I go, I like the "problem solving" aspect'.

Confidence is developed from being part of a group and the mutual interest and common goal lead to strong friendships being forged; members often socialise together outside the

Case study 7: (*cont.*)

project. When at the garden, there is no association with mental health: 'you are not labelled', it is 'not threatening' in any way, members are just seen as fellow gardeners by the other people who have plots there and mental health is not talked about unless it comes up in conversation. Involvement in the garden gives 'people dignity', the founding member acknowledged: 'I'd be much the poorer without it'.

More recently the half-plot next to the vegetable plot has been turned into a semi-wild community garden with a pond. The idea is that local schools and voluntary organisations can visit the garden to learn about growing produce and local ecology whilst concurrently integrating members into the broader community.

Further information: www.rethink.org

The two most developed countries internationally in relation to peer-run programmes are the USA[359] and New Zealand[91]. For example,[293]: 'There has been a quiet revolution happening in New Zealand. While the rest of the country has been paying attention to other things, support services run by and for people with experience of mental illness have been developing. There are now at least thirty-five or more of them' (pp. 4–5). Our next case study describes one such service – the Light House in Napier, New Zealand.

Case study 8: The Light House

In 1994, a group of people with experience of mental illness, meeting in each other's homes, began working together to get funding and a venue. In 1996, The Light House opened as a consumer-run community centre. The service now employs over 25 staff, many part-time, with a strong sense of shared ownership.

The aims of the service are to inspire recovery and reconnect people, and to be proactive. The service provides a range of services, including peer support and peer advocacy. The Hassle Free Clinic is a free medical clinic run by a local doctor every fortnight. The Whatever It Takes service provides home support for people with the highest needs who have no hope of recovery without peer support, advocacy and help in the community.

However, the vision is wider: 'to take over, govern and deliver services in order to minimise the impact of mental illness on generations to come'. The Light House centre is also the headquarters for political action, pushing for consumer participation at every level of planning and funding mental health services. This has involved coordination of hundreds of complaints about mental health services, filling consumer representative roles on a new mental health advisory group, and lobbying and media exposure.

Further information: www.lighthousetrust.co.nz

We now turn to another type of relationship which can be a major pro-recovery influence: the relationship between the consumer and the mental health professional.

13 Professional relationships

The focus in this chapter is on the relationship between the professional and the person with mental illness – *how* the clinician and the service user interact and work together. *What* they do is covered later, in Chapters 15 to 21.

Types of clinician–consumer relationships

Different types of relationship between clinicians and service users are possible. These can be understood as lying on a spectrum. At one end, there is a **real relationship**, defined as[388]:

> the personal relationship existing between two or more people as reflected in the degree to which each is genuine with the other and perceives the other in ways that befit the other.

A real relationship thus involves genuineness (being who one truly is, being non-phoney, being authentic in the here-and-now) and realism (perceiving the other in ways that befit him or her, rather than through a clinical or in other ways distorting lens). The importance of context is de-emphasised, and interpersonal authenticity is primary. This concept of a real relationship is long-standing[389], and not specific to mental health services.

In the middle of the spectrum of relationship types lie **partnership relationships**, which are defined by the mental health context and involve collaboration and joint working. Activation of both the expertise-by-training of the professional and the expertise-by-experience of the individual are necessary for a partnership relationship to be possible and to work.

At the opposite end lie **detached relationships**, which are highly context-based and involve therapeutic models. The relationship is filtered by the clinician through their particular model. A psychodynamic therapist will invoke concepts of transference and counter-transference to understand the relationship. A cognitive-behavioural therapist will understand the relationship in terms of interpersonal schema activation. A prescriber will use the relationship to assess symptomatology and compliance. The common features are that the discourse is driven by the clinician's agenda, and that assessment information flows from patient to clinician whereas expert knowledge passes from clinician to patient.

This spectrum broadly involves *being with* in a real relationship, through *doing with* in a partnership relationship, to *doing to* in a detached relationship. It is a spectrum rather than three distinct categories of relationship. For example, in Chapter 2 we identified that cognitive models emphasise collaboration and doing with the service user, and impose assumptions such as empiricism and giving primacy to rationality. So cognitive models are intermediate between partnership and detached relationships.

There is no best type of relationship – all can be of benefit and can involve high trust and alliance. The purpose of outlining this spectrum is to draw attention to the issue of power. A distribution of power lies at the heart of every relationship type. Power lies on a continuum, which in a mental health context has been conceptualised by the New Zealand Mental Health Commission as running from neglect and abuse, through paternalism and tokenism, to partnership and, finally, self-determination[292].

Detached relationships locate the power to interpret, understand, define and ultimately control the experience of mental illness with the mental health professional. The underpinning belief is 'I know what will help you'. At worst (as described in Chapter 7) this promotes neglect and abuse, and at best paternalism and tokenism. Modern approaches to clinical work emphasise involvement, but this remains inherently token – involvement is on the mental health professional's terms, with little expectation or openness to change in the professional as a result of the relationship.

Partnership relationships differ in that they involve a sharing of power – the expertise-by-training of the professional and the expertise-by-experience of the person with mental illness. In a partnership relationship, at times the patient is the expert and the clinician learns from or is changed by the patient. This kind of relationship thus promotes genuine co-working, and sets a context in which self-determination can develop. Real relationships have the potential to more directly promote self-determination.

In traditional mental health services, the primary emphasis is on detached relationships, with some importance attached to partnership relationships. Real relationships are normally seen as unprofessional.

In a personal-recovery-focussed mental health service, the centre of gravity shifts, so that greater emphasis is put on partnership relationships, and both real relationships and detached relationships are legitimised. To understand this statement, we need to elaborate the differences between a detached relationship and a partnership relationship.

Detached and partnership relationships

A partnership relationship differs from a detached relationship in where the decision-making power lies.

In a detached relationship, the power to make sense of what is said, to summarise (e.g. as a diagnosis or formulation), to identify realistic goals and available treatment choices, and to plan care lies with the professional. Decision-making power is nominally shared, but in reality held by the clinician. A key marker of this type of relationship is the resulting care plan:

- It contains professional jargon rather than the words of the patient
- The plan targets amelioration of deficits rather than strengths on which to build
- The goals concern avoiding bad things happening more than making good things happen
- Responsibility for the resulting actions lies more with mental health staff than with the patient
- It is authored by the professional, rather than the patient, their family or an advocate
- Collaboration is nominally demonstrated by the signature of the patient, or the patient having a copy of the care plan
- The care plan rarely creates ethical, organisational or behavioural challenges for the mental health system.

In a partnership relationship the service user is the ultimate decision-maker, other than where legal issues over-ride. This does not always mean that the professional does what the person says; clearly a professional cannot act unethically, or collude with an individual in damaging acts. But this is a quite different constraint to the paternalism discussed in Chapter 5. The basic orientation of a clinician in a partnership relationship is towards actively seeking to be led by the individual and their own wishes, goals and dreams[26]:

> Diagnosis becomes something other than the doctor defining the patient's world from the point of view of a detached expertise that arrives with its definitions and demarcations already in place. Instead, diagnosis becomes a process of exploration pursued by professional and patient together. It becomes an attempt to develop a framework of understanding and explanation that calls on different sorts of knowledge ... The patient's own understanding of his/her world moves centre-stage.
>
> (pp. 133–134)

This shift in power is easier in some cultural contexts than others. Sociopolitical and professional expectations that the health professional will understand and treat illness are difficult forces for the individual clinician or patient to resist. It may be no coincidence that the country with the most developed approach to recovery-focussed mental health services is New Zealand, which also has the most deeply embedded partnership model of any English-speaking country in relation to indigenous people. The Tiriti o Waitangi (Waitangi Treaty) was a founding document of New Zealand, and laid down the participation rights of indigenous Māori and Polynesian Islanders. This laid the cultural foundation for Māori concepts such as Whānau Ora ('Māori families being supported to achieve their maximum health and well-being'[390]) becoming integrated into mental health services.

A partnership relationship also differs from a detached relationship in the nature of listening undertaken by the mental health professional. Although all clinicians would agree about the importance of listening to the patient, in a detached relationship the listening is done in order to make a careful assessment, to monitor mental state and to plan care. The professional may try hard to understand the person, to find meaning in their experiences, and to openly acknowledge points of agreement and difference. However, an orientation at the heart of a detached relationship is that listening is done in order to fit the person into the clinical model, and not the other way round. This is not of course always inappropriate, but it differs from a partnership relationship. An unfortunate consequence of this type of listening is that the person may not feel understood. Bracken and Thomas propose alternative guiding questions[26]: What does this person, and this family, need at this stage? How can we help this person cope with this crisis without a loss of dignity? How can we help this person avoid compulsory interventions? If the goal of interaction is to answer this type of question, then the patient's values and preferences and strengths need to be established. This requires a different kind of discourse.

For example, there are lessons about engagement to learn from non-health sectors. In Case study 17 we will consider how challenging behaviour is responded to in an education context. Another sector which has developed skills in engaging with people is the hospitality industry. Key values, such as the importance of welcome, the customer always being right and the job being to provide help to meet the customer's needs, underpin the best interactions in this service industry. Hospitality workers are skilled in recognising how customers like to be engaged with – from face-to-face to elbow-to-elbow. Workers are not doing their job if customer care is poor. In the same way, a partnership relationship involves a warm welcome (because that makes the whole interaction more positive), listening to understand what the person wants, and then working with the person to identify options to meet their goals. How the person feels they were dealt with – called satisfaction with care in a mental health context – is a central, not peripheral, indicator of success.

A partnership relationship involves the clinician acting in accordance with three principles.

1. The experience of mental illness is normally meaningful

Meaninglessness enhances stigma and alienation: the sense of being 'other'. Detached relationships do not always emphasise meaning and understanding[83]. An expectation of meaningfulness leads the clinician to look for meaning. We elaborate on this aspect in Chapter 16.

2. A clinical model provides one of many ways to make sense of experience

In Chapter 2 we argued that a clinical model provides one coherent way of making sense of the individual's experiences, but should be treated as a hypothesis rather than revealed truth. Human experience cannot – in contrast to Enlightenment assumptions – be grasped using a technical idiom. This point has been made eloquently by many others[40;391;392], although normally as a starting point for an elaboration of another theory of how things really are. In this book we move away from an Enlightenment value of taming chaotic reality through technical rationality, and reject the claims of any theory as universally valid or foundational. A partnership relationship requires that the clinician has modesty in relation to the universality of their own theory. A hallmark of a partnership relationship is therefore a focus on consensus. This is challenging, because it involves genuine listening and negotiation. For example, if the predetermined question which structures the clinical interaction is 'What medication/therapy to prescribe?', then the relationship will not be one of partnership. A partnership relationship will involve asking 'Do you want help? If so, what kind?' and providing the information to support decision-making.

There is also a pragmatic reason to be focussed on the perspective of the person with mental illness. This is summarised in a conversation between service users about psychiatric nursing practice[393]:

> I think a lot of the time their [i.e. nurses'] training doesn't let them realise that the consumers know a lot about themselves and if they just took the time to get to listen to people they would realise that we know a heck of a lot about what has worked and what hasn't worked and they could circumvent a lot of trauma if they would just use the expertise that the person has about themselves.
>
> (p. 25)

Empirical evidence is consistent with this perspective[394]. The patient experience of being treated with respect and involved in decision-making is more predictive of good outcomes than the staff rating[395].

3. Only the individual can define their own best interests

A central value, discussed in Chapter 5, is that the individual is the person who can best define their own interests, and the job of the mental health professional is to support this process. This involves validating a service user who decides that their pathway to recovery lies only partly in, or totally outside, the mental health system.

Expertise-by-experience is highly valued in a partnership relationship. It comes closest to the essence of mental illness: subjective experience. What the person says may of course not accurately reflect their inner world: the experiences may not be expressible in words; they may not yet have processed the experiences sufficiently to be able to reflect on and describe them; or they may not trust the person asking them. But what people say, or otherwise communicate such as through art or poems, provides the best available approximation to their inner world. Lived experience is necessary because[128]: 'people with psychiatric disabilities – just like all those who do not have psychiatric disabilities – are the experts on the topic of their own experiences, needs, and preferences, and thus are best able to identify what would be helpful – or not – in promoting their own recovery'. When combined with the expertise of competent clinicians, this has the potential to ensure a power balance in the relationship because both clinician and patient contribute their own expertise. This synergy is captured in the TEAM acronym – Together Everyone Achieves More.

A term used to describe this type of partnership relationship is **mutuality** – the view that we have all recovered from challenges, and that it is helpful to emphasise this commonality[360]. The best recovery support occurs when the expertise of the professional and the self-knowledge of the individual are both given importance. Mutuality involves flexibility on the part of the professional and the service user. The professional needs to show modesty and humility about the universality of their clinical model, be prepared to work alongside and therefore be more exposed to the person, and to see their job as providing choices rather than fixing the problem. The service user needs to manage the anxiety and do the work associated with taking responsibility for one's own life, and learn to engage and do things that may involve risks and failures. Mutuality also involves both giving and receiving, so the clinician may be challenged, influenced and changed by the person – again emphasising commonality over difference.

Two key differences between detached and partnership relationships have been identified: power and listening. Partnership relationships have several advantages over detached relationships in relation to personal recovery: they generate hope; facilitate the development of meaning rather than imposing a clinical model; and support the service user to take personal responsibility.

Markers of a partnership relationship include:

1. At the team level, there is a concordance between what is said to the person and what is said about them. This is why unhelpful statements made within teams about people with mental illness should be appropriately challenged – not as politically correct point-scoring, but as a means of establishing, maintaining and owning a consistent set of values in the service.

2. It is acceptable for individual clinicians to discuss their own experience of mental health problems. This challenge to the them–us distinction implicit within detached relationships is only possible where there is genuine rather than nominal value placed on lived experience.

3. There is honesty about agreement and, more challengingly, disagreement between clinician and service user. Acknowledging difference is the bedrock of partnership, since it allows genuine collaboration between the professional with their expertise and the service user with theirs.

4. There is honesty about the power to change a situation. Although it gives short-term relief to promise cure, in the longer term it creates resentment and disillusionment with the system[4]. Sometimes a powerful antidote to the tendency towards a detached relationship, with its implicit expectations of cure through action by the clinician, is for an experienced mental health professional to admit 'I don't know', and to focus instead on their own commitment to supporting the person to take responsibility for their life.

The potential pay-offs are high. Partnership relationships characterised by collaboration and negotiation are associated with higher uptake of medication[253;255], lower 20-month hospitalisation rates[396], better prediction of in-patient violence during hospitalisation[397], and improved outcomes such as quality of life, symptoms and functioning in depression[398], schizophrenia[399] and case management[395].

Busy clinicians might argue that a partnership relationship is nothing new – the problem is resources, not willingness. Detached relationships take less time to develop and maintain than partnership relationships. If the mental health system is over-run with demands, then it may simply not be possible to offer anything other than a detached relationship.

This is true, so far as it goes. If the goal of mental health services is primarily to promote personal recovery, and if this is only possible where services are structured to support partnership relationships (with all the implications for more meeting time and greater staff continuity), then system structures may need to change. Although this is a comforting view, in the sense of absolving individual clinicians from the need to change, it is challenged in two ways.

First, the service user perspective is that partnership is not always experienced as the basic orientation in clinical encounters. In New Zealand, service users stated[292]:

Mental health professionals need to KNOW that:
- we are individuals with unique experiences
- we respond well to being treated with respect and accorded our basic human rights
- we respond well when we are listened to and understood (even when we are scared and angry)
- we respond well to having our concerns taken seriously. For example, when our concerns about medication side-effects are properly addressed
- our health improves more quickly if we are calmed rather than restrained
- we can manage our illness better if we are educated about it
- we can manage our illness better if we are given some help in identifying the issues in our lives that cause us stress
- we find it easier to manage our illness if we know about the kind of support groups that are available in the community
- we can participate more fully in the community if we are given some assistance with our social needs
- we can be assertive in our communities if we know our rights

(p. 45)

Second, working in a way which supports recovery is about more than resources (e.g. of time). Changing clinical focus from 'Why the system won't change' to 'What I can do' mirrors the consumer's journey from an entitlement to an empowerment perspective, which is at the heart of a recovery approach.

The writings of people who are in recovery from mental illness indicate that, sometimes, the critical contribution of a mental health professional occurs when there are elements of a real relationship. For example, this balance is noted by Ian Light, a mental health service user and academic lecturer[307]: 'In my own history of mental health service use, the nurses who have been most help to me have been those who have had the ability to respond both humanely and professionally to my distress' (p. 7). We turn now to what this means.

Real relationships

Working with a recovery focus challenges current conceptualisations of professional behaviour. In a real relationship, professionals relate to the individual exclusively as a person, and not at all as a person defined by mental illness. The next case study illustrates one approach to supporting real relationships in an acute in-patient mental health setting, and shows that there is no inherent contradiction between a therapeutic model (psychodrama, in this case) and a real relationship.

Case study 9: in-patient psychodrama group

Two one-hour sessions are held each week on the in-patient unit (in addition to one-to-one work using the psychodramatic framework with individual clients). The group is led by a psychodramatist (a psychotherapist trained in psychodrama). Each group involves a warm welcome from the director, clarifying of ground-rules, creation of a safe space to disclose, giving opportunities to all members to participate, and managing of time and emotional levels – all standard characteristics of a therapeutic group.

The group uses the psychodramatic framework[a]. Props are sometimes used to concretise – to develop an understanding about what's going on, to experiment with different and more adequate responses, and to develop more flexibility in relationships. Standard psychodrama techniques are used: doubling, role reversals and mirroring.

The key difference from most in-patient groups is that this group warms up both staff and patients to coming into the group as people first, in all their different roles. This means that staff in particular are asked to 'drop' their professional role and participate without differentiation. This creates a culture of 'we' rather than 'I–them', consistent with the psychodrama view that role-development is for everyone – we can *all* learn and grow from our encounters with each other.

The psychodrama group contains several elements that promote personal recovery:

- The language used by the director is non-pathological – the concept of lifefulness is frequently evoked, which differentiates between simply coping with adversity and embracing life by developing more adequate and engaging responses. This breaks down the stigmatising them-and-us implication of psychopathology language.
- Either the staff or the patient can bring their own issue and participate as the central actor, exploring and developing new approaches to responding. This has many benefits. It provides authentic role models for patients. It presents a human side of the professional. It fosters mutual respect between staff and patient, as both see the other as struggling to develop more adequate responses. Finally, it reduces the shame often experienced by patients about not being able to 'cope' – unlike most group situations, the boundary between participants who are coping and not coping is permeable.
- Metaphors for movement abound, starting with the greeting 'How are you travelling?'. This positions the group as process-focussed not outcome-focussed. It is not about obtaining the state of 'being better', but rather about the process of recovery.
- The group focus on the here-and-now. The founder of psychodrama, Jacob Moreno, said that the most important people in one's world are those who are in the immediate moment of the 'here-and-now'. This creates an invitation to come together and relate, which in turn positions what's going on in the group as real, supporting authenticity (being a person) rather than interpretation of transference (being a professional) in the relationship. This concords with consumer calls to 'be believed' when talking with professionals.
- A central theme is about trusting in your own creative genius. This makes explicit the view of the person as self-righting and having their own potent resources to find a way forward in their own life. It positions the actor as having responsibility for change, and gives permission to experiment and have fun. This contrasts with the passivity-inducing, risk-avoiding, humourless associations of traditional in-patient mental health services.

Further information: Lorraine Michael (lorraine.michael@svhm.org.au)

Note:
[a]Moreno JL. *Psychodrama*. Vols 1-3. New York: Beacon Press; 1972.

This change in relationship complicates decision-making about how to respond to attempts by the patient to move outside their prescribed role. The traditional clinical view is that this constitutes a boundary issue, and the professional response involves maintaining the boundary. Unfortunately, the implicit message in this strategy is to reinforce the role of patient. Boundaries evolved to protect service users, and this of course remains important. But we now know that many stories of recovery identify the contribution of staff who broke professional rules. For example[400]: 'After I worked for a month she gave me a rose' [gift from clinician to client]; 'Last month when I didn't have any money left, she let me borrow 100 crowns until the end of the month' [lending client money].

On the basis of qualitative interviews with 15 service users, Borg and Kristiansen identify five working practices which support recovery: conveying hope; sharing power; being available when needed; openness about the diversity of what can be helpful; and a willingness to stretch the boundaries of a professional role[401]. This last component is perhaps the most challenging. Examples given in their study included receiving gifts from patients, lending money and seeing the patient when off-duty. Of course, these can all be exploitative staff behaviours, so one approach is universal prohibition. But we are confronted by the reality that some patients experience rejection when we refuse a gift, however gracefully. What is needed when an expected cheque has not arrived is a loan of money. A small kindness of extra time goes a long way. How can professionals use this fact in their clinical work, whilst still acting ethically?

Reconstructing professionalism

Legitimising behaviours which lead to these kinds of benefit will involve re-negotiating the social construction of a professional relationship. Two approaches are to re-frame professional behaviour and to develop more individualised approaches to decision-making.

Alain Topor takes the first approach[402], by distinguishing between the two types of professionalism shown in Table 13.1.

The dangers of engaged professionalism are inappropriate boundary violations, such as financial or sexual or emotional exploitation. However, the dangers of detached professionalism are impeding recovery by keeping people in the patient role, and disempowering them by imposing and reinforcing a deficit-focussed discourse. Curtis and Hodge suggest that 'greater damage may be done by rigid enforcement of professional distance'[403] (p. 24) than by boundary violations.

The MHA Village (www.mhavillage.org) takes the second approach. They identify five criteria to be considered in deciding how to respond to the requests of members:

1. Ethical considerations – is the response exploitative?
2. Staff role – is the person competent to do the action, does the action fit within their role?
3. Member preference – is this something that the member wants?

Table 13.1 Characteristics of two types of professionalism

	Detached professionalism	Engaged professionalism
Time	Scheduled	Variable
Place	Predetermined	Flexible
I am … about my values and beliefs	Neutral	Explicit
Relationship	One-sided	Reciprocal

4. Staff preference – is the something the member of staff wants?

5. Clinical considerations – are there clinical reasons which over-ride other concerns.

In either approach, the consistent theme is that decision-making is explicit and visible – clinical supervision and team discussions make what would traditionally be an unethical professional response appropriate *for some people some of the time*. Sometimes, it is helpful to the person to have a hug, to have a lift, to know about the professional's spiritual beliefs, to give a token of thanks. Just like the issue of compulsion in the person's best interest discussed in Chapter 5, we cannot know for sure how to respond. The optimal approach avoids invariant solutions (e.g. No hugging, ever. No accepting of gifts, ever). We can simply do our best by exercising judgement.

That said, rule-breaking creates anxiety, whatever the motive. Staff want of course to not leave their behaviour open to question, for both benevolent and self-interest reasons. However, in a recovery-focussed service, there are changes in some expectations about behaviour. For example, there is less social distance between patients and staff, and patients are encouraged to take positive risks (see Chapter 20). The anxiety generated by these changes needs to be held by the system, not by individual workers within the system. A reasonable set of expectations is that staff responses are informed by:

1. An explicit values base, which the clinician can identify and apply

2. An understanding of the real (rather than constructed through custom-and-practice) non-negotiables: legislation, policy and professional codes of conduct

3. A belief that ethical challenges have individual rather than invariant solutions

4. An expectation that ethical dilemmas are discussed in teams and supervision rather than being individually resolved – with no licence whatsoever to covertly act outside accepted professional norms.

A means of recording the discussion and decision for future inspection is of course necessary.

A professional relationship

Working in a recovery-focussed way involves change for the professional. For example, the clinician's role as an expert is less prominent. The expert role implicit in a detached relationship remains as an important tool in the professional armoury. It is unhelpful to put expectations on a person who is still early in their recovery journey (what a professional might call acutely unwell) which they cannot even begin to meet. Sometimes people want an expert view – about diagnosis, prognosis and treatments. People who want to understand their experiences as a mental illness have a right to know the professional's opinion about what is wrong with them and what might help. We discuss this in Chapter 16. Similarly, sometimes people have lost the ability to look after themselves, and in the absence of any better option need an expert to provide guidance and to intervene, with compulsion when necessary. We explore this further in Chapter 21.

However, and it is a big however, in mental health services this should be one of many styles of interaction. In a service focussed on supporting personal recovery, it is likely that expert-style clinician–patient interactions will be the exception rather than the rule. Other interactional styles will more often be helpful and beneficial. It is noteworthy that the emphasis in evidence-based practice on *what* is to be done implicitly de-emphasises a focus on *how* it is done.

Raising awareness about clinician roles is a necessary first step towards reflective practice. Larry Davidson and colleagues identify established types of clinical roles which follow from alignment with different theorists, including as detective (Sigmund Freud), cultural anthropologist (Carl Jung), cheerleader (Carl Rogers), teacher (Aaron Beck), social control agent (E. Fuller Torrey) and (paid) friend (Peer Support Movement)[404]. A specific role which is prominent in a recovery-focussed service is as a coach[405]. In Chapter 12 we described this role for peers. For professionals, the advantages of a coaching approach are:

1. It assumes the person is or will be competent to manage their life. The capacity for personal responsibility is a given.

2. The focus is on facilitating the process of recovery to happen, rather than on the person. Coaching is about how the person can live with mental illness, and differs from a clinical focus on treating the mental illness.

3. The role of the coach is to enable this self-righting capacity to become active, rather than to fix the problem. This leads to amplification of strengths and natural supports, rather than of deficits.

4. Effort in the coaching relationship is directed towards the goals of the coachee, not the coach. The skills of the coach are a resource to be offered. Using these skills is *not* an end in itself.

5. Both participants must make an active contribution for the relationship to work.

Since clinical expertise is hard-won through years of training and supervised practice, being asked to let go of an expectation that this expertise will be given primacy is painful. More deeply, there is the challenge for the clinician of being asked to shift from a role as the person without problems towards a relationship involving two people struggling together to help one move on in their life. This transition requires emotional maturity and resilience. Competent clinical supervision is a key requirement for supporting pro-recovery practice. Professionals who do not feel they need clinical supervision are probably using automated and non-reflective problem-solving approaches in their work with clients, which is not consistent with an individualised recovery-focussed approach. The uncomfortable reality is that working to promote recovery will more often require professionals to reflect on their own values, boundaries and beliefs.

Real relationships are sometimes necessary for the reasons outlined above, but people come to mental health services wanting professional help, not just another human to have contact with. Detached relationships are also sometimes necessary, e.g. for people in the early stages of recovery, or where there are over-riding legal necessities. But detached relationships involve giving primacy to clinician imperatives. The centre of gravity in a recovery-focussed service is partnership relationships, in which the interaction is embedded in a clinical context.

Clinical expertise remains central to this type of relationship, although it is deployed to support self-management. The shift towards partnership relationships is not then a licence for the clinician to work less hard, or to abandon more easily, or to provide unfocussed or non-evidence-based treatment. It involves the use of clinical expertise in a different way. Larry Davidson and colleagues identify some of the lessons which mental health professionals will need to learn if they are to function as recovery guides[404]:

> Regardless of whether or not he or she sought your help, recognize that the client had already embarked on his or her own journey before meeting you … Your credibility and effectiveness as a recovery guide are enhanced to the degree that you are familiar with, and can anticipate, interesting sites, common destinations, and important landmarks along the way. . .Guides prepare for the journey by acquiring tools that will be effective in addressing or bypassing symptoms and other sequelae of the illness that act as barriers to the client's recovery.

(pp. 490–494)

This chapter is about the promotion of hope through relationships with professionals. These relationships provide one context in which hope can blossom, but the relationship itself is often insufficient – action is needed. The remaining chapters in this section are more concerned with the content of actions to promote recovery than with the relationship with the professional. Before coming to approaches to assess, plan and implement actions, and consistent with the recovery orientation of giving primacy to the person not the illness, we start with the promotion of well-being.

Chapter 14

Promoting well-being

In this chapter, we apply insights from the academic discipline of positive psychology, to suggest some approaches to promoting well-being in people with mental illness.

What is positive psychology?

Positive psychology is the science of what is needed for a good life. This is not a new focus – proposing qualities needed for a good life is an activity dating back to Aristotle's investigation of *eudaimonia*. But the emergence of a scientific discipline in this area is a modern phenomenon. Martin Seligman, often identified along with Mihaly Csikszentmihalyi as the founders of the discipline, suggests a definition[406]:

> The field of positive psychology at the subjective level is about valued subjective experiences: well-being, contentment, and satisfaction (in the past); hope and optimism (for the future); and flow and happiness (in the present).
>
> At the individual level, it is about positive individual traits: the capacity for love and vocation, courage, interpersonal skill, aesthetic sensibility, perseverance, forgiveness, originality, future mindedness, spirituality, high talent, and wisdom.
>
> At the group level, it is about the civic virtues and the institutions that move individuals toward better citizenship: responsibility, nurturance, altruism, civility, moderation, tolerance, and work ethic.

Findings from positive psychology are important to mental health services because its focus is as relevant to people with mental illness as to people without mental illness. Positive psychology is specifically relevant to personal recovery. Factors identified by consumers as important for their recovery include hope, spirituality, empowerment, connection, purpose, self-identity, symptom management and stigma[135]. All but symptom management were entirely absent from my professional training both as a clinical psychologist and – in the distant past – as a mental health nurse. Nor do they strongly feature in the training of other mental health professions[292]. By contrast, the concordance between the science of positive psychology and these priorities identified by recovered consumers first fuelled my interest in the applicability of positive psychology to supporting personal recovery. At least the focus of this science is pro-recovery.

An influential framework is Seligman's theory of Authentic Happiness, which identifies different types of good life[407;408]:

1. The **Pleasant Life**, which consists in having as much positive emotion as possible and learning the skills to prolong and intensify pleasures
2. The **Engaged Life**, which consists in knowing your character (highest) strengths and recrafting your work, love, friendship, play and parenting to use them as much as possible

3. The **Meaningful Life**, which consists in using your character strengths to belong to and serve something that you believe is larger than just your self

4. The **Achieving Life**, which is a life dedicated to achieving for the sake of achievement.

This framework points to the possibility of different types of good life – which means that a range of approaches to promoting well-being are needed. We will explore some of these approaches in this chapter.

Research centres are developing internationally, shown in the Appendix. Academic compilations of the emerging empirical evidence[409;410] and accessible introductions to the theory[411;412] and its applications[413] are becoming available. Three illustrative strands of work will be described, which are particularly relevant to personal recovery.

Illustrative strand 1: mental health and recovery

A central assertion in the positive psychology literature is that mental health is more than the absence of mental illness – they are not two ends of a single spectrum. Mental health is a distinct dimension from mental illness. This is not of course an original observation: the World Health Organization defines health as[414]:

> A state of complete physical, mental and social well-being and not merely the absence of disease or infirmity.

And mental health as:

> A state of well-being in which the individual realizes his or her own abilities, can cope with the normal stresses of life, can work productively and fruitfully, and is able to make a contribution to his or her community.

This distinction between mental illness and mental health is empirically validated, with only modest correlations between measures of depression and measures of psychological well-being, ranging from -0.40 to -0.55[415;416]. A more statistically robust approach is a confirmatory factor model, which showed that the latent factors of mental health and mental illness in a US sample ($n=3032$) correlated at 0.53, indicating that only one quarter of the variance between measures of mental illness and mental health is shared[417].

Why is this distinction important? Because it points to the need to support both the reduction of mental illness and the improvement of mental health. A conceptual framework is provided by the Complete State Model of Mental Health[418], proposed by Corey Keyes, and shown in Figure 14.1.

This model identifies two dimensions. Mental illness lies on a spectrum, from absent to present. Well-being also lies on a spectrum, from low to high. This conceptual framework provides a better match with the values of recovery. A perennial question about recovery is 'How can you be recovered if you still have the mental illness?'. Whatever answers are given (and there are many – see Chapters 24 and 25), they can be only partial answers since the term recovery is an illness term. By contrast, access to mental health is open to all. This provides an alternative frame of understanding for recovery:

> **Personal recovery** involves working towards better mental health, regardless of the presence of mental illness

People with mental illness who are in recovery are those who are actively engaged in working away from Floundering (through hope-supporting relationships) and Languishing (by developing a positive identity), and towards Struggling (through Framing and self-managing the mental illness) and Flourishing (by developing valued social roles).

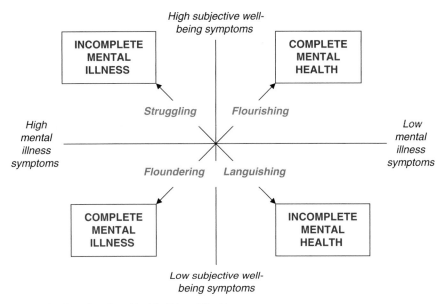

Figure 14.1 The Complete State Model of Mental Health.

This concept of mental health has been operationalised into 13 dimensions, across the domains of emotional well-being, psychological well-being and social well-being[417;419]. These dimensions have been empirically validated[415;420], and are shown in Table 14.1

Like mental illness, the concept of mental health can be expressed as a syndrome. Using the same diagnostic framework as DSM uses for major depression, the condition of Flourishing is defined as requiring high levels in Dimensions 1 (Positive affect) or 2 (Avowed quality of life) to be present, along with high levels on at least six of the 11 dimensions of positive functioning (Dimensions 3 to 13). Similarly, to be diagnosed as Languishing, individuals must exhibit low levels on one of the emotional well-being dimensions, and low levels on six of the remaining 11 dimensions. Adults who are neither flourishing nor languishing are said to be moderately mentally healthy. Finally, complete mental health is defined as the absence of mental illness and the presence of flourishing.

What is the prevalence of mental health, using these definitions? A cross-sectional assessment in the US population[419] (n=3032) is shown in Table 14.2.

A similar US study of youth (n=1234) found 6% of 12–14-year-olds Languishing, 45.2% with Moderate Mental Health, and 48.8% Flourishing, with respective proportions of 5.6%, 54.5% and 39.9% in 15–18-year-olds[421].

These results have two profound implications. First, careful consideration should be given to the balance between research into mental illness and mental health. Among US adults with no mental illness, one in 10 are languishing and fewer than 2 in 10 are flourishing. The implicit expectation that research into mental illness will promote mental well-being is neither empirically justified nor a cost-free assumption – the opportunity costs for an illness-dominated research agenda may be high. For example, Flourishing is aligned with concepts such as self-righting, self-efficacy and mastery as characteristics which critically impact on the ability to self-manage. As Keyes puts it[417]:

> In particular, is languishing a diathesis for, and is flourishing a protective factor
> against, the onset and recurrence of mental illness? Conceptually, one can think of

127

Table 14.1 Operationalisation, definition and examples of three domains of mental health

Domain	Dimension	Definition	Example
Emotional well-being	1. Positive affect	Regularly cheerful, interested in life, in good spirits, happy, calm and peaceful, full of life	*I feel happy and engaged in life most of the time*
	2. Avowed quality of life	Mostly or highly satisfied with life overall or in domains of life	*My life is good, and I wouldn't change it*
Psychological well-being	3. Self-acceptance	Holds positive attitudes toward self, acknowledges, likes most parts of self, personality	*When I look at the story of my life, I am pleased with how things have turned out so far*
	4. Personal growth	Seeks challenge, has insight into own potential, feels a sense of continued development	*For me, life has been a continuous process of learning, changing and growth*
	5. Purpose in life	Finds own life has a direction and meaning	*Some people wander aimlessly through life, but I am not one of them*
	6. Environmental mastery	Exercises ability to select, manage and mould personal environs to suit needs	*I am good at managing the responsibilities of daily life*
	7. Autonomy	Is guided by own, socially accepted, internal standards and values	*I have confidence in my own opinions, even if they differ from most other people*
	8. Positive relations with others	Has, or can form, warm, trusting personal relationships	*People would describe me as a giving person, willing to share my time with others*
Social well-being	9. Social acceptance	Holds positive attitudes toward, acknowledges and is accepting of human differences	*I believe people are kind*
	10. Social actualisation	Believes people, groups and society have potential and can evolve or grow positively	*The world is becoming a better place for everyone*
	11. Social contribution	Sees own daily activities as useful to and valued by society and others	*I have something valuable to give to the world*
	12. Social coherence	Interested in society and social life and finds them meaningful and somewhat intelligible	*I find it easy to predict what will happen next in society*
	13. Social integration	A sense of belonging to, and comfort and support from, a community	*My community is a source of support*

mental health as the continuum at the top of the cliff where most individuals reside. Flourishing individuals are at the healthiest and therefore farthest distance from the edge of this cliff; languishing places individuals very near the edge of the cliff. Hence, languishing may act as a diathesis that is activated by stressors that push individuals off the cliff and into mental illness.

(p. 547)

There is empirical support for this proposition. One validated approach involves training for optimism, by modifying the three components of explanatory style (permanence, pervasiveness, personalisation) through transforming negative thinking into positive cognitive processes that promote flexible thoughts and resilience. A study involving 70 children at high risk of depression showed that this technique reduced depressive symptomatology

Table 14.2 Prevalence of mental health and mental illness

Condition	Prevalence (%)
Mental Illness and Languishing	7
Mental Illness and Moderately Mentally Healthy	15
Mental Illness and Flourishing	1
Languishing (and no mental illness)	10
Moderate Mental Health (and no mental illness)	51
Complete Mental Health (Flourishing, no mental illness)	17

and lowered incidence rates at 2-year follow-up[422]. In a mental health service context, there is also emerging evidence that positive life events are important protective factors[330]. A study of 260 people with severe mental illness showed that an increasing ability to engage in pleasurable activities leads to the ability to regulate depressive symptoms to the point where they did not impact on identity by eroding self-esteem[423].

The second implication is that it is possible to be moderately mentally healthy, or even flourishing, despite the presence of ongoing mental illness. In other words, personal recovery is possible even in the presence of current symptoms. Cook and Jonikas label this process as thriving, in which individuals rebuild lives with qualities better than before their difficulties began[424]. Interventions which support the individual in moving towards mental health may be as important as interventions which address the mental illness.

Illustrative strand 2: hope

Hope is identified by many consumers as the starting point for their own recovery. Zlatka Russinova proposes that hope comprises three elements: perceived external resources, perceived internal resources and positive expectations[425]. She notes that generating hope in others requires a clinician to believe that such hopefulness might be justified.

From a psychological perspective, hope has progressed from meaning an overall perception that goals can be met to the more operationalised Hope Theory of C. Rick Snyder, in which hope is conceptualised as a bidimensional construct, comprising agency and pathways[426]. Agency (or a sense of will-power) involves the determination needed to begin and maintain the effort needed to achieve goals. Pathways (or a sense of way-power) involves belief in one's ability to generate successful plans, and alternatives when obstacles are met, in order to meet desired goals.

Hope is different to optimism – it involves not only positive expectancies and specific goals of agency, but also the flexibility to respond to obstacles by changing goals or methods. This distinction is illustrated by the response of Admiral Jim Stockdale when asked which people did *not* survive the Vietcong prisoner-of-war camps[427]: 'Oh, that's easy. It was the optimists. They were the ones who said we were going to be out by Christmas. And then they said we'd be out by Easter and then out by the Fourth of July and out by Thanksgiving, and then Christmas again . . . You know, I think they all died of broken hearts' (p. 48).

An intervention based on Hope Theory has shown beneficial impact. The intervention focussed on setting and working on reasonable goals, discussing the process and using homework, with the goal of increasing the production of pathway and agency thoughts. When tested as a group therapy with depressed older adults, hopelessness and anxiety reduced, hope increased and (in comparison with a reminiscence therapy control) depressive symptomatology was reduced[428]. A 5-week hope-focussed orientation group for people starting to use a community mental health centre led to benefits in relation to well-being, functioning, coping and symptomatology, especially for clients with lower initial hope[429].

This is relevant to mental health practice, because people with high hope are more likely to have positive expectations that they can cope with future adversity[430], and indeed hopefulness moderates the relationship between unanticipated stressors and successful coping[431]. Clinical implications emerging from this research are the importance of using coaching[405] and cognitive therapy skills to help people find alternative goals when faced with goal blockage (rather than unproductively ruminating)[432], and the need to help the person develop a supportive network of high-hope confidantes to whom they can turn for advice[433].

Illustrative strand 3: flow

The positive psychology literature has addressed the question of how to lead an engaged life. A key emergent concept is flow, which Nakamura and Csikszentmihalyi identify as requiring two conditions[434]:

(a) Perceived challenges that stretch (i.e. neither over-match nor under-utilise) existing skills – a sense that one is engaging challenges at the level of one's capacities

(b) Clear proximal (short-term) goals and immediate feedback on progress.

They define being **in flow** as:

> the subjective experience of engaging just-manageable challenges by tackling a series of goals, continuously processing feedback about progress, and adjusting action based on this feedback
>
> (p. 90)

In terms of flow, a good life is one that involves complete absorption in what one does.

Flow is an important concept for mental health professionals to understand, since it is the structural opposite of positive emotion. Flow is a subjective experience, but unlike positive emotions it is not defined by feelings. Rather, it results from doing activities we like. Indeed, 80% of people report that when in flow, feelings and thinking are temporarily blocked[434]. This means that **feeling good is not always necessary for a good life**. Consequently, an automatic focus on taking away experiences of unhappiness (such as symptoms of depression) may be counter-productive. It is possible to experience authentic happiness by living a meaningful life that comes through full engagement. This of course has implications for how mental health services work – the goal may not be to help the person to feel better, but to re-engage in their life. What this means for mental health services is that a *central* challenge is supporting reasonable goal-setting and goal-striving. These goals need to be:

1. *Personally relevant, rather than meeting the needs of staff*

   There may of course be other reasons for staff-based care planning, but care plans focussed on clinical risk, medication compliance, relapse prevention and symptom reduction will not promote personal recovery.

2. *The right level of challenge*

   The concept of a reasonable goal captures the balance in setting goals which are neither too easy (leading to boredom and distraction) nor too difficult (leading to anxiety and heightened self-awareness). A good life is not achieved by simply lowering expectations, as commentators from both left-wing politics (who want more justice) and right-wing politics (who want more excellence) have noted[435]. But nor is it achieved by raising expectations too high – recovery should be a journey, not a tread-mill.

3. *Proximal rather than distal*

Short-term goals provide more opportunity to become engrossed in the experience, and make engaged goal-striving more likely.

4. *Structured so that feedback is immediate and authentic*

It is this immediate feedback loop that promotes full attentional awareness on the challenge.

One approach to increasing well-being is therefore to support personally relevant goal-setting and goal-striving activity. This approach is used in the Collaborative Recovery Model.

Case study 10: Collaborative Recovery Model

The Collaborative Recovery Model (CRM)[a] is a staff training programme, based on the principles of positive psychology and its derived coaching practices. The training comprises two one-day workshops followed by one-day booster sessions six months and one year later. The content aims to develop skills in promoting autonomy and self-determination, and in creating a recovery vision – in other words, to help staff to use evidence-based skills to promote personal recovery. It is organised into six modules – two on guiding principles and four on specific skills.

The first guiding principle is a focus on personal recovery, identifying the centrality of hope, identity, meaning and personal responsibility[b]. The second guiding principle is collaboration and autonomy support. The importance of collaboration is underpinned by the empirical evidence linking working alliance with positive outcomes. Autonomy support means assisting people to make *their own* choices and is derived from self-determination theory, which recognises that being autonomous does not mean being isolated or independent of others[c].

The skills modules are:

1. Change enhancement using motivational interviewing
2. Collaborative needs assessment, to identify unmet needs
3. Collaborative goal-setting and striving, comprising the development of a personal recovery vision and identification of measurable, important and potentially attainable 3-month goals to progress towards the vision
4. Collaborative task assignment (referred to as homework) and monitoring, comprising review, design and assignment, along with development of strategies for overcoming identified obstacles.

Overall, the approach teaches the goal-striving cycle using what is called Collaborative Goal Technology[d]. It is based on adult learning principles, which are not specific to mental health, and therefore provide a normalising framework. The focus on goals provides a practical approach to improving hope, since goals require hope. A key training point is an awareness of the balance between meaning and manageability[e] – personally more meaningful goals are associated with lower manageability in people who currently lack self-efficacy (as is common in mental illness). Separating distal goals (the personal recovery vision) from more proximal goals (the 3-month plan) has three advantages. First, more proximal goals tend to have higher manageability. Second, the presence of the distal goal increases meaning for the proximal goal – commitment is higher because plans are for a purpose which is important to the consumer. Third, it supports staff engagement in the proximal goal (e.g. 'I will not be in bed during the day'), even if the distal goal (e.g. 'I will run my own business') appears to the clinician to be unrealistic.

Further information: Lindsay Oades (loades@uow.edu.au)

Notes:
[a]Oades L, Deane F, Crowe T, Lambert WG, Kavanagh D, Lloyd C. Collaborative recovery: an integrative model for working with individuals who experience chronic and recurring mental illness. *Australasian Psychiatry* 2005; **13**(3):279–284.

Case study 10: (*cont.*)

[b]Andresen R, Oades L, Caputi P. The experience of recovery from schizophrenia: towards an empirically-validated stage model. *Australian and New Zealand Journal of Psychiatry* 2003; **37**:586–594.
[c]Sheldon KM, Williams G, Joiner T. *Self-Determination Theory in the Clinic: Motivating Physical and Mental Health.* New Haven: Yale University Press; 2003.
[d]Clarke SP, Oades LG, Crowe T, Deane F. Collaborative goal technology: theory and practice. *Psychiatric Rehabilitation Journal* 2006; **30**(2):129–136.
[e]Little BR. Personal project pursuit: dimensions and dynamics of personal meaning. In: Wong PTP, Fry PS, eds. *The Human Quest for Meaning: A Handbook of Research and Clinical Applications.* Mahwah, NJ: Lawrence Erlbaum; 1998. 193–235.

The approach emphasises key recovery values of autonomy and self-determination[436], and builds on an established evidence base around personal goal-setting and goal-striving[437]. Preliminary evaluations of CRM are positive, showing improvements in staff attitudes (e.g. hopefulness) and knowledge[438]. A 10-site randomised controlled trial across three Australian states is under way.

We now consider more directly the implications of positive psychology research for promoting well-being in people with mental illness.

Interventions to promote well-being

What interventions increase levels of well-being or amplify existing strengths?

Cognitive behavioural therapy (CBT)

This psychological intervention will be familiar to most clinical readers, so no introduction will be given. Competently provided CBT is aligned with many elements of promoting recovery and personal well-being:

- It has the flexibility to be focussed on personally valued goals, rather than service-valued goals
- Responsibility for change lies with the patient, not the therapist
- A key therapeutic strategy is the development of meta-cognitive awareness – an awareness of thoughts being distinct from self. This creates the context in which a positive identity can flourish, despite the presence of ongoing symptoms of mental illness
- It trains self-management skills and reinforces interdependence and independence rather than dependence, leading to sustained gains after the end of the formal therapy
- The emphasis on homework, reality testing and learning opportunities contributes to keeping the person in their life
- If unhappiness is caused by a mismatch between self and ideal-self images, then CBT has the potential to focus on the environmental reality as much as the personal interpretation of experience. This reduces the distortion due to a focus on intrapsychic assessment, and allows (although this is not yet fully exploited in current CBT approaches) action planning around changing the environment.

Mindfulness

Meditation is 'a family of techniques which have in common a conscious attempt to focus attention in a non-analytical way, and an attempt not to dwell on discursive, ruminative thought'[439]. Teaching meditation to members of the public increases self-reported happiness and well-being, changes which are corroborated by healthier EEG readings, heart rates and flu immunity[440].

Meditation has been applied to mental health issues, such as anger[441] and – in the form of mindfulness-based cognitive therapy (MBCT) – depression[442]. Mindfulness is a form of meditation which involves attending non-judgementally to all stimuli in the internal and external environment but to avoid getting caught up in (i.e. ruminating on) any particular stimulus. Mindfulness requires a different mind-set to the quick-fix of a magic pharmaco-logical or psychological bullet. Just as becoming a top-class violinist requires 10 000 hours of practice with a competent teacher[443], so too mindfulness needs to become a way of life if it is to transform identity. It involves changing habits:

- enhancing meta-cognitive awareness by noticing what one is thinking about
- developing the ability to urge-surf by noticing but not being caught up in rising cognitions
- developing cognitive fluidity – taking habits from one space and using in another (e.g. using metaphors: thoughts as passing cars; thoughts as clouds; hare brain, tortoise mind)
- paying attention to a wider range of the available percept or experiences.

The pay-off in terms of well-being is high. Mindfulness has the potential to lead to a reconstructed, more complex identity, in which self and thought are separated. Develop-ment of a watching self gives a different means of responding to (i.e. framing) and working on (i.e. self-managing) experiences of mental illness. Developing habits of greater occupa-tion of the available attention reduces rumination and increases being in the moment – the flow concept we discussed earlier[444]:

> by increasing the amount of time a person spends thinking grateful and calming thoughts, there is simply less time to think upsetting and 'unhelpful' thoughts. Assuming that attention is a zero-sum game, the most efficient way to reduce negative and increase positive thoughts and emotions may be to focus on increasing the positive.
>
> (p. 28)

Overall, the personal qualities cultivated through mindfulness practice are nonjudging, nonstriving, acceptance, patience, trust, openness, letting go, gentleness, generosity, empathy, gratitude and lovingkindness[445] – qualities which are highly relevant to the personal recovery journey of people with mental illness.

Narrative psychology

A further clinical approach emerges from a sub-discipline called *narrative psychology*, which investigates the value of translating emotional experiences into words. This brings together insights from three strands of research[446]:

1. Inhibition – not talking about emotional trauma is unhealthy
2. Cognitive – development of a self-narrative allows closure
3. Social dynamics – keeping a secret detaches one from society.

One approach involves asking people to write about (or in other ways generate an account of) their experiences, as a means of making sense of their own story. The most beneficial story content includes placing the story in a context appropriate to its purpose, the transformation of a bad experience into a good outcome, and the imposition of a coherent structure[447]. Developing stories about growth, dealing with difficult life events and personal redemption

Box 14.1 Weekly exercises for group positive psychotherapy

Week 1. Using your strengths
Use the Values in Action Inventory of Strengths[a] to assess your top five strengths, and think of ways to use those strengths more in your everyday life.

Week 2. Three good things/blessings
Every evening write down three good things that happened that day, and why you think they happened.

Week 3. Obituary/biography
Imagine that you have passed away after living a fruitful and satisfying life. What would you want your obituary to say? Write a 1–2-page essay summarising what you would most like to be remembered for.

Week 4. Gratitude visit
Think of someone to whom you are very grateful, but whom you have never properly thanked. Compose a letter to them describing your gratitude, and read it to the person by phone or in person.

Week 5. Active/constructive responding
An active/constructive response is one where you react in a visibly positive and enthusiastic way to good news from someone else. At least once a day, respond actively and constructively to someone you know.

Week 6. Savouring
Once a day, take the time to enjoy something that you usually hurry through (such as eating a meal, taking a shower, walking to class). When it's over, write down what you did, how you did it differently, and how it felt compared to when you rush through it.

Note:
[a]Peterson C, Seligman M. *Character Strengths and Virtues*. New York: Oxford University Press; 2004.

all contribute to a positive narrative identity[448]. Empirical evidence suggests that this approach is particularly beneficial for groups who, as a whole, are not as open about their emotions: men[449], people with high hostility[450] and people with alexithymia[451].

Positive psychotherapy

An approach which brings together several of these methods is positive psychotherapy (PPT)[452]. The focus in PPT is on increasing positive emotion, engagement and meaning. For example, groups for depression undertake a series of weekly exercises, shown in Box 14.1.

These exercises are intended to tap into Seligman's proposed components of Authentic Happiness[407]. Randomised controlled trials of group PPT with mild to moderately depressed students ($n=40$) and individual PPT with severely depressed mental health clients ($n=46$) both showed gains in symptom reduction and happiness, with moderate to large effect sizes and improvement sustained at one-year follow-up[452].

We have described how some findings from positive psychology can be applied to work with people with mental illness. This requires knowledge and skills in the mental health workforce which are not, in general, currently present. So we turn now to current mental health practice, and how the processes of assessment, goal-planning and treatment for mental illness can support recovery.

15 The foundations of a recovery-focussed mental health service

What is the primary purpose of mental health services? In Chapter 2 we identified the many problems arising from a belief that the aim of mental health services is to treat mental illness. We argued that the primary purpose should be to promote personal recovery, and provided five rationales for this view in Chapters 4 to 8.

If the primary goal of mental health services is to promote personal recovery, then what does this mean for clinical processes? How do we recognise a recovery focus in a mental health service? How can the effectiveness of such a service be evaluated? In the next eight chapters we explore these questions. Our focus is on the day-to-day values, processes and work of mental health professionals.

Recovery starts with discomfort. For the consumer, this discomfort may involve experiencing the tension between professional expertise and lived experience. What fits? What doesn't? It is not enough to be passively compliant with treatment recommendations – active work is needed. For the professional, the journey towards working in a way which supports recovery also involves discomfort, at the level of values. A recovery-focussed professional has a fundamental orientation towards supporting the process of recovery in the consumer. It is fundamental in the sense of emerging from core values and informing every aspect of practice. Working in a recovery-focussed way therefore starts with a consideration of values.

Values

Whether or not explicitly stated, values underpin all behaviours by clinicians. Assessment asks about some topics and not others. Goal-planning prioritises what matters. Any intervention, including a decision not to intervene, has embedded values and creates ethical dilemmas. Reducing risk involves taking away choices. Protecting the public means segregating people with mental illnesses. Increasing effectiveness by tailoring services to local needs reduces equity of service provision. Respecting confidentiality means not being fully open with family carers. Clinical actions always involve placing a greater weight on one value than on another.

A consistent theme in services which have developed expertise in relation to recovery is that values are both explicitly identified and used to inform daily decision-making. This contrasts with the technical rationality described in Chapter 4, in which nomothetic evidence is intended to underpin clinical decision-making. This is what is meant by the call for ethics before technology[26]. To make this change requires three processes: making values explicit, embedding them in daily practice, and tailoring practice using performance feedback.

The first process is to **make values explicit**, and hence amenable to debate. This involves identifying and making visible the permeating organisational values in a live, rather than paper-based, way. This is different from the traditional organisational mission statement

---

Box 15.1 The four critical recovery values of the Center for Psychiatric Rehabilitation

1. **Person orientation**
   The service focuses on the individual first and foremost as an individual with strengths, talents, interests as well as limitations, rather than focusing on the person as a 'case', exhibiting indicators of disease
2. **Person involvement**
   The service focuses on people's rights to full partnership in all aspects of their recovery, including partnership in designing, planning, implementing and evaluating the service that supports their recovery
3. **Self-determination/choice**
   The service focuses on people's right to make individual decisions or choice about all aspects of their own recovery process, including areas such as the desired goals and outcomes, preferred services used to achieve the outcomes, preferred moments to engage or disengage in services
4. **Growth potential**
   The service focuses on the inherent capacity of any individual to recover, regardless of whether at the moment he or she is overwhelmed by the disability, struggling, living with or living beyond the disability

---

which is of little relevance to front-line staff, and to which they often have minimal sense of connection.

What are the guiding values of a recovery-focussed mental health service? They don't have to be complex. Bill Anthony has proposed the transcendent principle of personhood[453]:

> People with severe mental illnesses are people
> (p. 205)

This provides a fundamental orientation for mental health services. People with mental illness want to work, love, play, make choices, be citizens – all the normal entitlements, roles and responsibilities of being a person. The task of mental health services is to support progress towards these goals.

This single principle is a helpful summary for those staff who easily connect with recovery values, but many professionals will find a slightly expanded approach more helpful. At the Center for Psychiatric Rehabilitation (CPS) at Boston University (www.bu.edu/cpr), four recovery values are identified[454], which underpin their approach to promoting well-being described later in Case study 17. These are shown in Box 15.1.

These four values have profound implications for how the service works[455;456]. Person orientation means the service promotes access to resources outside the mental health system where meaningful, socially valued roles can be attained, rather than limiting people to mental health ghettoes. Person involvement means 'nothing about us without us': meaningful involvement of consumers at all levels of the system, including designing and delivering services. Self-determination/choice involves the opportunity to choose one's own long-term goals, rather than experiencing coercion which has the effect of diminishing rather than strengthening the self[121]. So, for example, it means that a student's choice to give up a new work role because 'the other people didn't like me' is validated rather than pathologised. This doesn't preclude discussion about what happened, consequences, costs, benefits and learning points, but the choice itself is supported. Finally, growth potential means a commitment to creating and maintaining hopefulness in people using and working in services, through selection, training, supervision and programme development processes.

Box 15.2 Recovery values at the MHA Village

1. **Client choice**: a menu approach is used to provide services based on the individual's own goals
2. **Quality of life**: the services focus on areas that address all parts of individuals' lives (e.g. work, education, finance, social goals)
3. **Community focus**: living, learning and working should be done through integration rather than segregation
4. **Whatever it takes**: services are available on a continuous basis, and follow a 'no-fail' approach – individuals are not transferred out because of the challenges they pose

Box 15.3 Ten recovery principles of the Yale Program for Recovery and Community Health

1. Care is recovery-oriented
2. Care is strengths-based
3. Care is community-focussed
4. Care is person-centred
5. Care allows for reciprocity in relationships
6. Care is culturally responsive
7. Care is grounded in the person's life context
8. Care is relationally mediated
9. Care optimises natural supports
10. It (really) is your job

As an alternative, some of the recovery-promoting values used at the MHA Village (www.mhavillage.org) are shown in Box 15.2.

Again, the impact of working in accordance with these values is profound. Client choice means that the response to a client who does not take up an intervention may be to identify the need to develop new menu items (i.e. support and intervention approaches), rather than labelling the client as non-compliant. Quality of life means that staff supported someone who wanted a sexual relationship to use a dating service. Community focus means that real-life work expectations are placed on individuals, as outlined later in Case study 18.

The Yale Program for Recovery and Community Health (www.yale.edu/prch) has published ten principles for recovery-oriented community-based care[404], shown in Box 15.3.

Their last principle addresses their experience that many clinicians, even when stating agreement with all the previous principles, do not change their own practice.

My own suggested core values for a recovery-focussed mental health service are shown in Box 15.4.

These values point to the need for a new balance, with less responsibility for and more responsibility with the person. Taking responsibility for the person outside situations of crisis atrophies the person's knowledge of being responsible for their own life, and reduces their capacity to take personal responsibility and self-manage. Taking responsibility with the person means explicitly negotiating and collaborating within a partnership relationship, holding a rapidly reducing share of responsibility as the clinical focus moves as soon as possible from doing to (during crisis), through doing with, to the person doing for themselves. It also involves values-awareness by the clinician – a self-knowledge about personal and clinical values.

The second process is to **embed values into the daily life and working practices of the mental health system**. This is a major challenge, since training in values does not easily

Box 15.4 Proposed values for a recovery-focussed mental health service

Value 1: the primary goal of mental health services is to support personal recovery
Based on the five rationales presented in Chapters 4 to 8, supporting personal recovery is the first and main goal of mental health services. Treatment goals are important but secondary.

Value 2: actions by mental health professionals will primarily focus on identifying, elaborating and supporting work towards the person's goals
If people are to be responsible for their own life, then supporting this process means avoiding the imposition of clinical meanings and assumptions about what matters, and instead focussing on the person's life goals.

Value 3: mental health services work as if people are, or (when in crisis) will be, responsible for their own lives
It is not the job of mental health professionals to fix people, or lead them to recovery. The primary job is to support people to develop and use self-management skills in their own life. The instinctive response of clinicians to any situation needs to be *'You can do it, we can help'*:

- *You can do it* because of a genuine belief in the immense potential for self-righting and taking personal responsibility within each person and their wider community
- *We can help* because of a simultaneous belief that professional training has high value for many people, especially when Value 2 is followed

impact on practice[309]. It involves both bottom-up and top-down ownership, and requires skilled leadership and system transformation. People working in recovery-focussed services need to know and own the organisational values around recovery, have the ability to link values with behaviour, and feel empowered to address discordance. In Chapter 13 we explored how values impact on the relationship between professionals and consumers, and identified the need for changes to the social construction of a professional relationship. Later in this chapter we will outline the contribution of values-based practice to recovery.

The third process involves **tailoring practice through performance feedback**. Without good information about success, the natural tendency is to assume all is well (or, at least, to focus attention on the many other pressing demands). For example, working practices at the CPR (whose values were outlined in Box 15.1) are tailored using the Stop – Start – Continue approach: using evaluation data to identify what needs to stop, to start or to continue to amplify the presence of the intended values in the organisation. In their education program (described in Case study 17), evaluation showed a slow throughput of clients. This led to a questioning of whether the service was fully supporting the value of each person having growth potential to reclaim valued social roles. As a result, they re-oriented their programmes towards a greater location in the community, with more opportunities for community participation.

As another example, UK training in Wellness Recovery Action Planning (WRAP)[351] has evolved using feedback from participants about the presence of specific values in the training, including:

> Self-determination, personal responsibility, empowerment and self-agency are key aspects of these sessions
>
> All 'peers' are treated as equals with dignity, compassion, mutual respect and unconditional high regard
>
> Sessions are based on the premise there are 'no limits' to Recovery
>
> It is understood that each person is the expert on her or himself

Clinical reality can make it difficult to follow values. Sometimes people say they want things which are hard to understand or even seem harmful, or they say they want no help even though their lives seem, to the observer, highly impoverished. The challenge is developing approaches to responding which are concordant with explicitly stated values. There is much existing expertise in the mental health system to build on. We now identify some established clinical approaches which can contribute to a recovery focus.

Evidence-based practice as a contributor to recovery

The development of evidence-based practice (EBP) is to be welcomed. The systematic evaluation of interventions before their widespread introduction will reduce the likelihood of damaging practices such as those outlined in Chapter 7. The development and dissemination of clinical guidelines[142;165] to increase consistency and quality of treatment is a key achievement of mental health services in the twentieth century. Clinical practice should always be informed by this knowledge base.

However, the limitations of EBP are also important to understand. This relates to the limitations of nomothetic knowledge, outlined in Chapter 4. For example, Whitwell highlights the changing nature of what is seen as effective, with each generation of clinicians believing that their approaches, unlike previous treatment regimes, are scientific and evidence-based[22]. He raises the null hypothesis issue – that no specific treatments are effective, and concludes that in fact each new treatment only has an effect due to nonspecific factors such as positive expectations, contact with a support system, positive human values, support with basic necessities, human contact and restoration of physical health. Whilst admiring the modesty involved in this stance, this view goes too far. Treatments are effective, for some people, some of the time.

The central limitation of EBP is the tendency to reduce rather than amplify meaning. The more central EBP becomes, the more decontextualised, objectified and divested of meaning the patient becomes. So whilst EBP has an important contribution, in a recovery-focussed service it is a tool rather than a clinical imperative. As Whitwell comments[22], EBP supporters:

> see it as a way of cleansing medicine from messy subjectivism. Its advocates use the results to produce protocols for treatment – so that decisions made will conform to 'best practice'. This however is only a short distance away from the old ideas of compliance – except now not only should the patient comply, but also the doctor.
>
> (p. 131)

Working to support recovery means that the expert clinician offers knowledge about best available evidence for treatments as a resource within a partnership relationship. In general (with exceptions discussed in Chapters 20 and 21), trying to convince the patient they need clinician-specified treatment or imposing treatments in the patient's best interest is a sign that the professional is getting in the way of the person's recovery. Forced treatment is oxymoronic, and doing things to the patient is more likely to promote passivity, dependency and other anti-recovery effects.

One antidote to the EBP tendency to remove meaning is offered by narrative-based medicine.

Narrative-based practice as a contributor to recovery

An approach to blending group-level nomothetic knowledge and patient-level idiographic knowledge is found in narrative-based medicine, in which the aim of listening is to understand what the patient is saying[457]:

> Even the most pompous professors have been known to warn their students, 'Listen to the patient: he or she is telling you the diagnosis'. A more sophisticated view holds that when doctors take a medical history they inevitably act as ethnographers, historians, and biographers, required to understand aspects of personhood, personality, social and psychological functioning, and biological and physical phenomena.
>
> (p. 49)

Narrative-based medicine highlights the role of literature in giving insights into the human condition[458], and can act as a balance to the reductionism of evidence-based medicine[459]:

> Narrative is endemic to medicine, but has been excluded in the rise of EBM (evidence-based medicine). It remains to be seen whether narrative's ecumenicalism will be rebuffed or reconciled with EBM's fundamentalism, but there are signs of convergence. . . . There is an emerging image of the mature and experienced clinician of the future, who will have the capacity to integrate narrative- and evidence-based perspectives, quantitative and qualitative methods, and have a balanced awareness of the contributions and limitations of both as a sound basis for clinical judgements.

Narrative is important. Comparing self-reported and clinical accounts of an experience indicates the profound difference between clinical and subjective perspectives[4;110]. For example, Mary O'Hagan wrote[122]:

> Today I wanted to die. Everything was hurting. My body was screaming. I saw the doctor. I said nothing. Now I feel terrible. Nothing seems good and nothing good seems possible.
>
> I am stuck in this twilight mood
> Where I go down
> Into a lonely black hole
> Where there is room for only one.

Her contemporaneous admission file recorded: 'Flat. Lacking in motivation, sleep and appetite good. Discussed aetiology. Cont. LiCarb 250mg qid. Levels next time.'

Lodge differentiates between the use of science to uncover generalisable insights and laws, and the use of literature to describe the 'dense specificity of personal experience'[460]. As Whitwell puts it[22]: 'narrative is not some second-rate homely account, to be disregarded once science has caught up. It is the closest we can come to the unknowable reality of the experience of other people' (p. 59). Understanding is a matter of narrative, and the application of scientific treatments needs to be consistent with the patient's narrative. This integration provides a vehicle for placing the patient's meaning centre-stage. Why should we want to do this? The answer is a matter of values.

Values-based practice as a contributor to recovery

A third established approach is values-based practice – the theory and skills base for effective health care decision-making where different (and hence potentially conflicting) values are in play[309]. Ten pointers to good process in values-based practice, developed by Bill Fulford[309] and with names suggested by Glenn Roberts[461], are shown in Table 15.1.

Values-based practice highlights that the application of technology (e.g. assessment processes, treatments, outcome evaluation) is not a neutral activity. Awareness of and debate about implicit values is as important as discussion about the optimal treatment strategy. It points to the primacy of the patient's values, the importance and limitations of evidence-based practice, and the centrality of language, communication and negotiation.

Table 15.1 Ten principles of values-based practice

Principle name	Description
The 'Two feet' principle	All decisions are based on values *and* facts, including decisions about diagnosis
The 'Squeaky wheel' principle	We tend to notice values only when they are diverse or conflicting and likely to be problematic
The 'Science-driven' principle	Increasing scientific knowledge creates choices, which brings the full diversity of human values into play
The 'Patient-perspective' principle	The first source of values information is the perspective of the patient
The 'Multi-perspective' principle	Conflicts of values are resolved by balancing legitimately different perspectives, not by reference to a predefined rule
The 'Values-blindness' principle	Careful attention to language use raises awareness of values
The 'Values-myopia' principle	First-hand narratives, survey, media and social science reports can all improve our knowledge of other people's values
The 'Space of values' principle	Ethical reasoning is employed to explore differences of values, not to determine 'what is right'
The 'How it's done' principle	Communication skills are central to conflict resolution and clinical decision-making
The 'Who decides' principle	Decisions are taken by patients and professionals in partnership

A mental health service using a values-based practice approach necessarily places great emphasis on the dreams, aspirations and goals of the person. This approach therefore promotes a focus on personal recovery.

Perhaps the most developed approach to working in a pro-recovery way has emerged from the rehabilitation part of the mental health system.

Rehabilitation as a contributor to recovery

Rehabilitation services work longer-term with people who have severe and enduring mental illness. There is a difference between rehabilitation and recovery[462]:

> Rehabilitation refers to the services and technologies that are made available to disabled persons so that they may learn to adapt to their world. Recovery refers to the lived or real life experience of persons as they accept and overcome the challenge of the disability.

Rehabilitation services are concerned with bridging the gap between an individual and their aspirations, through effective treatments, skills training and practical and emotional support. These are key pro-recovery skills, which perhaps accounts for the close alignment between rehabilitation and recovery[463]. See for example uspra.org. However, not all rehabilitation values support recovery. This is evident in the best current text-book on rehabilitation psychiatry[21]. On the one hand, the rhetoric is highly pro-recovery:

> The central ambitions of contemporary rehabilitation services are to rekindle hope and to open routes to personal recovery, while accepting and accounting for continuing difficulty and disability. Best practice pivots on a mature and creative

balance of optimism and realism, and requires the ability to tolerate protracted uncertainty and remain curious and hopeful.

(p. xv)

On the other, traditional assumptions leak in:

In truth, many if not all people with psychotic and other severe mental illnesses do have 'long-term conditions' for which long-term thinking and strategies are appropriate.

(p. xvii)

Table 15.2 Differences between traditional and recovery-focussed services

Traditional approach	Recovery approach
Values and power arrangements	
(Apparently) value-free	Value-centred
Professional accountability	Personal responsibility
Control-oriented	Oriented to choice
Power over people	Awakens people's power
Basic concepts	
Scientific	Humanistic
Pathography	Biography
Psychopathology	Distressing experience
Diagnosis	Personal meaning
Treatment	Growth and discovery
Doctors and patients	Experts by training and experts by experience
Knowledge base	
Randomised controlled trials	Guiding narratives
Systematic reviews	Modelled on heroes
Decontextualised	Within a social context
Working practices	
Recognition	Understanding
Focus on the disorder	Focus on the person
Illness-based	Strengths-based
Based on reducing adverse events	Based on hopes and dreams
Individual adapts to the programme	Provider adapts to the individual
Rewards passivity and compliance	Fosters empowerment
Expert care co-ordinators	Self-management
Goals of the service	
Anti-disease	Pro-health
Bringing under control	Self-control
Compliance	Choice
Return to normal	Transformation

> We were not able to recruit as broad a contribution as we would have wished from service users to give a view about user-led services. At present we can look in vain for a mental health equivalent of the League of Friends[a] that characterises patient involvement in general hospital.
>
> (p. xix)

> This then raises such familiar, mundane but essential issues such as how to get someone out of bed, how to get day and night in their proper places, how to ensure that the person is dressed appropriately, has adequate personal hygiene and is taking necessary medication.
>
> (p. xx)

Assumptions of chronicity, acceptable types of user involvement and doing-to may be deeply entrenched views within rehabilitation services: values which will need to change if rehabilitation approaches are to fully support recovery. A key challenge to mental health practitioners will be to provide best possible recovery-oriented rehabilitation services, whilst simultaneously recognising that, for some people, their journey to recovery is primarily or exclusively outside mental health services.

British readers will be familiar with the saying *Don't throw the baby out with the bath-water*, meaning that it is important during any change process to identify what to keep, as well as what to let go of. Whenever calling for change, it is easy to denigrate the old and idealise the new. This is not the intention in this book. Traditional mental health services have developed much expertise which supports personal recovery. We have identified four existing approaches which should feature prominently in any pro-recovery mental health service: evidence-based practice, narrative-based practice, values-based practice and rehabilitation. We now turn to the bath-water aspects: the points of difference.

Differences between traditional and recovery-focussed services

The central differences between a recovery-focussed approach and traditional clinical practice have been considered by several authors with experience of trying to implement pro-recovery change[143;464–467]. In Table 15.2 we summarise some points of variation.

Table 15.2 provides a summary of some key differences, and is consistent with the Personal Recovery Framework of Chapter 9. We now make the summary more concrete, by outlining how recovery-focussed services work in practice. We start with assessment.

---

[a]A voluntary organisation in UK general hospitals, typically staffed by ex-patients and informal carers, which fund-raises and provides practical support to patients – but as an adjunct to the clinical services rather than as a peer-led service

Assessment

How can assessment promote recovery? In Chapter 13 we described partnership relationships, and distinguished them from detached relationships. In a partnership relationship
there are two experts in the room, and the process is characterised by two-way conversation
rather than one-way examination. We turn now to the content of this conversation.

The aims of assessment differ from the traditional clinical goal of identifying the illness
and planning the treatment. Aims of a recovery-focussed assessment include:

1. To promote and validate the development of personal meaning
2. To amplify strengths rather than deficits
3. To foster personal responsibility rather than passive compliance
4. To support the development of a positive identity rather than an illness identity
5. To develop hopefulness rather than hopelessness.

In considering how assessment can meet these aims, the intention is not to provide a
comprehensive how-to-assess guide. Rather, the goal is to provide resources and pointers to
good practice which can be integrated, in different ways, into the work of individual
clinicians.

Using assessment to develop and validate personal meaning

The development of personal meaning is central to recovery, but 'most people find little in
the way of meaning or purpose in fulfilling the role of mental patient'[330] (p. 156). How can
clinicians assess the person in a way that avoids imposing meaning and hence getting in the
way of recovery?

In the Personal Recovery Framework presented in Chapter 9, we identified the central
distinction between the person experiencing the mental illness and the mental illness itself,
and the consequent importance of a primary focus on the person, not the illness. Consistent
with this stance, our first consideration of meaning should be at the level of the person, and
their search for a meaningful life. Can we define the ubiquitous term meaning of life?
A conceptual framework is provided by Baumeister[468], who differentiated between four
needs for meaning. These are shown in Table 16.1, along with their implications for clinical
practice.

This framework is not specific to people with mental illness – it applies to anyone. All
four needs for meaning are important. The meaning of life is normally not singular, but
emerges from a constellation of domains including family, love, work, spirituality and
personal projects[469]. Multiple sources of meaning are also buffers, reducing the impact of
losing one source and relieving the pressure on any individual domain to satisfy all four
needs for meaning[447].

Reflective practice is relevant to the assessment process, because assessment is action: in a
socially constructed world, questions shape the emergent meaning. Applying this framework

Table 16.1 Four needs for meaning

Type of meaning	Definition	Implication for working practices in mental health services
1. Purpose	Present events draw meaning from their connection with future events	Listen for personal meaning and meaning-making approaches in accounts of past and current events
Two types:		
(i) Goals	An objective outcome, such as job promotion, having a child	Identify personal goals, provide goal-setting and goal-striving support. Facilitate access to mainstream opportunities (employment, education, leisure, social)
(ii) Fulfilments	A subjective anticipated state of future fulfilment, such as being in love, going to Heaven	Encourage optimism and hopefulness. Ask future-oriented questions – 'Where would you like to be in 5 years?', 'How can I support you to work towards that dream?'
2. Values	Lends a sense of goodness or positivity to life, can justify certain courses of action	Support spiritual development by facilitating access to religious, faith, humanist, cultural or political groups. Avoid undermining the individual's values by imposing personal or professional values (e.g. a clinical model, the importance of empiricism, societal norms)
3. Efficacy	A belief one can make a difference	Identify and amplify times of well-being, when person showed mastery and coped with unanticipated difficulties. Plan ahead. Identify personal and social resources. Support the development of crisis plans
4. Self-worth	Reasons for believing one is a good, worthy person	Actively encourage the person to take on 'giving back' roles – voluntary work, co-running a group, writing about their experiences, becoming a peer mentor. Foster affiliation with high-status groups (especially outside the mental health system)

in a mental illness context orients the clinician towards key reflective practice questions. Do I know this person as s/he sees her/himself? Do I know what is meaningful to this person? Am I working to support the person to transcend their illness experience, to meet personal goals and fulfilments, to live in a value-concordant way, to be empowered, and to experience giving as well as receiving?

To make this more concrete, the empirical evidence suggests that staff working in mental health services hold stigmatising views about mental illness[70]. How might this change? One approach is to increase cultural competence, the ability to work with people without imposing culture-based filters of meaning on the interaction[188]. In relation to recovery, cultural competence can be viewed as a means to an end. The end is working with each person as an individual, rather than defining the person in terms of stereotypes and group norms. The development of skills in cultural competence can be an important step towards that end. The Yale Program for Recovery and Community Health (www.yale.edu/prch) teaches five cultural tenets:

1. Working with clients is inevitably a cross-cultural enterprise
2. Becoming culturally competent is a process not an end point
3. A central part of working effectively across cultures is becoming aware of our personal cultural filters

4. Group-specific information can be used as a starting point for exploring individual experiences

5. Stereotyping is a natural part of the human perception process, but is one we need to be aware of and challenge.

For the patient, integration of the direct meaning of the mental illness into personal and social identity is a key step on the journey of recovery. It is also a very personal process – it cannot be done to the person, so assessment involves working with the person to help them develop their own explanation. The process of integration normally starts with the quest for direct meaning – making sense of what has been, and is, happening. A desire for many patients will be to reduce anxiety by wanting an answer from the expert. Therefore part of the assessment will involve collecting enough information to be able to offer a clinical perspective, and to develop treatment goals (which we cover in Chapter 17). This perspective will be an important resource for some patients, for whom receiving a diagnosis can be immensely helpful:

> It just made sense of not sleeping, waking up early and not being able to get to sleep and not being able to eat, being constantly worried about what was going to happen.[186]
>
> It is impossible for any sane person even to begin to imagine how I felt. It is also obvious to anyone with a shred of common sense that I was ill. Any characterisation of my behaviour as 'bizarre', that such an 'illness' attribution would then be an act of social control (to empower the medical profession), is clearly absurd.[67]
>
> I found it kind of liberating. For a while I could receive the absolution I needed for failing to do the things I usually did. My relationships with friends and family improved: I had not simply become lazy, unreliable and extremely irritable, now there was something 'wrong'.[76]

There should be no withholding of a view about diagnosis, but there should also be a tentativeness in how it is used in the assessment process. It is a resource to offer to the patient, not 'the' answer. The anxiety containment achieved through a diagnosis can be real, in showing that others have experienced similar things. But it can also be illusory if the patient thinks a diagnosis is an explanation (when it is a description), and can actively impede recovery if the patient expects the expert, who now knows what's going on, to cure them. For many, perhaps most, people with mental illness, there is no magic bullet, despite what they may hope for from the clinician. The reality is that recovery involves innumerable small acts. Nothing more. And nothing less. Tentativeness in communicating a clinical perspective therefore needs to be genuine, rather than a therapeutic manoeuvre to soften the blow of diagnostic reality.

Recovery-focussed clinicians know that the meaning of choice is the choice of meaning. If recovery is 'a manifestation of empowerment'[470], then it potentially 'involves the individual rejecting labels linked to psychiatric disabilities and regaining a sense of personal integrity'[333]. Nurturing this process of empowerment involves a willingness to accept that clinical explanations may not be helpful for every individual, and to actively support the person to access other sources of meaning, such as spirituality (discussed in Chapter 10) or self-help groups (Chapter 12). A marker that the focus is on personal rather than clinical meaning is when the idea of a *Coming Off Diagnosis* group to support users of mental health services to develop their own framing of their experiences is understood rather than ridiculed.

In practice, this all adds up to a clinical assessment involving a stance of enquiring about, and expecting to find together, some meaning in the experience, whilst giving primacy to the views of the patient not the professional. This does not of course imply that what the person currently believes is necessarily true in an objective sense, but that the basic orientation of the assessment process is towards helping the patient and the clinician to understand the experience, rather than to explain the cause. Glenn Roberts identifies three approaches in relation to experiences of psychosis[83]:

1. Finding specific and concrete meanings

This involves listening without filtering through a clinical model, to understand the developmental and autobiographical context in which experiences take place. In psychosis, for example, the guiding question might be 'Has this in some sense actually happened to the person?'. Most commonly the experience that is clinically seen as a delusional belief won't have literally happened, but may have happened in a different context or time, such as the person experiencing persecutory delusion who was abused as a child. Making sense at this level is directly and powerfully therapeutic, in creating a space to develop non-psychotic ways of engaging with the underlying issue.

2. Understanding metaphoric or thematic associations

This involves following the feeling, or emergent themes, in the way the person talks about their experiences – viewing delusions as unlabelled metaphors[471]. The level of meaning might be a pervasive sense of powerlessness, guilt, shame or lack of value, or identification with the role of victim. The advantage of this approach is that it both normalises the experience – you don't have to have a mental illness to have unresolved issues – and provides an opportunity to support the person in developing self-awareness and new identity formation.

3. Understanding the purpose and significance of an individual's elaboration of their psychosis

This final approach involves setting aside entirely the issue of where the experiences have come from, and focussing instead on what maintains and reinforces the person's interpretation. The guiding question might be 'Is this a helpful way for the individual to make sense of their experiences?'. The advantage of this approach is that it leads to a hope-promoting focus on making the future better, rather than a hope-destroying account of the individual as incomprehensible. As Roberts puts it[83]:

> there is a perennial risk that this backward search for meanings can become endless, and a problem in its own right. Any gardener knows that digging up the roots is not a good way to promote growth . . . [T]he purpose of understanding is not to 'crack the code', but always in the service of supporting the individual's journey in recovery and getting on with life.
>
> (p. 94)

Three levels of understanding are thus being differentiated:

- Understanding the meaning *of* madness – how does it arise?
- Understanding meaning *in* madness – either specific or metaphorical
- Understanding meaning *through* madness – existential considerations.

This effort to understand can offer a buttress against the damaging clinical tendency to pathologise. For example, when confronted with someone hearing voices, the traditional instinctive clinical response is:

- To give primacy to voice-hearing, and hence ignore the social context, other problems the person is experiencing, and their strengths and abilities
- To link voice-hearing with schizophrenia, when other explanatory frameworks exist[42]

- To assume that medication is necessary, when alternative responses exist[472]
- To define the experience as a mental illness, and consequently to locate the person in a role as a person with a mental illness, despite its stigmatising consequences.

  Many consumers report feeling pathologised by mental health services[473]:

  > Some people will try to tell you that your anger is a symptom of mental illness. Don't believe them. Anger is not a symptom of mental illness. Some people may even try to medicate you in order to make your anger go away. This can be dangerous – by extinguishing someone's anger we run the risk of breaking their spirit and of wounding their dignity . . . Your anger is not a symptom of mental illness. Your angry indignation is a sane response to the situation you are facing.

The outcome of the individual's quest for meaning may or may not be consistent with a clinical perspective. A recovery value is that it doesn't matter! Most people have idiosyncratic views which would seem odd to some external observers. It is not the job of mental health services to make people rational. Nor is it their job to make people normal; mental health services overvalue the bland. As Pat Deegan put it[474]:'The goal of the recovery process is not to become normal. The goal is to embrace our human vocation of becoming more deeply, more fully human'. Self-awareness about values and avoiding the implicit prioritisation of rationality and normality are difficult tasks for clinicians. Pragmatic suggestions to support this process include:

1. Involving people with lived experience as workers in mental health services is an aid for mental health professionals in engaging in a recovery-supporting way with patients, as we discussed in Chapter 12.
2. Developing new scripts which validate personal meaning. For example, responding to 'I have schizophrenia' with 'I'm wondering if that's what you think or what other people have said about you?'.
3. Creating opportunities for the professional to meet voice-hearers:
   a. who accept the voices as being real, e.g. through the Hearing Voices Network (www.hearing-voices.org)
   b. outside the normal clinical context, e.g. through trialogues (Case study 26)
   c. who are further along in their recovery journey, e.g. as colleagues in consumer-employee roles.
4. Applying cognitive-behavioural insights based on social rank theory[475] to understand that the relationship between the voice-hearer and their voice is a social relationship, and so issues of victimhood, power, fear and empowerment are valid assessment topics.
5. Experimenting in asking about strengths as well as deficits, to challenge the confirmation bias involved in a deficit-focussed assessment.

For example, understanding the person's behaviour as an effort to cope with their experiences rather than as a symptom of mental illness can be helpful. The study of approaches to coping has a long history. Much of the work is influenced by the Cognitive Appraisal Model (also known as the Transactional Model) of Richard Lazarus. In this model, coping is defined as[476]:

> constantly changing cognitive and behavioral efforts to manage specific external and/ or internal demands that are appraised as taxing or exceeding the resources of the person.

(p. 141)

Coping strategies are cognitive and behavioural responses intended to reduce either the gap between reality (environmental outcomes) and wants (ideal self-image), or the threat (cognitive dissonance) associated with the gap. The model proposes that people do not unthinkingly react to change, e.g. symptoms. Rather, coping responses are generated by: (i) appraising the situation, e.g. in terms of demands, threats, opportunities; (ii) identifying the available resources for managing the situation; and (iii) estimating the consequences of different responses. Therefore, coping responses are influenced by appraisal (e.g. controllability, relevance) and may have effects on motivation, cognition, emotion or interpersonal functioning.

The model is of course limited – no one is always rational and the person may be stuck in unhelpful response patterns. However, the merit of the model is that each element provides a potential point of clinical action. For the anxious person, developing skills in reducing hyper-vigilance to threat alert will enhance coping ability. For the depressed person, exploring beliefs about support available from others may increase the available resources. For the person with a substance abuse problem, motivational interviewing to identify all effects of the behaviour may increase motivation to change.

There is no shortage of lists of coping strategies, from 161 derived from existing measures[477], to 66 different cognitive and behavioural strategies to deal with negative events[478]. Two relevant superordinate groupings have been proposed. The first grouping differentiates between the focus of the coping response[476]. Problem-focussed coping involves changing the environment, to remove obstacles blocking successful striving. Emotion-focussed coping (also known as reorganisation strategies[479]) involves intrapsychic change to reduce the mismatch or perceived threat. Meaning-focussed coping (also known as reappraisal coping[479]) involves re-framing the meaning of the event or situation to make it more compatible with beliefs and goals. These categories have predictive value. For example, perceiving a diagnosis of HIV/AIDS as a challenge (i.e. amenable to change) is associated with experiencing more control over the illness (meaning-focussed coping), using more problem-focussed coping and social support, and better emotional well-being[480].

The second grouping is into avoidance versus approach strategies[481]. This distinction refers to whether the focus is towards or away from a problem or negative event. Approach strategies deal with a mismatch between self and environment by actively confronting the problem. Avoidance strategies either deny the mismatch or seek to escape the damaging consequences.

Combining these two groupings gives four classes of coping response, shown in Table 16.2.

The final column of Table 16.2 indicates how these coping responses can be interpreted clinically. The fact that these are all negative labels may stand out, although this is inevitable when clinical terminology describes deficits and not strengths. What from the outside can appear to be symptoms of mental illness can be interpreted very differently. Understanding normalises these processes, which otherwise would be pathologised.

We now identify approaches to a balanced assessment of strengths and deficits.

Using assessment to amplify strengths

In Chapter 2 we identified how a clinical model leads to a negative bias in assessment. We noted that clinical assessment should focus on four dimensions[57]:

1. Deficiencies and undermining characteristics of the person
2. Strengths and assets of the person
3. Lacks and destructive factors in the environment
4. Resource and opportunities in the environment.

Table 16.2 Coping styles

	Coping response	Thoughts	Feelings	Behaviours	Clinical interpretation
Emotional avoidance	Emotionally withdraw from a too-painful reality	'There's no problem'	Drained, dead inside, wrung out, heavy, anxious, depressed	Drug and alcohol over-use Social isolation Day-dreaming Excessive sleep Giving up	Disengaged Amotivational Affective blunting Passivity Lacking insight
Re-framing	Try to make sense of the situation in a way that fits with current beliefs	'I can make sense of what's happened without changing myself'	Suspicious, anxious, afraid, alone, uncertain, angry	'Odd' behaviour Increased religious activity	Paranoid Delusional Reasoning bias Lacking insight
Active engagement	Try to change the world to fit with beliefs	'I can change the situation without changing myself'	Engaged, angry	Challenging	Non-compliant Manipulative
Integration	Change beliefs, values and goals to better fit reality	'This is how things are. So now what . . .?'	Acceptance, combined happiness and sadness	Ventilation of feelings Use of social support	

Assessing a person in a way which does not overly focus on negatives is difficult, for several reasons. First, it is hard work. Each dimension is dynamic and changing, and interdependent in complex ways. Holding this complexity is intellectually demanding, and requires a tentative stance and openness to changing understanding. It is much easier and in some ways more rewarding to be the clinical expert, who can summarise the problems of the person (i.e. Dimension 1) with a pithy piece of professional language. This issue will reduce with the development of a shared taxonomy and language for Dimensions 2 to 4. This is beginning to emerge. For example, the concept of character strengths has been disaggregated into six core virtues of wisdom, courage, humanity, justice, temperance and transcendence[482]. Similarly, positive affect has been disaggregated into Joviality (e.g. cheerful, happy, enthusiastic), Self-Assurance (e.g. confident, strong, daring) and Attentiveness (e.g. alert, concentrating, determined)[483].

Second, the expectation in the mental health system that it is the person who is going to be treated inevitably leads to a focus of attention on the individual. This of course is a consequence of clinical (and patient) beliefs about what the job is, and doesn't have to be the case. The importance of the wider context is considered further in Chapter 23.

Third, the clinician's illusion means that professionals don't see people as often when they are coping[323], so they gain the false impression they cannot cope or self-right. So Dimension 1 (and to some extent Dimension 3) tends to dominate clinical interactions. Case study 25 includes strategies to address this issue.

Finally, the questions clinicians ask impose a structure on the dialogue, and influence content. The highly practised deficits-focussed discourse of taking a history systematically identifies all the deficient, inexplicable, different and abnormal qualities and experiences of the person. This focus on deficits (and the other Ds: difficulties, disappointment, diagnosis, disease, disability, disempowerment, disenfranchisement, demoralisation, dysfunction) reinforces an illness identity, and the person disappears. Up close, nobody is normal: a deficit-focussed discourse will always elicit confirmatory evidence for an illness-saturated view of the person. Since illness is a negatively valued state, this bias adversely shapes how the person is seen by themselves and others.

Deficits, risk and symptoms are important, and so structured approaches to their assessment are an important clinical skill. However, there is no established structured dialogue, equivalent to a mental state examination, to identify a person's strengths, values, coping strategies, dreams, goals and aspirations. What might this look like? This will involve assessment of mental health. In Box 16.1 a Mental Health Assessment is proposed, with the equivalent elements from a standard history-taking interview shown in square brackets. The assessment is consistent with the Complete State Model of Mental Health[418] introduced in Chapter 14, and informed by empirical research reviewed in Chapter 2.

Of course, this discourse would be irrelevant for a clinician who sees their job as diagnosing and treating, and irritating for a patient who wants the clinician to tell them what the problem is and how to address it. So role expectations are central, and recovery-focussed clinicians hold different expectations about the primary purpose of their role.

The Mental Health Assessment is also clearly one-sided, systematically ignoring the negative part of the story and unlikely to yield a balanced picture. This is, of course, the point – problems and deficits should not be the *only* dimension assessed. The more we seek out and elaborate actual and potential mental well-being, the less we see (and support, and create) mental illness. A balanced approach is needed, and Box 16.1 is intended to provide a corrective to the conventional imbalance.

Another approach is embedded in the Appreciative Listening Cycle[484]. This contrasts with the Problem Focus Cycle, shown in Figure 16.1.

The Problem Focus Cycle has two anti-recovery features. First, it focuses on problems, thus reinforcing an illness identity and neglecting the innate, growth-oriented capacities and strengths of the individual. Its orientation is towards objectifying the person, by seeing the problem as primary. Hence there is great attention paid to compliance, with the embedded assumption that non-compliance is undesirable. Yet for people without a mental illness, there is much greater ambivalence about challenging rules – sometimes opposition and independence are highly valued.

Second, by starting with a professional imposition of meaning, the remainder of the process (no matter how sensitively done and patient-focussed) is inevitably clinician-led. For example, clinicians of course differ in the extent to which they involve the patient in decision-making, but the consistent assumption built into this process is that the clinician knows the best solution: the intervention may need to be tailored to the patient, but starts with and is based on clinical expertise rather than the expertise of lived experience.

In a recovery-focussed service, certain assumptions are turned on their head. This is one. In a partnership relationship, the assumption is that the patient knows the best solution – it is after all their life. Of course, their view may benefit from the input of clinical expertise. But this characteristic of a paradigm shift – what was previously of peripheral interest (the patient's view) becomes central – is present in a recovery-focussed system. We discuss this further in Chapter 26.

In the Appreciative Listening Cycle, the starting point is called the consumer's passions. This is shown in Figure 16.2.

Box 16.1 Mental Health Assessment

Current strengths and resources [History of the presenting illness]
How are you making sense of what's going on in your life at present? What keeps you going? How have you found the strength to get this far? What do you have going for you? Consider spirituality, social roles, cultural/political identity, self-belief, life skills, toughness, resilience, humour, environmental mastery, support from others, ability to take a philosophical approach to life or to express emotion artistically.

Learning from the past [Precipitating events]
Was there a time when it became more difficult to cope? Why was that, do you think? What would turn the situation around? What have these experiences taught you? Are there any positive ways in which you have changed or grown as a person? Consider gratitude, altruism, empathy, compassion, self-acceptance, self-efficacy, meaning.

Personal goals [Risk assessment]
How would you like your life to be different? If you woke up tomorrow and the problem had gone away, how would you know? What would you notice had changed about yourself, and what would others notice about you? What are your dreams now? How have they changed?

Past coping history [Past psychiatric history]
How have you got through the tough times in your life? What supports have you found useful? What do you wish had happened?

Inherited resources [Genetic background]
Is there any history of high achieving in your family? Any artists, authors, athletes or academics?

Family environment [Family environment]
When you were growing up, was there anyone you really admired? Who was the most kind person to you? Who taught you the most? Who did you want to be like? What important lessons did you learn during childhood?

Developmental history [Developmental history]
What was life like for you when you were growing up? What did you enjoy? What's your best memory? What skills or abilities did you discover you had? What came easily to you?

Valued social roles [Occupational history]
How would you describe yourself? How do other people see you? What would someone who knew you really well and liked you say? What would you like them to say? How are you useful or of value to others?

Social supports [Relationship history]
Who do you lean on in times of trouble? Who leans on you?

Personal gifts [Forensic history, drug and alcohol]
What is special about you? Has anyone ever paid you a compliment? What do you like about yourself? What things that you've done or ways that you've behaved make you feel really proud of yourself?

Personal recovery [Premorbid personality]
Do you have a sense of who you were before these problems? How did you feel about that person back then? Do you want to go back to how you were, or become someone new? What bits of yourself then would you hold on to?

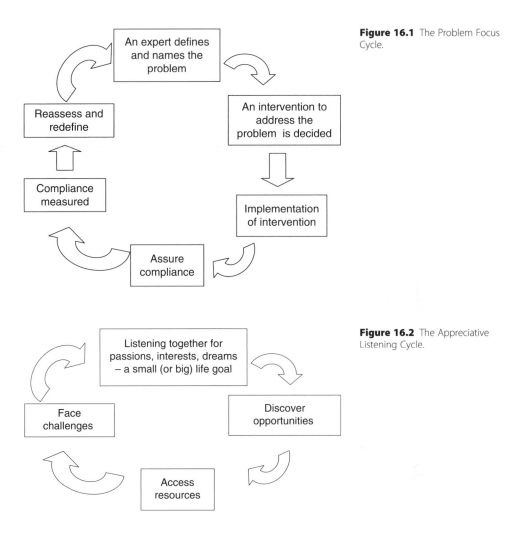

Figure 16.1 The Problem Focus Cycle.

Figure 16.2 The Appreciative Listening Cycle.

The approach emerges from the appreciative listening enquiry field, in which the four steps are labelled as Discover, Dream, Design and Destiny[485]. It starts by identifying something – anything – that matters to the individual, and then working together towards that goal. The slips along the road to meeting the person's goals become normalised as challenges, rather than compliance issues. Setbacks become the jumping-off point for new growth and learning, rather than treatment failures. Of course, some setbacks may relate to mental illness, but the key difference is that they are not the start point. Pharmacological and psychological treatments for mental illness often will be one means of facing a challenge, but this is in service to the person's goals – a means, not an end.

The Appreciative Listening Cycle does something the Problem Focus Cycle does not: it locates the responsibility for change with the individual. This does not mean the person is unsupported or abandoned. There may be substantial effort going into skill-building and staff-intensive support may be needed to reach the goal and deal with setbacks. But it creates the possibility of generating surprise: 'I did it!'. This type of surprise is the bed-rock of resilience.

Another assessment approach builds on the character strengths concept introduced in Chapter 14. These comprise one's highest strengths, and have been disaggregated into virtues of wisdom, courage, humanity, justice, temperance and transcendence[482]. This framework underpins the Values in Action Inventory of Strengths (VIAS)[482], which is available as a 240-item online questionnaire at www.viastrengths.org. After completion, the respondent is presented with a list of their five top 'signature' strengths. Consistent with its origins, the questionnaire reflects US values, and under-emphasises strengths valued more highly in other cultures such as patience and forbearance[486]. It also focusses on individual-level strengths, thus neglecting familial and cultural strengths such as connectedness. However, a 54-country study involving 117 676 internet respondents demonstrated a high level of consistency in the profile of character strengths internationally[487], and VIAS provides a theoretically based and empirically established counterbalance to assessment of deficits.

The VIAS has been used by a psychiatric rehabilitation centre, with very positive findings[342]:

> The survey creates a mindset of serious and effortful self-appraisal . . . at the conclusion . . . most participants report feelings of pride and expansiveness, with the discovery of a self that is invariably better than expected . . .
>
> Some . . . report a sense of accomplishment and mastery from merely completing the assessment. Most report that their mood improves after receiving their results and they think more positively about themselves.
>
> (p. 121)

The general principle across all these approaches is a stance of expecting to find more than just problems. The importance of nurturing a non-illness-based identity is central to the accounts of many people experiencing recovery[330]:

> Having joy is one way to stay out of depression.
> It was just realizing . . . that life isn't one big horror.
> At least [now] I've got something to think about other than to think about the bad part, the lonely part. At least I know I can think about: I'm going to go out with [my friend]. It's only lunch, but it'll be good.
>
> (pp. 154–155)

One aim of identifying strengths is to activate the person's capacity to take responsibility for their own life.

Using assessment to foster personal responsibility

An unintended consequence of clinicians working so hard to look after people with mental illness can be a reluctance to allow individuals to take responsibility for their own life. Clinicians need to get out of the way of the person's recovery. This means supporting the individual to take as much personal responsibility as possible, rather than assuming responsibility for them. The clinical job is to support and amplify the individual's efforts towards recovery, by avoiding as far as possible detached relationships, deficit-focussed assessments, doing-to treatments, and drip-feeding responsibility back to the person. This transition in responsibility needs to be managed in a skilful rather than abandoning way, a balance understood by people using mental health services[55]:

> Over the years I've realised that support services can do too much as well as too little. I have learned to recognize when to stop my reliance on the support of professionals.

If I hadn't taken risks to get well in the past, I might still be in a sort of low-level state.
I might have had only one spell in hospital rather than a dozen, but I doubt
I would be where I'm at today.

(p. 56)

This can be difficult for clinicians, who are generally highly caring and want the best for the people with whom they work. They will have experience of people being allowed to make their own choices with damaging consequences. Staff may need support to work in a responsibility-promoting way, e.g. by linking this behaviour with the values of self-determination and personal responsibility.

This is one area where rehabilitation services and CBT both have relevant expertise, in their emphasis on the ability of the individual to make a difference to their life, rather than being a passive victim of an illness or recipient of treatment. Clinical communication skills remain central. For example, with some service users it may be more helpful to talk about personal resourcefulness (which points to creativity) than personal responsibility (which some people may feel is imposing expectations on them).

What practical difference does this orientation make? One example is in goal-setting activity. Many people experience difficulty in developing purposive activity. Clinicians can support this by using person-centred questioning: 'When have you most felt alive?', 'When did you last have fun / laugh out loud?', 'What would make a difference in your life?', 'What are your dreams?', 'What do you want in life?', 'What would make your life better?', 'What would give your life more meaning?', 'What would make your life more enjoyable?', etc. The challenge is then *not* to get in the way by assuming responsibility, for example through helping the client to decide whether the goal is realistic, or identifying *for the person* the steps towards their goal. This is not of course to argue that people don't need support – of course they do. Rather, it is arguing that the instinctive response needs to be locating the responsibility for change with the person.

The antidote to the clinical tendency to assume responsibility is to use coaching skills for supporting partnership relationships: 'What would it take to meet this goal?', 'What would happen if you challenge the rule that says you're not allowed to do that?', etc. Mental health clinicians need expertise in facilitating, not in doing. The resulting authentic and mutual relationship with the consumer has greater potential for healing than a relationship focussed on treatment and cure.

Using assessment to support a positive identity

One thing professionals know is that the experience of mental illness will almost certainly change the person. Researchers asking people about recovery found that[488]: 'some of the participants talk about becoming *different* people as a result of their illness, others talk about becoming *better* people' (p. 239). Changes in identity during personal recovery are as individual as any other recovery process[489]. However, two broad types of change can be distinguished: redefining existing elements of identity (identity re-definition) and developing new elements (identity growth). Some examples of identity-transforming beliefs in relation to direct and indirect meaning are shown in Table 16.3.

Identity transformation is presented in Table 16.3 by describing new beliefs, but it is of course a much deeper process, involving a core sense of who the person is. Recovery-focussed clinicians know that this identity work begins as soon as possible: focussing solely on cure of the mental illness gets in the way of supporting people to live good lives now. Health is not promoted simply by reducing illness, just as life cannot be lived just by minimising dysfunction.

Table 16.3 Identity redefinition and identity growth

	Identity change	Examples of transformative beliefs	Why this helps
Direct meaning of mental illness	*Redefinition*	My mental illness means I cannot function *some of the time*, rather than all the time	I can lead my life the rest of the time
		I have more control than anyone else over my mental illness	Increased agency and empowerment
	Growth	My mental illness has led me to understand myself in new ways	(a) increased self-knowledge; (b) value and meaning placed on experience
		Other people have been like me and recovered	(a) normalising of experience; (b) hope-promoting
Indirect meaning for the person	*Redefinition*	My mental illness has happened because of my childhood	(a) life becomes more meaningful; (b) development of coherent personal narrative
		My mental illness means I am in touch with my creativity	Increased value associated with self as a whole person, rather than self-image as being damaged
	Growth	I am more compassionate to others now	(a) becoming a 'better' person is socially valued; (b) being compassionate with others can lead to greater self-compassion
		My mental illness has given me a job, teaching about mental health issues	(a) development of a social role; (b) using own experiences; (c) benefiting others

It can be difficult to see the person when the illness is very prominent. One approach is to draw from non-mental-health approaches to amplifying a positive identity (e.g. www.bluesalmon.org.uk). Another approach is to use a time-line to help put the person as they are now into the broader context of their own life. Even though the person may be currently struggling to exercise personal responsibility, it is helpful for the clinician to know about their best efforts and successes – creating a shared belief that the person can be expected to re-engage in their life in the future. A third approach is to deliberately increase involvement with the person when well, so that the worker can hold a picture of the well person during crisis (see Case study 25). All of this takes time. A mental health system which only has capacity for a short, symptom-focussed assessment of the patient is a structural impediment to the efforts of clinicians to support recovery.

Assessment at the level of indirect meaning is important, in giving the person a chance to process and make sense of what the mental illness means for them as person. For the clinician, this involves giving the patient an invitation to open up the conversation. Whilst the content of the illness experience may be of central importance to the clinician, for the patient the main concern may be the wider social and temporal context – what does it mean for the person in their environment, and for their past, and their future? This is of course highly individual, but fits with the focus on contextualised meaning rather than decontextualised description. Talking about indirect meaning is a different task from discussing prognosis, which is a component of direct meaning understood within a clinical model. Conversation about indirect meaning also helpfully differentiates between the person and that part of them which is experiencing mental illness.

Using assessment to develop hope

Change at the level of identity is a frightening prospect, and reassurance about the possibility of recovery may be vital. How can this hope for the future be realistically supported, when we cannot know what the future holds for an individual patient?

An organising theoretical model of hope and consequent set of strategies is provided by Russinova[425]. In conjunction with findings from elsewhere[4;426], it is possible to identify values, attitudes and behaviours in mental health professionals which promote hope in the people they work with. These are shown in Table 16.4.

Although this list initially looks very difficult to disagree with, it provides challenges for traditional clinical practice. For example, 'Trust in the authenticity of what the person says' is not compatible with assessing in relation to a predefined clinical model. It requires the cognitive flexibility in the clinician to both value the client's interpretation and to bring professional expertise to bear. This is why the concept of insight is so toxic for personal recovery – it indicates a cognitive stance which views one person (the professional) as right and the other (the patient) as wrong unless they agree. This is not just making the obvious point that it should always be remembered that a delusional belief might be right, no matter how far-fetched it sounds. This is making a more challenging and values-based point, that in a recovery-focussed service the professional perspective does not have automatic primacy over the patient perspective. In a partnership relationship, based on the constructivist

Table 16.4 Strategies for promoting hope

	Using interpersonal resources	Activating internal resources	Accessing external resources
Values	Valuing the person as a unique human being	Failure is a positive sign of engagement, and contributes to self-knowledge	Target efforts towards supporting the person to maintain relationships and social roles
	Trust in the authenticity of what the person says	To be human is to have limitations – the challenge is to exceed or accept them	Find or build an audience to the person's uniqueness, strengths and best efforts
Attitudes	Believing in the person's potential and strength	Losses need to be grieved for	Housing, employment and education are key external resources
	Accepting the person for who they are	The person needs to find meaning in their mental illness, and more importantly in their life	Employ recovered consumers in services as role models
	View set-backs and 'relapse' as part of recovery		
Behaviours	Listening non-judgementally	Support the person to set and reach personally valued goals	Facilitate contact with peer role models and self-help groups
	Tolerate the uncertainty about the person's future	Support the person to develop better approaches to coping	Be available in crisis
	Express and demonstrate a genuine concern for the person's well-being	Help the person to recall previous achievements and positive experiences	Support access to a full range of treatments and information
	Use humour appropriately	Support and actively encourage exploration of spirituality	Support close relationships

epistemology described in Chapter 4, there is no single correct interpretation of reality. Rather, what matters is working together to find an explanation which is helpful to the patient. Recovery begins with hope, and is sustained by acceptance. Hope, not acceptance, is the starting point[474]: 'How can we accept the illness when we have no hope. Why should one pile despair on top of hopelessness? The combination could be fatal. So perhaps people are wise in not accepting the illness until they have the resources to deal with it.'

In practice, this means the assessment conversation between clinician and consumer in a recovery-focussed service may look different, in two ways. First, the topic of interest is the person not the illness, and promotion of well-being is as important as treatment of illness. Therefore the content is not solely about deficits. Second, the discourse is not a one-way relationship, focussed on the clinician assessing the patient and then providing expert advice. Rather, the discourse is as much about helping the consumer to learn about themselves as giving the clinician the information they need. This requires coaching skills, and modesty and tentativeness from the clinician about the limits of their expert knowledge. It will even involve the clinician learning from the consumer.

We close this discussion of promoting hope with two concrete suggestions. First, perhaps the biggest weapon of depression is that it is a killer of hope. Addressing experiences of depression can be an important step towards the person being able to take personal responsibility. Second, it is helpful for clinicians to talk about recovery. The very existence of the concept in clinical discourse has transformative potential, and acts as a counterbalance to the alternative implicit message that long-term contact with mental health services is the norm.

Messages to communicate through assessment

To summarise, mental health services can support recovery during assessment by communicating several messages, shown in Box 16.2.

These messages may differ from what is communicated to people using traditional mental health services. They may to the seasoned clinician even sound naïve, especially in relation to people in crisis. The intention is not to be unrealistic. Chadwick draws on his own experience of psychosis to suggest that[67]: 'when dealing with a newly admitted deluded

---

Box 16.2 Professional-to-patient assessment messages which support recovery

1. The experience you are going through is meaningful, and part of your journey in life. I will use all my expertise to support you to make sense of what is happening to you, working with you to help you to find your own way forward. I don't know what will happen to you, but I do know that many people with similar experiences have recovered their life.
2. Some people with similar experiences find it helpful to make sense of what is going on as a mental illness. Others develop their own meaning through contact with others who have been through similar experiences. Some make sense of what has happened to them in spiritual terms, or in other ways entirely outside the mental health system.
3. Whatever sense you make of it, you will over time increasingly fit this experience into the bigger picture of who you are as a person. Although you may change as a result, you will control the direction of this change. A point may come where you can even identify good things that have come out of the experience
4. It's fine to hope for miracles, but don't expect them! As you become ready, the challenge will be for you to make decisions about your own life. This is going to be hard work – but you won't be alone.

patient the terms on which you think the interaction is taking place are not anything like the terms as seen from the patient's perspective . . . the patient is literally living and behaving in a different world from you.'

The clinical skill during crisis is to provide a map back to experiencing hope and personal responsibility. If a map is to be of use for navigation, it needs to include the current location, orientation and terrain markers. The skilled recovery-focussed clinician:

- Connects with the person where they are, accepting that their unusual beliefs, statements and behaviour are meaningful. Accepting involves not imposing an explanatory model, but offering alternative explanations in a tentative and non-authoritative way. This is difficult if you believe that you know for certain what is going on, and professional training which treats as revealed truth one model of understanding will actively impede this skill.

- Will offer pointers for the direction of travel. This can involve discussion about help and support which is available now or when the person is ready, overt discussions about power ('for the moment I have had to take control over your life, and this is what needs to happen for me to give this power back'), positive goal-setting, being a holder of hope for the person when they are hopeless, or being a spring safety-net instead of a sagging safety-net by actively easing the person back into their life.

- Will use their expertise-by-training as a resource for the client. This might involve 'Other people I have worked with have found X useful', or 'Although it's hard right now to even think about talking about what you are going through, as soon as you do manage to disclose even a small part you may well experience a real sense of achievement. It will probably still hurt, but it will be the pain of healing'.

Sometimes the view is put forward that professional expertise is devalued in a recovery-focussed service. In fact, it is realistically valued. It is not treated as revealed truth – but then nor should it be. It is an important resource for service users to draw on.

The purpose of assessment is to develop goal-oriented action plans, to which we now turn.

Chapter 7

Action planning

In a mental health service focussed on personal recovery, assessment leads to the identification of two types of goal: those arising from the person; and those arising from societally imposed behavioural constraints or perceptions by others (e.g. clinicians) about best interests. It is helpful to distinguish between goals that are important *to* the person and goals that are important *for* the person[490].

Recovery goals are the individual's dreams and aspirations. They are influenced by personality and values. They are unique, often idiosyncratic. They are forward-looking, although they may of course involve the past. They harness approach motivation (focussing on what the person actively wants) rather than avoidance motivation (focussing on what the person wants to avoid). Recovery goals are strengths-based and oriented towards reinforcing a positive identity and developing valued social roles. They can be challenging to mental health professionals, either because they seem unrealistic or inappropriate, or supporting them is outside the professional role. They sometimes involve effort by the professional, or they may have nothing to do with mental health services. They always require the consumer to take personal responsibility and put in effort. Recovery goals are set by the consumer, and are dreams with deadlines[491].

Treatment goals arise from the societal requirements and professional obligations imposed on mental health services to constrain and control behaviour and improve health. The person with a history of severe self-neglect may need regular clinical assessment. The person who becomes rapidly unable to cope with the responsibilities of child-care may need assessment by social services. The person who is actively suicidal may need to be assessed for compulsory hospitalisation. The person who becomes dangerous due to command hallucinations may need compliance with antipsychotic medication to be monitored. Treatment goals are set by the clinician, on the basis of societal, legal and professional requirements. These goals will normally relate to serious harmful risk, symptoms, medication and lifestyle choices. They will be about minimising the impact of an illness and avoiding bad things happening, such as relapse, hospitalisation, harmful risk, etc. The resulting actions will often be doing-to tasks undertaken by the clinician. Treatment goals and associated actions provide the basis of defensible practice, and are important and necessary. They may be signed off by the consumer to show they have seen them, and the consumer will be as involved in the process as possible, and may negotiate specific elements, but they are not the consumer's goals.

Recovery goals and treatment goals are different. A simple exercise to highlight this difference is to ask a group of clinicians to each highlight three things which keep them well, and help them to cope with stresses in life. Then compare this list with care plan items. It is likely that the clinician-generated list will focus on well-being and natural life supports (e.g. family, friends, spirituality, work, love, nature, personal interests), whereas the care plan list will focus on treatment of illness. This highlights the assumption that people with mental illness need treatment, whereas everyone else needs well-being – a perspective of fundamental otherness which needs to change before a recovery focus is possible. Recovery goals look like the goals of people with no mental illness. They are based on approach-motivation, and support flourishing and thriving – rather than compliance-oriented treatment goals which use avoidance-motivation with the aim of surviving and getting by.

This dichotomy is potentially unhelpful, in two ways. First, it suggests that clinical and consumer priorities are intrinsically opposed. This is not the case. Sometimes a recovery goal and a treatment goal are the same – reducing distress might be the individual's and the clinician's goal. Sometimes the person will agree with a treatment goal as a means towards a personally valued end – taking medication in order to be able to concentrate at work. But sometimes there is no overlap between these two types of goal. Second, it creates the impression that working in a recovery-focussed way can be done by getting someone else to develop recovery goals with the consumer whilst the clinician continues with traditional treatment planning. This is not the intention – supporting recovery is the job of clinicians!

Distinguishing between recovery goals and treatment goals has several advantages:

1. **It is honest**
   It does not maintain a pretence that everything in a care plan is necessarily in the person's interest.

2. **It promotes a focus on values**
   More clearly identifying actions professionals have to do makes power, choice and control issues more explicit and hence amenable to debate – both at the individual clinician level (through an increased emphasis on reflective practice) and at the sociopolitical level.

3. **It promotes a focus on the patient's aspirations and preferences**
   Trying to make the recovery goals of the patient explicit highlights the need to support the person to identify their goals and preferred methods of goal attainment. This places their views at the heart of action planning.

4. **It reduces compulsion**
   For the clinician, a stronger orientation towards promoting self-determination leads to a corresponding orientation away from overruling the individual in their choices. For the service user, the more that clinical effort is directed towards recovery goals, the less the person offers resistance.

5. **It promotes partnership**
   Identifying treatment goals as 'the beast to feed' (i.e. externalising this imperative as something to which both parties are subject and which requires certain actions, irrespective of personal opinions) positions doing-to tasks as a joint problem – allowing clinicians and patients to work towards a joint goal of reducing monitoring and compulsion.
   A professional orientation towards supporting recovery goals means that it is not for them to decide what is realistic, although they may raise this concern where applicable and work with the service user to break down the recovery goal into smaller steps.

The process of developing treatment goals needs no elaboration, since it is at the heart of traditional clinical practice. But how can recovery goals be explored? A range of simple questions can be used:

- Ask the person what they want from life, and validate their response
- Ask the person about their dreams when they were younger – what did they used to want before the mental illness? Do they still want it, or have they changed towards other goals?

- Ask what life would be like without the mental illness: 'If you could wave a magic wand and wake up tomorrow without this illness, how would you know it has gone? What would be different? What could you do tomorrow that you can't do today?'

We now describe some more systematic approaches (among others[491;492]) to support the identification of recovery goals.

Working to recovery is a work-book developed by Ron Coleman and colleagues, which provides a personal planning tool for recovery[493]. Initial topics are: What recovery means to me; About myself; My needs; and My strengths. It covers stepping-stones to recovery, including relationships with others (such as 'map makers' to recovery) and with the four selves (confidence, esteem, awareness and acceptance). It helps identify positive and negative feelings about the mental illness, and looks at choices and experiences during the mental health career, including experiences with the care planning process, medication, other mainstream treatments and complementary therapy. It finishes with a personal development plan, identifying priorities, goals and anticipated support needs.

Pathways to recovery is a work-book which supports the journey of exploration, self-discovery and planning[494]. It focusses on the domains of life which people need to thrive, such as a sense of home, increasing knowledge and education, finding work or volunteer activities that bring satisfaction, developing meaningful relationships with others, achieving intimacy and enhancing sexuality, attaining higher levels of wellness, and exploring spirituality. An important feature is the inclusion of over 30 first-person accounts of recovery. It is intended to support the development of a positive non-illness identity.

The focus in **Wellness Recovery Action Planning (WRAP)** is on self-managing mental illness[351]. WRAP was developed by Mary-Ellen Copeland, and now widely used in many countries (see www.mentalhealthrecovery.com for more information). It involves a personal process of action planning, covering the following elements:

- What keeps me well
- Patterns of wellness over time
- Personal triggers/buttons
- Early warning signs and action plan
- Ways of coping and self-management
- Support systems
- Crisis planning/advance directives
- Ways of building wellness.

A key feature is that the starting point is wellness. This positions illness experiences as the exception, which can be addressed both through amplifying wellness and through activating extra support if needed. This is consistent with the emphasis on identity in the Personal Recovery Framework.

Most commonly, WRAP is facilitated by people with their own experience of mental illness, either in individual work with clients or in a group-based (e.g. eight-session) training format. Structures supporting the completion of WRAP vary, from being offered by an entirely separate service (e.g. Case study 17) to being a culture change approach (e.g. Case study 25). It can also serve as a required gateway to other programmes (e.g. Case study 24). Some services provide a continuous rolling WRAP training programme, which consumers can start at any point. Requiring all service staff to undertake this training, in which they process something from which they are recovering, can promote experiential learning and reduce stigmatising distinctions.

Some established recovery-focussed services have separate routes for developing recovery goals and developing treatment goals, e.g. Case study 13. By way of contrast, our next case study illustrates an approach to integrating recovery and treatment goals into a single planning process.

Case study 11: person-centred planning

The Yale Program for Recovery and Community Health trains clinicians in person-centred planning[a]. Two key principles inform the process:
1. Personally valued goals are the starting point. They are not the thing to focus on *after* clinical goals such as medication compliance, abstinence and symptom reduction are achieved. For example, referral to supported employment is not delayed until clinical stability is obtained. The planning process is therefore strengths-based, because a deficit-based assessment leads to a crossing off (temporarily or permanently) of many valued social roles (mother, worker, spiritual person).
2. Meeting goals through personal effort and natural supports is preferable to meeting goals through mental health service effort. This reinforces a positive identity, maximises personal responsibility and keeps the person in their life. Focussing on service interventions reinforces the mental patient identity and allows the community to continue discriminating.

Person-centred planning starts by the person identifying goals which promote their recovery, self-determination and community integration. This involves helping the person to connect with their own dreams – either now or when younger. The focus is on identifying goals which promote well-being and thriving, rather than avoiding illness problems and getting by. Identified goals are often big, and always meaningful. Goals are never about receiving treatment as a goal in itself, but will often involve treatment as a component of progressing towards personally valued goals.

Objectives or stepping-stone actions are then set for each goal. Every objective is linked to specific goals – everything for a purpose. Objectives have deadlines, to create a sense of momentum and an expectation of progress. They should be achievable and, as far as possible, enjoyable. They are positive: 'The person will . . .' rather than 'The person will not'. Person-first language ('person with depression' rather than 'depressive') emphasises the personhood rather than the illness identity.

Objectives harness strengths. For example, a person who takes their medication irregularly may be viewed as 'non-compliant', with a resulting action of 'Monitor to ensure medication is taken as prescribed'. Viewed from a strengths-based perspective, this person might be seen as 'making use of alternative coping strategies such as exercise and relaxation to reduce reliance on medication', leading to an action 'Work collaboratively to develop a contingency plan for when medications are to be used on an "as-needed" basis'. Agency is amplified, because there is a huge difference between someone who uses medication as a recovery tool and someone who requires medication for clinical stability.

In developing objectives, the orientation is towards actions the person can do for themselves, or can achieve by harnessing existing or new natural supports in their life. If the person's goal is intellectual stimulation, then the objective might be going to a book-reading in a bookshop, rather than attending a service-based current affairs group. If the goal is spiritual development, then going to (say) a church may be more supportive of a positive identity than attending a spirituality group specifically for consumers labelled with mental illness. Only when personal resources and natural supports are insufficient is consideration given to a service response – because it is better to get the support from the system than not at all.

Case study 11: (*cont.*)

Structural approaches can help to support person-centred planning. For example, having three parts to the intervention section of each plan: actions to be done by the consumer, ways in which the person's natural supports will contribute, and actions the mental health service will take.

Further information: Janis Tondora (Janis.Tondora@yale.edu)

Note:
[a]Tondora J, Pocklington S, Osher D, Davidson L. *Implementation of person-centered care and planning: From policy to practice to evaluation.* Washington DC: Substance Abuse and Mental Health Services Administration; 2005.

As a final word on assessment, there is as noted earlier no fundamental incompatibility between recovery goals and treatment goals. The consumer may align precisely with the clinical perspective, or the professional may set treatment goals on the basis of the individual's aspirations. However, this agreement should not be assumed, and consumer involvement in the care planning process has often been nominal, e.g. shown by them signing the plan. The consumer's perspective needs to take primacy if the direction of travel for subsequent action is to be as focussed as possible on promoting personal recovery. In a clinical context, where power is unequally distributed, it is especially important to ensure the consumer's voice is heard. This is why the identification of recovery goals needs to be an explicit focus within the assessment process.

One joint aim can be focussing clinical effort on the goals of the individual. It is self-evident that this will produce greater engagement than targeting clinical imperatives. And yet it will require a shift in values[330]: 'Neither the person's efforts nor our own as professionals should be limited to reducing symptoms and dysfunction. Just as life cannot be lived by minimizing dysfunction alone . . . recovery is not achieved solely through minimizing illness' (p. 160).

A second joint aim can be to reduce the number of treatment goals to zero. This is not to imply that treatment goals are bad – it is not a bad thing to stop someone from, say, harming themselves or others. The point is that where the person is taking responsibility for their own behaviour as part of their recovery goals, there is no need for the professional to manage risk as a treatment goal. Where the person is managing their own symptoms using a variety of approaches, the professional no longer needs to focus on medication compliance. The paradox at the heart of this book is that when the person finds effective ways to get on with their life, there is less need for treatment. Providing effective treatments is therefore not the best starting point. Life is about recovery goals, not treatment goals.

Where the professional and the consumer are solely working towards recovery goals, there is closest alignment and greatest possibility of a partnership relationship. This scenario makes clinical work more effective for the consumer – everyone is pulling in the same direction. Perhaps paradoxically to those who may view the profession of psychiatry as the problem, it also makes the clinical interaction more similar to what takes place in other medical areas. Since most mental health clinicians don't enjoy compulsion, this partnership relationship is also more enjoyable for the professional. A recovery approach is in this sense liberating for both consumers and clinicians.

Once the recovery goals and the treatment goals are identified, action follows.

Chapter 18

Supporting the development of self-management skills

Mental health professionals support recovery by offering treatments and interventions which amplify the person's self-management skills. This chapter includes ideas and suggestions as a resource to inform the development of reflective practice. Many of the ideas discussed will not be new to experienced clinicians. The aim is to highlight how offering treatment with an aim of promoting self-management (rather than compliance) can provide a vital resource for supporting recovery.

The offering of treatment

In a recovery-focussed service, access to competently provided effective treatments is a vital support for many people's recovery[120]. However, providing treatment is not the primary purpose of mental health services. A recovery-focussed service supports people to use medication, other treatments and services as a resource in their own recovery[474].

This means that evidence-based treatments are (with two exceptions) offered not imposed. Most professionals have highly developed skills in working with individuals who may be ambivalent or antithetical towards engagement. The challenge is to utilise these professional skills to support the person to engage in *their own life*, rather than in addressing clinical preoccupations. The challenge is to work with (not on) the person: services on tap, not on top.

The secondary functions of treatment are to meet treatment goals and to deal with crises. These are the two exceptions to the principle of offering rather than imposing treatments. Meeting these functions may involve compulsion – things being done to the consumer in a non-negotiated way. Treatment goals will typically relate to issues of risk (discussed in Chapter 20) and safety (Chapter 21).

Mental health services should as much as possible be focussed on recovery goals. The aim of treatment is to foster the development of self-management skills, not to fix the problem. This orientation is based on an assumption that the person has, or will have, capacity to take responsibility for their life. Clinical work starts with supporting the person to work towards their goals, through the development of self-management skills.

Supporting self-management

The primary clinical job is to support the development of self-management skills. A definition of self-management is that it involves[56]:

> The systematic provision of education and supportive interventions by health care staff to increase patients' skills and confidence in managing their health problems, including regular assessment of progress and problems, goal setting, and problem-solving support

(p. 27)

A consumer definition would also emphasise the importance of empowerment, hope, exposure to role models, and working towards personally valued recovery goals. Taking personal responsibility for transforming from an identity as a person with a mental illness to a person in recovery is repeatedly identified in consumer narratives as a necessary step in the recovery journey[120;123;495]. For example[116]:'Recovery is not a gift from doctors but the responsibility of us all . . . We must become confident in our own abilities to change our lives; we must give up being reliant on others doing everything for us.' Taking personal responsibility reduces the experience of victimhood, and increases the person's experience of empowerment[320;332]. It also creates the possibility of success, surprise and transformation – *First you leap, then you grow wings*' is the motto of the Yale Program for Recovery and Community Health (www.yale.edu/prch).

Two implications arise from this perspective. First, it provides an insight into why some people might be reluctant to give up the role of patient – taking responsibility for one's own life can be scary. Second, it shows that (just like recovery itself) responsibility is something that is taken by the person, not given to the person. Mental health services can only work in ways which support an individual to take personal responsibility for their life – they cannot give responsibility to someone who is unwilling to take it. Yet self-management is a goal worth striving for. There is robust evidence of the benefits of self-management approaches in mental illness[496], including depression[497], anxiety[498] and psychosis[499].

Supporting self-management is a central clinical contribution to recovery. Services need to be engineered towards this goal. For example, role expectations are set from initial contact with a service. If the first contact involves an expert assessing someone in the context of a detached relationship, this sets a trajectory of passivity and responsibility for change being taken by the clinician. Similarly, if the environment is unpleasant or the welcome is unfriendly, this creates a negative impression which is difficult to change. This message is well understood by the customer service industry, which emphasises the central importance of the customer having a positive experience during so-called moments of truth – those few interactions where customers have a high level of emotional energy invested in the outcome. Many recovery-focussed services pay particular attention to how people are welcomed. Simple expedients such as a pleasant rather than oppressive welcoming environment are important. The Yale PRCH is based in a space which contains art exhibits, creating a very different environment for both visitors and workers. Displaying stories of recovery rather than medication information in the waiting room creates different expectations. Providing fresh fruit and drinks costs little, and communicates a message of respect. The first personal contact is also important. Club-houses hire greeters to welcome new members[500]. The Living Room service uses a peer-led triage service, so the first contact of someone in crisis is with a peer rather than a professional worker (see Case study 14).

To understand how self-management can be supported, we need to disaggregate the concept of self-management into agency beliefs, empowerment (behaviours arising from agency), goal-setting and motivation to change.

Supporting the development of agency

A necessary requirement for self-management is a sense of agency: a self-belief that the person can impact on their own life. It can be a difficult process precisely because mental illness often takes away agency, as described by the person with schizophrenia who said all she could do to improve her situation was 'just take my medicine and pray'[501]. Asking someone to take responsibility for their lives before they have that capacity will not benefit the person. This is not making the case for low expectations – people do often rise to the challenge. It is making the case for support which fits the person's stage of recovery.

Developing a sense of agency can be a painful process for the consumer, often starting with accepting that they have an illness or in other ways finding a direct meaning that fits. This acceptance can involve changes to how the person thinks about and understands challenges in life[118]. Because it can be a painful process, consumers may take time to come to the point of doing that work. The resulting avoidance often expresses itself as a wish to be rescued, fixed, made better – for someone else to take responsibility. Consumers at this point in their recovery cannot identify goals, never overtly disagree with their clinician, and are emotionally, and sometimes physically, disengaged.

Unfortunately this behaviour pattern can create a toxic cocktail with clinical responses. When viewed through a clinical lens, it is easy to pathologise the avoidant behaviour as a personality trait or illness symptom. Responses which potentially decrease agency include focussing on compliance; imposing rather than offering treatments; responding to disagreement with compulsion rather than validation; communicating that the clinician knows the solution to the person's difficulties; and trying to fix the person. These responses get in the way of recovery.

One way of avoiding these responses is through self-awareness by the clinician. Professional training does not sufficiently emphasise the fostering of self-management skills, but clinicians normally have substantial expertise to draw on – from their own life. Awareness of personal experiences of a path being walked in life suddenly coming to an end can foster consciousness about how difficult the ensuing processes can be.

Although the development of a sense of agency by the consumer can be a painful process, it also leads to the paradox of recovery: 'in accepting what we cannot do, we begin to discover who we can be and what we can do'[119]. Over time, these limitations become 'the ground from which spring our own unique possibilities'[502]. If the person currently has a minimal or absent sense of agency, then the development of agency is the goal.

Clinicians can do many things to increase agency: foster hope; identify strengths and dreams; support goal-striving; set the person up to experience achievement; encourage them to give back to others; create opportunities to access mutual self-help groups; employ peer support workers; give voice to role models of success; support access to experiences of pleasure; amplify personal success; and aid the integration of positive experiences into personal identity.

Even if the consumer has some sense of being able to impact on their life, they need to be able to act on this. So we turn to empowerment.

Supporting the development of empowerment

Empowerment behaviours emerge from agency beliefs. Although much of the literature on empowerment stems from a Western (especially USA) individualistic perspective, we will use empowerment here in its broader sense of behaviours which impact on one's life, whether or not this is at the level of personal identity or other levels, such as spiritual empowerment or social identity.

There are some structural approaches to increasing empowerment. Within services, this can include getting the complaints procedure in place and working, having the option to change clinician, having advance directives in place and routinely used, offering easily accessible WRAP training, and supporting access to self-management resources (e.g. www.glasgowsteps.com). Since the consumer movement is self-advocacy in action, exposure to peers and other consumers who can model empowerment and demonstrate experience in self-managing can be profound experiences.

Graham Thornicroft identifies strategies to promote empowerment[56]:

1. Ensuring full participation in formulating care plans and crisis plans[503]
2. Providing access to cognitive behavioural therapy to address negative self-stigma[504]
3. Creating user-led and user-run services[500]
4. Developing peer support worker roles in mental health services[505]
5. Advocating for employers to give positive credit for experience of mental illness[506]
6. Supporting user-led evaluation of treatments and services[507].

At the individual clinician–consumer level, empowerment requires skills in self-advocacy: the ability to stick up for yourself. Therefore assertiveness is necessary. Clinicians can support assertiveness by teaching the DESC script – Describe the problem, Explain how it makes you feel, provide a Solution and state the Consequence of the solution[508]. But supporting empowerment involves more than skills training. For example, where a previously passive patient begins to assert their views and priorities, this changes the relationship dynamic: 'When I see a different psychiatrist every time, it makes me feel irritated that I have to tell my story from the start again. I would prefer to see the same person, so that I can build up a trusting relationship with them over time'. The response to this assertion attempt will enhance or hinder the person's efforts towards empowerment. There may be lessons to learn from other areas of life. For example, in education disagreement is valued as integral to learning, and validating approaches have been developed for managing student–teacher differences (see Case study 17). Also, an individual's efforts to self-manage may lead them to try non-mental-health types of help, such as spiritual support or a cultural ceremony. Clinicians need to support rather than pathologise this development.

How can staff practise fostering rather than impeding empowerment? A team-level approach is to allocate a recovery hat to an individual in each clinical team meeting. That person's role is then to be an advocate for patients being discussed, with input focussed on how services are supporting the individual's recovery. It is helpful to rotate the role because: (a) otherwise the person who volunteers is likely to be the in-team recovery champion and their views can be easily marginalised; (b) this ensures everyone practises a recovery perspective, and so it has a cross-team impact; (c) it holds clinicians back from being too negative about the recovery perspective if they will be the person putting it at the next meeting; and (d) it becomes owned by the whole team. This gives clinicians a chance to practise responding to assertion in a validating rather than disempowering way, and links with the discussion in Chapter 16 about understanding the behaviours of patients as attempts to cope with their problems, rather than through a lens of pathology. This approach of reframing behaviours as coping attempts carries over into interventions to support empowerment. COPE is a widely used scale to assess coping behaviours[509], and its sub-scales are shown in Table 18.1.

What can we learn from research using COPE and other measures of coping in relation to recovery? Three clinically relevant findings emerge from research in the UK[510] and USA[511]. First, individuals in recovery often undertake community-based activities, especially in impersonal public settings such as shopping centres and fast-food restaurants which are characterised by brief (and perhaps superficial) social interactions. This points to a clinical focus on supporting the person to remain connected into their community, discussed further in Chapter 23. Second, a focus on spirituality is common. This can range from occasional meditation or prayer, through attending uplifting religious or secular

Table 18.1 Coping mechanisms and associated behaviours

COPE sub-scale	Behaviour
1. Active coping	Taking action or exerting efforts to remove or circumvent the stressor
2. Planning	Thinking about how to confront the stressor, planning one's active coping efforts
3. Seeking instrumental social support	Seeking assistance, information or advice about what to do
4. Seeking emotional social support	Getting sympathy or emotional support from someone
5. Suppression of competing activities	Suppressing attention to other activities to concentrate on dealing with the stressor
6. Religion	Increased engagement in religious activities
7. Positive reinterpretation and growth	Making the best of the situation by growing from it or viewing it more favourably
8. Restraint coping	Coping passively by holding back one's coping attempts until they can be of use
9. Resignation or acceptance	Accepting the fact that the stressful event has occurred and is real
10. Focus on and venting of emotions	Awareness of one's emotional distress, a tendency to ventilate those feelings
11. Denial	An attempt to reject the reality of the stressful event
12. Mental disengagement	Disengagement from the interfered-with goal, e.g. daydreaming, sleep, self-distraction
13. Behavioural disengagement	Giving up, or withdrawing effort from, efforts to attain the interfered-with goal
14. Alcohol/drug use	Using alcohol and other drugs as a way of disengaging from the stressor
15. Humour	Making jokes about the stressor

activities or an active sense of connection with a Higher Being, to the impressive level of adaptation of one man who founded and led a congregation following the tenets of a religion he created[409]. A spiritual perspective specifically fosters separation of the mental illness from the person, and strategies to support this approach were identified in Chapter 10. Third, linguistic strategies are common. One informant who characterised himself as withdrawn stated that 'I would rather stay home ... one has to find satisfaction in oneself ... before, I was always after people to get something'[128]. The term 'withdrawn' is thus re-framed as intentional and beneficial. This indicates the need to pay close attention to language.

In a recovery-focussed service, there is an orientation towards viewing resistance to change as reasonable, understandable and normal. This leads to a helpful response to people who seem to refuse to take responsibility for themselves, and carry on with apparently damaging behaviours. The traditional clinical approach has been to view the person as the problem. The fundamental shift in a recovery perspective is to see the person as part of the solution. A recovery-focussed approach assumes the person has capacity to take responsibility for their life. The question then moves away from how the clinician can stop the damaging behaviour, and becomes how to support the person to get to a point where they want to stop. The WIIFM Principle motivates the behaviour of most people – What's In It For Me? The challenge is to identify what personally valued recovery goal is being undermined by the behaviour. If this proves impossible, then the behaviour (such as disengaging from services which are not targeting the individual's goals) may be entirely rational and nothing to do with illness.

So there are many challenges to working in an empowering way, but again this is a goal worth striving for. Services which promote empowerment by working respectfully and with high consumer involvement in decision-making produce better recovery outcomes[395].

The next two steps that arise for an agency-experiencing and empowered consumer are then the identifying of personally valued recovery goals, and initiating movement towards these goals. We discussed how to identify recovery goals in Chapter 17. The only further point to note here is that the development of agency and empowerment do not always precede goal-setting – sometimes the person tries something they don't believe they can attain, and when successful experiences increased mastery and competence.

We turn now to how professionals can support work towards recovery goals.

Supporting the development of motivation

The approach of motivational interviewing addresses how to initiate movement towards recovery goals[512]. Motivational interviewing is a person-centred approach to supporting changes in behaviour through the exploration and resolution of ambivalence, and is oriented towards collaboration, evocation and autonomy. It is based on the trans-theoretical model of change, which distinguishes between precontemplative, contemplative, action and maintenance phases of change[513]. This a relevant distinction in mental health services, because of how common it is for precontemplative and contemplative people to be assumed to be in the action phase. The patient who does not take medication is prescribed an injectable depot to enhance compliance. The patient with abnormal sleep patterns is told to attend a morning activity. The patient who shows problem drinking is put through a detox programme. Treating (literally) a person who is not ready to change as if they are has two toxic consequences. First, it means the action is clinician-centred rather than person-centred, and may not be the type of action the person themselves will ultimately find beneficial. Second, it means that the mental health service and the person are pulling in opposite directions, with the service focussing on compliance, and the patient disengaging, becoming resentful or angry or giving up and exhibiting passivity and dependence. Motivational interviewing offers a more person-centred approach, using techniques for eliciting and amplifying motivation to change such as:

- Ensure person-centredness by using reflective listening to test the hypothesis about what is heard against what is meant: 'It sounds like you . . .', 'You're feeling . . .', 'So you . . .'
- Focus on *why* the person might want to change, not *how* they will change.
- Focus on pro-change motivations: 'Think of your recovery goal. Rate readiness to change behaviour towards the goal on a scale from 1 (not ready) to 10 (fully ready). Why wasn't your rating lower?'
- Undershooting (e.g. 'So your cutting doesn't cause any problems at all for you?')
- Overshooting (e.g. 'So it seems like there's no chance whatsoever you'll be able to meet your goal?')
- Questioning to increase motivation – 'What makes you think you can do it?', 'If you succeed, how will things be different?', 'What were you like before the problem emerged?', 'What worries you about this situation?', 'What's the worst that could happen if you don't make a change?'
- Explore values – 'What are the most important things in your life?'. Note behaviour–value contradictions.

In terms of the clinician–consumer relationships outlined in Chapter 13, motivational interviewing where trust is present promotes a partnership relationship rather than a detached relationship. Recovery is supported where the consumer experiences the resulting treatment as person-centred, enhancing of natural supports, strengths-based and community-focussed[404].

Motivation is created through agency and empowerment and goal-striving, but it is sustained through success. This points to the need to create new rituals in the mental health system. A focus on degradation ceremonies in which a diagnosis is awarded (often many times, as the diagnosis changes) and reinforced through deficit-focussed discourse at out-patient appointments does not support personal recovery. There is a need to create celebration rituals. The next case study shows how one service seeks to make success highly visible.

Case study 12: the Golden Ducky award

At the MHA Village, a high value is put on noticing and celebrating success. This is at its most public in its annual high-profile Golden Ducky awards ceremony. The ceremony involves as much fanfare as possible – organisations are approached to sponsor limousines, red carpets and other accoutrements of awards ceremonies. Attenders dress to impress, with clothing and manicures provided where needed by the Village.

Over 750 members, graduates, staff and other guests receive 100 Golden Ducky awards. The award is based on a video shown to all members, featuring the Sesame Street character Ernie who wants to learn to play the saxophone, but has to learn that he first has to put down his rubber ducky. The need to let go of the mental illness identity is at the heart of the evening, which involves public celebration of achievements by people in the Village 'family' and community heroes from outside who have worked towards this goal.

Awards include:

- Financial Independence – for development of skills in budgeting and money management
- Educational – for completing a formal educational course
- Employment – for maintaining a community employment role for more than 10 months
- Family Booster – for re-connecting with a family, or making a financial, emotional or practical difference
- Living Free – for abstinence from substances
- Independent Living – for maintaining a community apartment for more than a year
- Community Involvement – for making a positive impact on the community.

In 2008 there were 40 graduates, who received Highest Achievement graduation awards at the high-profile ceremony, which includes acceptance speeches, choirs and a reception.

Further information: www.mhavillage.org

We have argued that the basic orientation in a recovery-focussed service is towards the promotion of self-management. What does this mean for the traditional clinical imperatives of medication, risk management and compulsory treatment or hospitalisation during relapse? In the next three chapters we consider these important issues.

19 The contribution of medication to recovery

Medication and choice

In a recovery-focussed mental health service, a full range of psychotropic medication is available. However, the job of the service is not to get medication taken, whatever the cost. The job, of course, is to support personal recovery. This may or may not involve use of medication for an individual at a particular point in their life journey. So medication is one potential recovery support, among many. But prescribing of psychotropic medication is almost universal in current mental health services[208;209;213]. Using medication as a resource to promote personal recovery will require new values, beliefs and working practices.

A shift in beliefs and consequent working practices may be helped by exposure to unbiased empirical evidence about psychopharmacological effectiveness. This was reviewed in Chapter 6, which also identified that people decide not to take their medication for a wide range of reasons. For example, David Whitwell suggests the following causes for non-adherence: loss of autonomy; accepting something of which they disapprove; taking tablets to deal with mental suffering is seen as weak, stupid and superficial; viewing it as being prescribed to shut them up; link with coercion; direct side-effects, toxic effects, stigma, uncertainty about effectiveness[22].

The language of prescribing systematically understates or ignores these diverse and understandable reasons. It euphemises the harm caused by medication as 'side-effects', when these effects may be of central importance in the person's decision-making. It also assumes that normality is a desirable goal, a view that is challenged in many recovery narratives. Peter Chadwick describes the impact of medication as leading to more organised thinking but with less colour and flamboyance in life[67]. Richard McLean describes his life as 'less interesting' on medication[514]. Elyn Saks, a professor of law and psychiatry at University of Southern California, differentiates between medication which kept her alive and psychoanalysis that helped her find a life worth living[515]. Overall, automatically assuming that a decision not to take medication as prescribed is irrational, unhealthy, indicative of impaired insight and not in the person's best interest is a belief that gets in the way of supporting recovery.

New values are needed. For psychiatrists and other prescribers, an embedded current value is that the job is to prescribe – failing to prescribe would be negligent[22]. Since every diagnosis has an associated drug treatment, this need-to-prescribe becomes a permeating assumption applied to all mental health service users. This value creates the context in which a person who decides not to take their medication is labelled as lacking insight and non-compliant. This is an attributional bias, in two ways. It valorises the behaviour negatively (i.e. as a bad thing), when it may be a sign of empowerment, or of rational decision-making about costs and benefits of medication use. It also locates the cause internally to the patient, rather than considering external attributions – 'non-compliant patient' is a more common term than 'ineffective medication' or 'incorrect prescription'.

These attributional biases work against personal recovery. They create the beliefs that taking medication is always a good thing, when it is not. They foster a focus on passive rather than active compliance, by sending the message that just as it is the job of the prescriber to prescribe, it is the job of the patient to take the prescribed medication. Passive compliance is antithetical to personal responsibility.

Clinical responses based on this attributional bias also hinder recovery. Since most clinicians are altruistic people who do not want to treat patients compulsorily, a curious distortion of the more benevolent term 'choice' has occurred in relation to medication. It has sometimes been distorted to mean that patients are given choices, but only within a narrow range of predefined constraints decided by the prescriber: for example, the choice of which of two antipsychotics to take, or whether to have a marginally higher or lower dose. Another distortion is when informed choice is promoted through the use of psychological interventions (e.g. compliance therapy[516]) which use principles from motivational interviewing to improve compliance, i.e. the predefined aim is to get the patient to take the medication, rather than to aid decision-making. Another strategy is providing psychoeducation involving propagation of a biomedical model as if it is uncontested, normally involving the assertion that mental illness is caused by – and therefore necessarily treated by restoration of – neurotransmitter disturbance[239]. The development of approaches to compelling people to take treatment (the euphemism which almost always means medication) is the logical next step, with many countries considering or implementing legislation for compulsory treatment in the community, despite the clear evidence that the approach is at best inadequately researched[517] and at worst ineffective[518]. All these approaches to trying to make people take their medication get in the way of personal recovery; they disempower the patient, they take away responsibility from the individual for their own well-being and they promote passivity and dependence.

It is worth noting that there is an opposite danger. I have spoken to several prescribers who recount narratives of being personally aware of issues with over-prescribing, encouraging patients to reduce or come off medication, and then seeing them rapidly relapse with disastrous consequences. As much skill and partnership with the patient needs to be brought to a decision not to prescribe as to a decision to prescribe.

The job of the clinician is to give genuine choice and control about medication to the service user. This means that the person may decide to use medication as the prescriber recommends, or may modify the recommendations of the prescriber, or may decide not to take medication. Genuine choice is available only where any of these choices is allowable, which is why prescribing levels are a litmus test for a recovery focus[519]. The content of the individual's decision about medication is in a sense irrelevant – what matters is the extent to which the person is taking personal responsibility for their well-being.

Medication and recovery

So what does a recovery-focussed approach to medication look like? Of course, many clinicians will place great importance on medication. Their psychopharmacological expertise may be well-developed. This is an important resource to bring to the decision-making process. The change in a recovery-focussed service is that this expertise is meshed with the consumer's expertise about their own values, beliefs, goals and preferred approaches to meeting challenges. In a partnership relationship, the job of the clinician is to help the person come to the best choice *for them*. The clinician does not know what is the best choice, because they only have half the story. They do not know what is in the person's best interest (despite the common legal and social expectation of this being a core part of the professional's role). Even if medication always impacted beneficially on symptoms (which it does not), individuals vary widely in the importance they attach to symptom reduction. This is illustrated by a survey of the views of people taking psychotropic medication[268]:

> Without major tranquillisers myself and my family feel I may not have survived, as hyperactivity and starvation led to rapid weight loss as well as psychological symptoms.
>
> The drugs block out most of the damaging voices and delusions and keep my mood stable.
>
> Injections seem to dampen down the voices. They decrease the voices but not altogether, and the side effects are unpleasant.
>
> They do not cure the cause of conditions; they have the side effects of making you unnaturally doped, enormously fat.
>
> With major tranquillisers, I feel as if I'm in a trance. I don't feel like myself.

Medication may or may not be necessary for recovery – the journey of recovery involves finding out whether it has a part to play. Since medication will be a tool for many people, at points in their life, it is often important to discuss. The discussion needs to focus on what will be helpful for the individual, and in order to have that discussion the first thing that needs clarifying is the person's recovery goals. Once it is clear what the person is trying to achieve in life, then the role of medication can be discussed in a more focussed way. Some people will want to be prescribed medication, and it should be fully available. Some people will experience decisional uncertainty, and the clinical task is then to support decision-making through crystallising questions, providing unbiased information and supporting the person to plan and undertake experiments. This will involve truly shared decision-making – two experts in the room, jointly undertaking information exchange and (always) clarification of values. Decisions about medication, just like any other form of treatment, are personal not medical decisions.

How is this done? This is an area where mental health services can learn from innovative approaches to supporting the decision-making process in general medicine (e.g. www.dhmc.org/shared_decision_making.cfm, http://decisionaid.ohri.ca/odsf.html). Some of these decision-support approaches are now being evaluated in mental health services, e.g. CommonGround[520]. One such approach is to reframe medicine – in the sense of things that help you to feel better – as much more than solely pharmacological. Pat Deegan's notion of personal medicine[521] includes all the things that people do to feel better: laughter, love, hope, caffeine, exercise, chocolate, etc. In other words, medicine is what you do, not just what you take. Pill medicine (i.e. psychotropic prescribed medication) is then a sub-set of personal medicine. This approach is of course already used, such as when prescribing exercise[522], nutrition therapy[523] or bibliotherapy[524]. This has two implications. First, the prescriber is not the arbiter of the best medicine – only the consumer can judge what medicines are helpful. This is facilitated by the development of what Deegan calls power statements which reflect the person's goals for using psychiatric medication[525]:

> For example, a husband developed the following power statement to share with his psychiatrist:
>
> My marriage is powerful personal medicine, and is the most important thing in my life. I don't want paranoia or sexual side effects from medication to stress my marriage. You and I have to find a medication that supports me in my marriage so that my marriage can support my recovery.

> Notice how the power statement contextualizes the use of medication within the overarching goal for recovery. Also, notice how the power statement acts as an invitation to collaboration and shared decision-making between the prescriber and the client.
>
> (p. 67)

Second, it highlights that finding the balance between pill medicine and other forms of personal medicine is central. If the most important medicine *to the individual* is pill medicine, then a focus on medication is appropriate. If, by contrast, the most important medicine (i.e. what gets and keeps the person well) is some other form of personal medicine, then a focus on psychopharmacology will hinder recovery. The medication trap occurs where the focus on pill medicine inadvertently undermines the person's efforts to find their own personal medicine. Finding a balance between personal medicine and pill medicine is an essential ingredient of recovery.

For some people, pill medicine becomes a central issue. In a recovery-focussed service, there is an orientation towards supporting the person to take responsibility for their own lives. One implication is that people will be supported to come off medication. This of course will involve the normal approaches of giving expert information from a clinical perspective about advantages and disadvantages. It will also involve identifying alternatives – continuing with medication for a fixed period and then re-reviewing, identifying early warning signs and joint crisis plans before stopping, graded withdrawal, etc. However, it will also involve giving primacy to the individual's wishes, by validating their decision even where it differs from the prescriber's view. The work then is to support the person to plan ahead, and to identify alternative sources of support. This requires a partnership relationship, in which taking responsibility for one's life is viewed as more important than taking prescribed medication. Both prescribers and consumers will benefit from exposure to the resources which are becoming available to support people who want to come off their psychiatric medication, including web-sites (e.g. www.comingoff.com), booklets published by voluntary sector groups[526;527] and books[528–530].

A recovery-promoting approach is thus to view medication as an 'exchangeable protection against relapse'[531], in which pharmacological and psychosocial approaches both buffer the individual against relapse. For example, framing medication as a potential tool for sustaining well-being creates a very different dialogue[351]. The advantage of this view is that it creates a focus on promoting resilience (which definitely matters) rather than on medication (which may or may not matter). Resilience can be supported by working with the consumer to identify answers to the statements 'I have . . .' (external supports of people and resources), 'I am . . .' (inner personal strengths) and 'I can . . .' (social and interpersonal skills)[292]. (See www.resilnet.uiuc.edu for more on resilience.) Medication is thus one potential external support, alongside a whole range of other types of resilience-promoting supports, skills and strengths.

Chapter 20

The contribution of risk-taking to recovery

An important clinical issue raised by a shift towards individuals having responsibility for, and control over, their own lives is risk. What if the person chooses to do things which are a danger to themselves, and hence create anxiety in the clinician? At present, the tension is often resolved by reducing clinical anxiety, as noted by Glenn Roberts:

> Deegan's rallying call that 'professionals must embrace the concept of the dignity of risk, and the right to failure if they are to be supportive of us'[474] seems completely at odds with the risk-averse climate in which we live and work, where, for instance, patients may have to be medically vetted before an occupational therapist can take them for a cycle ride.[466]

(p. 28)

As well as risk of harm to self, there is a high expectation on mental health services that they will manage risk to other people. Clinical language has evolved to support this demand. Concepts such as *medical responsibility*, *clinical responsibility*, *best interests* and *under the care of* all support the belief that it is possible for mental health services to be responsible for the lives of others. The personal and professional consequences of tragedies on clinicians are also highly aversive, such as being questioned in the coroner's court to identify whether everything that could be done was done (who can really meet that threshold?) to save someone's life, or being pilloried for poor practice in the media or by public enquiries following a high-profile homicide.

This political and professional reality influences the mental health system towards risk avoidance. Does this matter?

Two types of risk

A focus on risk avoidance matters because people need to take risks to grow, develop and change. In everyday language, taking risks is a necessary part of being human. The conflation of these two uses of the term risk – something necessary and something to avoid – is unhelpful. In a recovery-focussed service, there is a clear separation of the two meanings.

Harmful risk relates to behaviours which are illegal or not socially sanctioned. Into these categories fall homicidal and suicidal acts, anti-social and criminal behaviour (such as assault, aggressive begging and theft), personal irresponsibility (such as out-of-character promiscuity or financial profligacy), self-harming patterns of behaviour (such as violent partner choice or self-neglect) and relapse of mental illness. (Note that in Chapter 2 we discussed the potential positive aspects of mental illness, but here assume that relapse of mental illness is undesirable for most people.) Harmful risk is to be avoided. Treatment goals focus on reducing harmful risk. Avoidance of harmful risk can also be part of a recovery goal, although this is avoidance for a reason: 'My marriage means such a lot to me that I want to avoid threatening it through sexually disinhibited behaviour when I am unwell'.

Positive risk-taking relates to behaviours which involve the person taking on challenges leading to personal growth and development. This includes developing new interests, trying something you're not sure you can achieve, deciding to act differently in a relationship, and developing and consolidating a positive identity. There is nearly always benefit from this – even if it all goes wrong, the learning is valuable. Resilience is developed through trying and failing – whether it be the common things like dating, employment, sex and religion, or the idiosyncratic things like singing, archery, political activism or dress, we all learn from mistakes. People with mental illness are (of course!) no different. Positive risk-taking – risk for a reason – will be needed to meet many recovery goals.

Recovery-focussed services are mindful of several issues in relation to risk. First, this is a political as well as scientific domain. A recent review concluded that the lifetime prevalence of violent behaviour (defined as use of a weapon such as a knife or gun in a fight and engaging in more than one fight that came to blows) is 16% in people with severe mental illness, compared with a population prevalence level of 7%[532]. The low base rate of severe mental illness means the attributable risk is only 3–5%. The same study concluded that the lifetime prevalence of violent behaviour among people who abuse drugs or alcohol is 35%, and in those with comorbid mental illness and substance abuse is 44%. There are also risk factors for injury which have much higher base rates, such as driving with two or more passengers (Odds Ratio 2.2, 95%CI 1.3–3.8) or using a mobile phone whilst driving (OR 4.1, 95%CI 2.2–7.7)[533]. Singling out people with mental illness for special risk management attention is not the actuarial place to start, but the logical places – such as pubs and the school run – are not politically acceptable targets. Risk management in mental health services is discriminatory.

Second, disinterested scientific enquiry is difficult in this domain. The part of the academic system which is most focussed on the issue – forensic mental health – has (as a statement of fact rather than as a judgement) a vested interest in finding higher levels of harmful risk to others. Research from this perspective inevitably amplifies the link. This is not because of fraud, but because researchers tend to find more of what they are looking for than what they are not looking for. Studies by geneticists amplify the extent of genetic influences on behaviour. Research by psychologists amplifies the impact of intrapsychic influences, etc. Coupled with biased media portrayals[534;535], this can create a highly distorted picture. Unfortunately, some professionals reinforce this distortion: the person dubbed by the *Washington Post* as 'the most famous psychiatrist in America' writes that[536]: 'the typical citizen is well aware that untreated mentally-ill individuals can be dangerous, whether professionals want to speak about it or not. All he need do is open his morning paper.' The belief that schizophrenia is a chronic deteriorating condition was only challenged when individuals and more recently research studies began appearing which provided a weight of evidence that recovery is possible. There is no equivalent expert group with a vested interest in finding lower levels of harmful risk to others, who could provide an academic counter-balance to this tendency towards amplifying the link. Consumer-led research may be one future correcting influence[537].

Third, the goal of eliminating harmful risk is both an illusion and damaging. It is an illusion stemming from the technical rationality and Apollonian views of the world outlined in Chapter 4. The underpinning assumption is that if we had the right risk assessment and management technologies, and the right clinical guidelines and rules, we could stop tragedies from happening. In fact, the only definitive trial ($n=1445$) of schizophrenia treatment examining community violence as an outcome showed very modest results: under intention-to-treat analysis violence across all treatment groups declined from 19% to 14%, but no difference by medication was found[538]. Because risk cannot in fact be eliminated, the danger is that the endless quest to manage risk consumes an ever-greater proportion of clinical resources. Focussing on harmful risks creates the same issue as the approach of treating until well and only then getting on with life. It fosters a cycle of disengagement (because the service is focussed on what it thinks matters, rather than what the person thinks matters) and compulsory intervention (to reduce risk). Inadvertently, this can be a feature in services which aim to provide highest-quality care. Detailed assessment processes involving consideration of multiple components of risk meet the clinical need for best practice, but the message they can inadvertently send is that they are there to stop the person from doing things, rather than support the person towards a better life. Engagement with, and productive use of, mental health services is much more likely if recovery goals rather than treatment goals are given primacy.

Fourth, a clinical emphasis on risk management can be unintentionally counterproductive, by reducing skills in risk self-management. People (whether they have mental illness or not) avoid acting on harmful impulses because they have valued social roles they don't want to jeopardise, a positive identity they don't want to threaten, and the ability to recognise and self-regulate emotions and their behavioural sequelae. A focus on avoidance of harmful risk through action by clinicians creates a culture which may in fact *reduce* the extent to which people develop skills at taking responsibility for their own actions.

Fifth, any approach to risk needs to be organisationally mandated, with responsibility held by the service rather than the individual worker. Defensive practice is inevitable if consumer choice equates to clinician risk. A realistic professional concern is that, despite the rhetoric, if a tragedy happens involving a patient being seen by mental health services, the individual clinician will be blamed[466]: 'Clinicians may wonder whether, when things go wrong, the principle of risk-sharing will extend to the trust board, and it may be a wise early step to seek endorsement from senior management in developing recovery-based services where choice and risk are significant issues' (p. 33).

Finally, risk management involves power, and so is an ethical issue. Most mental health services have expertise in managing this ethical tension, but focussing on recovery will make this tension more explicit. The person who is not actively trying to do anything poses fewer ethical dilemmas than the person who is striving towards recovery goals. For example, a client at a service which was attempting to implement the Strengths Model[72] identified riding a motorbike as a personal goal. This new skill clearly had the potential for personal growth, but also raised clinical anxiety, since the client was on high-dose anti-psychotic medication and had a long history of symptoms of schizophrenia. If the service had given primacy to avoiding harmful risk, the client probably would not now be running a motorbike group for other consumers. A recovery-focussed mental health service must be prepared to experience this uncomfortable tension, which in increasingly litigious societies may be especially anxiety-provoking.

A recovery-supporting approach to risk

Taking all these issues into account, some features of a recovery-focussed approach to risk management can be identified:

- Audited and organisationally supported systems are used to assess, develop and document actions focussed on reducing harmful risk. The consumer understands that these treatment goals are necessary for the professional – it is not *necessarily* done for the consumer. The development of treatment goals is led by the professional

- Audited and organisationally supported systems are used to assess, develop and document actions involving positive risk-taking in the service of recovery goals. The professional understands that this is about the recovery goals of the consumer – it is not *necessarily* agreed with by the professional. The development of recovery goals is led by the client
- There is a greater focus on positive risk-taking than on avoiding harmful risk, because this is what develops risk self-management skills
- Actions to reduce harmful risks are as far as possible decided collaboratively with the consumer. Differences are discussed openly, and where treatment goals need to be set because of the level of risk, this is acknowledged and explained, and a consensual middle ground sought
- Clinical decisions are where possible made by multiprofessional teams rather than individual clinicians. This allows for distributed responsibility for decision-making rather than anxiety being held by an individual worker.

A balanced approach values both minimising harmful risks and maximising creation of positive learning opportunities. In terms of the tension between what the person and the clinician wants, the challenge is clear[491]:

> Providers need to learn to comfortably exist in a 'conflict zone' somewhere between unacceptable provider control and unacceptable risk by the individual and family. Objectives need to be selected with awareness of and sensitivity to this underlying dynamic. Most individuals learn and grow from taking risks and learning from both their successes and failures . . . individuals and families on the road to recovery should not be unreasonably denied the same opportunities.
>
> (p. 150)

This balance is embedded in the approach to enhancing autonomy rather than creating dependency which is described in our next case study. The aim of the Strengths Model is to help people to achieve the goals they set for themselves, by moving from a deficit-based to a strengths-based approach to care[72].

Case study 13: the Strengths Model

The Strengths Model is being implemented in the adult rehabilitation and continuing care services at St Vincent's Mental Health statutory sector services in Melbourne, Victoria. The service uses three care-planning types of document:

1. **Professional treatment plan**

    This outlines treatment goals, with a particular focus on medication, psychological treatments, early warning signs and risk – akin to a treatment plan in a traditional mental health service. It is written by the case manager, in collaboration where possible with the consumer. It incorporates the early warning signs elements from WRAP[351]. The advantages of separating treatment plans from goals are (i) it makes more explicit the clinical responsibilities of the case manager – the treatment plan is a component of care, but not the main work; and (ii) it allows a more transparent negotiation about clinical versus client priorities.

2. **Strengths assessment**

    This identifies the person's strengths and current situation – What's going on today, what can I do now, what has worked for me in the past? The assessment requires new skills in clinicians, as they learn how to move from a deficit-focussed mental state examination to skills

Case study 13: (*cont.*)

in systematically identifying strengths. Assessment includes previously ignored areas, such as spiritual well-being. The process leads to shifts in attitude, from 'mental patient' to 'struggling and engaged person'.

3. **Goal plan**

   This is led by the consumer and co-written with the case manager. It uses the individual consumer's unique journey of recovery as a springboard to identify goals, and to establish an agenda for the work with the case manager. The goals may be short-term stepping-stones (who will do what, by when) or longer-term goals – a personal vision or dream for the future. An important value is that all goals are recorded, regardless of whether they are 'realistic'. This is a value because it communicates that it is wrong for professionals to decide what is realistic. Goals set and attained by clients, who are all long-term users of the service, include riding a motorbike, going fishing, gaining a fork-lift truck licence and obtaining employment.

   Workers in the service identify the following changes arising from the change in model:

- **Expectations** – from the modest (and often impoverished, such as 'maintenance') expectations of treatment to big dreams and 'audacious' goals
- **Planning** – from the case manager driving the plan to the consumer as the director of their own life
- **Anxiety in the consumer** – taking control of their own life can be scary and initially undesirable. The intention is that this anxiety reduces with increasing self-efficacy and self-esteem
- **Anxiety in the case manager** – empowering the consumer raises anxieties about risk. The intention is that experiencing the consumer as the director of their own life reduces the case manager's anxiety, as they learn that they cannot be responsible for the person's life
- **New ways of talking** – the clinical discourse is less negative and more sophisticated, seeing the person in the round rather than through a deficits filter. The content is more developmental and community-focussed, with fewer implicit expectations of mental health care always being needed. There is less use of black humour (the euphemism for prejudicial views) – pejorative casenote descriptions such as 'WOO' (Waste Of Oxygen) are no longer tolerated
- **New ways of being** – different ways of working with the consumer are needed, which change the implicit power structures and approaches to relating, e.g. 'moving from an interrogation mode to a conversational mode'[72] (p. 119)
- **Medication** – from being a high priority for the case manager to a more negotiated part of the support package
- **Risk** – from being a central element of the (only) treatment plan to being more obviously a care manager – rather than consumer – priority
- **Service links** – from a primary focus on other mental health and social care services to a focus on mainstream community services.

   Change is sustained in several ways. For example, group supervision involves all case managers (i.e. no service managers or psychiatrists), with an expectation of attendance. The content is goal-directed, focussed on strengths and intended to inform the assessment and goal-planning processes. The facilitator is called a strengths supervisor, and their role is to support participants to make the transition from seeing deficits to seeing strengths in the client. Other change approaches include local leadership, ongoing involvement from an external expert site (see Case study 23), regular audit and formal and informal consumer feedback.

   Further information: Bridget Hamilton (Bridget.hamilton@svmh.org.au)

Risk is best addressed proactively. Lines of behaviour crossed once are more easily crossed again, and stress is more easily contained if diverted rather than allowed to grow to crisis point. From a recovery perspective, this means that harmful risks are reduced by: (i) harnessing motivation through focussing on approach rather than avoidance motivation; (ii) amplifying rather than minimising risk self-management skills, and (iii) intervening early. The development of recovery goals which involve positive risk-taking may therefore, paradoxically, reduce harmful risk. They give someone a reason not to self-harm or self-neglect or be violent. Focussing on strengths creates possibilities, rather than focussing on illness deficits, which creates a compliance and passivity context in which the anger of disenfranchisement and disempowerment are more likely.

We turn now to the sharp end of the mental health system: how to work with people in crisis.

Recovery through crisis

Language is important. The experiences that professionals might understand as relapse are referred to here as crisis. The advantage of this more neutral term is that it avoids the assumption that the experience has to be understood in illness terms. A recurrence of psychotic symptoms can follow from interpersonal conflict, work problems, loss of housing, existential or spiritual crises, decisions about medication, loss of natural supports, unhelpful behavioural responses, self-medicating with alcohol or cannabis, and many other reasons. Labelling the experience as a relapse orients clinical attention towards symptom reduction, rather than the bigger picture of the person. Labelling as a crisis has more helpful connotations, in which the experience also has potential to be a learning opportunity, or a turning point.

Compulsion

Compulsion during crisis is sometimes necessary in recovery-focussed mental health services. For someone who is unable to take personal responsibility for their lives, and consequently at risk of harming themselves or others, their views are temporarily subordinated to wider societal values. **A focus on personal recovery is not a charter to stand back and let tragedies happen because the person didn't ask for or want help.** So compulsion during crisis is acceptable, if other options have been exhausted.

The traditional service response to a person presenting in crisis has been hospitalisation. However, many people experience admission negatively[201]. For example, in the UK a survey of 343 people who had experienced an admission found 45% reported a negative effect on their mental health, compared with 27% reporting a positive effect[539]. Only 18% of respondents reported talking to staff for more than 15 minutes per day. When asked what help is needed in a crisis, only 2% of 401 UK service users identified hospital admission[540]. The situation is no different in other countries. A US survey concluded[541]:'Participants reported that [hospital] settings cause them to lose their living skills, and re-traumatise them. The lack of access to the outside world gives a sense of being a citizen and a community member.' In New Zealand, services are similarly characterised[295]: 'The main interventions in acute units are medication and containment. Many people are there under the Mental Health Act and the vast majority are on medication. Typically, there are few other treatments or services available to people' (p. 9).

Traditional acute in-patient units are particularly challenging settings for a recovery focus because:

- they are often located within institutions, with consequent organisational and professional resistance to change
- there is a historical expectation of compulsion and a subordination of the wishes of the patient to the overarching aim of risk management
- the oppressive and counter-therapeutic atmosphere of many in-patient units and the use of chemical or physical restraints to ensure safety are in themselves traumatising

- the person is removed from their context, and illness-related behaviour is prominent, leading to deindividuation and a negative bias (described in Chapter 2).

This has long-term effects – over a third of people with mental illness report avoiding mental health services because of fear of coercion[542].

On the other hand, the capacity for psychiatric rescue through the ability to make clear plans along with the authority to carry them out is a major strength of mental health services. The system is a better safety net than any currently available widespread alternative. Receiving mental health care during a crisis is better than receiving nothing, and better than being dealt with by the criminal justice system.

Whilst hospital may be a good safety net, the challenge is to make the net springy rather than saggy. Consumers report a 'lack of springiness in the net to allow me to get back on the tightrope'[143]. As Glenn Roberts put it[466]: 'Service users want rapid access to help in a crisis, but once it has resolved they do not necessarily wish to be caught up in long-term involvement and monitoring, however well intentioned' (p. 30). The key challenge is creating the springiness in the safety net. What would a recovery-focussed in-patient service then look like? An overview is provided by the New Zealand Mental Health Commission, which mapped candidate elements[295] shown in Box 21.1.

Box 21.1 Features of a recovery-focussed in-patient service

1. A safe normalising environment
An open-door policy, a home-like environment, and containing fewer than 15 people. Avoiding admission where possible: 'while general hospitals may be well located in the community, they still represent a symbolic exit from community life'[295] (p. 15).

2. Recovery values
A shift from segregation to social inclusion, from paternalism to self-determination, and from 'the dominance of medical approaches . . . to more holistic approaches' (p. 15). Crisis is not only a time of risk, but an opportunity for personal growth.

3. Egalitarian culture
Power structures are different, with more mingling between staff and patients. Talking, negotiating and self-responsibility are emphasised. Participatory approaches to decision-making dominate, rather than authoritative approaches to control.

4. A well-matched mix of people
The service is responsive to the cultural and developmental needs of the individual. This means recognising, for example, that a unit catering predominantly for the needs of a group of older adults with chronic mental illness may *in itself* be traumatising for a young person experiencing a first episode of psychosis[125]. A wide range of accessible staff from health and other backgrounds (e.g. peer support workers, chaplains)

5. A broad range of competencies
Both pharmacological and psychosocial expertise are available to all in-patients. A focus remains on encouraging and amplifying self-directedness and self-advocacy, rather than 'being compelled into dependency and compliance or resorting to rebellion' (p. 16).

6. A broad range of interventions
Available forms of support include medication, complementary treatments such as homeopathy, physical treatments such as massage, self-help approaches and psychosocial approaches such as counselling, practical assistance, peer support or therapeutic communities.

The orientation in recovery-focussed mental health services is towards avoiding unnecessary crises and responding helpfully to crises when they do occur. What does this involve? A recovery-focussed approach to crisis has four aims:

(i)   to prevent unnecessary crises;

(ii) to minimise the loss of personal responsibility during crisis;

(iii) to maintain hope during crisis;

(iv) to support identity in and beyond the crisis.

We now consider each aim.

Preventing unnecessary crises

The best way of reducing the likelihood of a crisis is through the development of self-management skills. These lead to agency, empowerment and the resilience to cope with set-backs. The general approach to supporting self-management skills was described in Chapter 18. An important type of self-management skill is the ability to recognise and respond to the symptoms of mental illness.

Early warning signs work supports the person experiencing psychosis to identify their relapse signature[543] – the general and idiosyncratic symptoms which occur in a specific order over a particular period, and for that individual are indicative of impending psychotic relapse. The approach aims to develop a collaborative relationship, to enhance self-management skills and to predict relapse. The fortnightly use of standardised symptom measures can predict psychotic relapse with a sensitivity of 50–79% and a specificity of 75–81%[544], and higher if more individual changes are also considered. This mirrors the finding that regular assessment using standardised measures reduces hospitalisation[545]. The challenge in relation to recovery is to undertake early warning signs work in a way which enhances the person's ability to self-right, rather than creating anxiety about, and over-vigilance for, relapse. Clinical skills are needed to communicate two things to the consumer.

First, not all of life's bumps are indicators of potential relapse. Difficult feelings like anger, hurt, suspicion and guilt can be psychologically healthy responses, and not necessarily an indicator of impending relapse. Furthermore, everyone has good and bad days – and the goal is to create a virtuous cycle by recognising strengths and achievements, rather than a vicious cycle of hyper-vigilance to prodromal symptoms. At least as much clinical effort needs to go into the promotion of self-efficacy and flourishing, orientations which equip the person with the skills to engage in life and an attitude of being able to deal with (rather than avoid) adversity. This is like the difference between learning to stand still so as to avoid falling over, and learning how to get up after a fall. Life is a lot more fun when movement is possible!

Second, relapse, in the sense of going backwards, is normal. People struggling to break free from previous behaviour or emotional patterns experience set-backs. It may be helpful to communicate that most abstinent smokers have made 12–14 previous quit attempts[546], or that most millionaires have experienced bankruptcy or near-bankruptcy 3.2 times[547]. Set-backs are normal and necessary in life – they are a sign of health, not illness. The response to these set-backs is the critical factor. It is to the role of mental health services during this part of a person's life that we now turn.

Minimising the loss of personal responsibility during crisis

The orientation in a recovery-focussed service is towards making as few decisions for the person as possible. Services and treatment processes are geared towards minimising the impact of the crisis on hope and the consumer's ability to take responsibility in the future.

This is done by keeping the process of decision-making as close to the person as possible. Ideally, people make their own decisions. Where they have temporarily lost this ability, their previously elicited views are used, or proxy decision-makers make decisions on their behalf. Only where these avenues are not available can it be justified for a clinician to make decisions in the person's best interests.

A key approach to reducing loss of autonomy is therefore the use of advance directives. These allow people to express in advance their preferences for what they want to happen during a future crisis. They are designed for people with psychiatric or other disabilities who anticipate periods of decisional incapacity associated with symptom exacerbation. They can take many forms[548], but broadly fall into two categories: advance instructions including statements of acceptance or rejection of certain treatments, and identification of a proxy decision-maker to make decisions on the person's behalf[549]. The legal standing of advance directives varies by country, but for example in the USA there is related legislation in most states[550], and developing interest in New Zealand (www.mhc.govt.nz). In England and Wales, the Mental Capacity Act (2005) requires consideration of 'the person's past and present wishes and feelings (and, in particular, any relevant written statement made by him when he had capacity)'.

Advance directives reduce rates of compulsory hospitalisation[503], and are popular with consumers[551;552]. Although only between 4% and 13% of individuals in a large ($n=1000$) US study had an advance directive, between 70% and 83% were interested in one if they had support[553]. Advance directives offer many pro-recovery features, including self-direction, empowerment, strengths-based assessment and promoting respect for the individual's wishes[554]: 'You know what the doctor said to me? [He said] "You've got rights and it's great that you know you have them . . . Now you know your rights and we'll try to respect those completely"' (p. 72). Greater use of peer-led interventions to support individuals to complete and use advance directives has been suggested[554], building on evaluations of peer-led approaches in New York[552] and Washington[555].

Clinicians hold mixed views about advance directives. Identified barriers include the intrinsic complexity (e.g. legal language, finding witnesses, filing with providers) and the systemic barriers impacting on provider access to the advance directive when the person presents in crisis[554;556]. They also note (and perhaps this is the real issue) the ethical dilemma of being asked to follow the advance directive if they do not perceive this as in the person's best interest[557;558]. In a recovery-focussed mental health service, advance directives are not something that get in the way of providing good-quality crisis care. They are routinely developed and acted on precisely because **advance directives give the information the clinician needs to do their job – which is keeping the person and their values centre-stage during crisis.**

Advance directives are what makes a partnership relationship possible during crisis. Therefore they need to be a joint undertaking, in which the consumer educates the clinician about their preferences, and the clinician provides empirical, ethical and procedural information to inform the consumer's decision-making. If there is disagreement between the clinician and patient perspectives, then it is clearly better discussed in advance than when in crisis.

Other approaches to reducing the likelihood of disempowerment during crisis include shared care agreements[559] and patient-held records[560]. What these approaches all have in common is that there is randomised controlled trial evidence to support their use, and they all orient the individual towards taking responsibility for their own lives and what happens to them in crisis.

A central challenge for mental health services is recognising when treatment is helping and when it is hindering. In a crisis situation, the job of services may be to hold people up (in the supportive sense). During the rest of the person's life, the job of services is to avoid holding people up (in the constraining sense). This balance involves constantly maximising self-determination. A key element of self-determination is the ability to state preferences and for those choices to be honoured by mental health services in times of crisis or hospitalisation[561]. An explicit focus on self-determination is important[333]: 'Because it is the individual with the psychiatric disability who recovers, it is this person who must direct his or her own goals by identifying a life path and determining desired steps to take along that path, choosing from various options and designing a unique life journey' (p. 11).

Once the person is in crisis, how can services respond in a way which minimises loss of autonomy? A change is needed in relation to the construct of capacity. Like other apparently binary concepts such as insight and compliance, it is often used as if it is unidimensional and discontinuous. A more nuanced view of capacity as multidimensional and continuous has the advantage of pointing to a goal of maximising what the person can decide for themselves during crisis. Being involved in apparently small day-to-day decisions can provide a way of sustaining the personal responsibility muscle during crisis. There are many domains in which even people who are compulsorily detained and treated can take responsibility, such as food, activities, personal hygiene, keeping their bedroom clean and tidy, etc. This is of course difficult for people in crisis – which is exactly where skilled professionals can be a great support, when they are oriented away from a doing-to style of working and towards doing things with the person and supporting the person to do things for themselves. Reinforcing success, e.g. through praise for getting up when this is a struggle, is an important intervention.

If, as we have argued, hope is vital for recovery, how can hope be maintained when in crisis?

Maintaining hope during crisis

We noted in Chapter 3 that hope is a problem for mental health services. Maintaining hope in a crisis is even more difficult, because the clinician's illusion makes it difficult to see crisis as an exception rather than the norm[323]. For clinicians who work only with people in crisis, this illusion expresses itself in two ways:

(a) If the clinician only sees people with a diagnosis of schizophrenia when they are in crisis, then the available evidence will suggest that schizophrenia is always associated with high levels of distressing, disabling and unmanageable symptoms. This provides a context in which symptom-oriented rather than person-centred treatment flourishes. Addressing this aspect involves exposing the clinician to people with a diagnosis of schizophrenia who are not in crisis, either by bringing role models into the crisis setting or taking the clinician out (e.g. by rotating between crisis and community work settings)

(b) If the clinician only sees an individual during crisis, then it is difficult not to form a view that this is how they are all the time, leading to therapeutic pessimism, and a decontextualised understanding of the person which underestimates their strengths and normal self-management skills. In Chapter 16 we identified time-lines as one approach to putting the crisis into a temporal context. Another approach is for clinicians to work with an individual both during crisis and during the rest of their life, rather than having separate crisis teams (see Case study 25).

A key resource is the experience of peers, and a peer-run residential crisis service is described in the next case study.

Case study 14: the Living Room

Since 1996 Recovery Innovations has run one of the two crisis centres in Phoenix, Arizona (population over 3 million). The service has two components – a relatively traditional locked sub-acute unit with eight beds, and a sub-acute eight-bed alternative called the Living Room. More than 500 people per month come to the centre, either voluntarily or brought by others (including 14% by the police). On arrival, they are met by a peer triage worker, so their first contact is with someone who has lived experience of mental illness. This creates a positive initial experience, which is especially important since this is the first contact with mental health services for 40% of attenders. The focus in the peer triage is on the individual's needs, and the peer may share some of their own story. The goal is to communicate a 'chronic message of hope'. The peer may then act as an advocate in the subsequent psychiatric assessment.

Following this process, the person may be discharged, admitted compulsorily to the locked unit, or admitted voluntarily to the Living Room. Only 6% of people brought by the police require compulsory admission. Criteria for staying in the Living Room include being able to take some responsibility for oneself, but guests often include people brought to the centre in handcuffs by the police.

The Living Room is staffed by three shifts of two peer support crisis specialists. They influence the environment, which is intended to be supportive to those in crisis – guests have full access to things such as food, drinks, television and videos, and plants and other decorations reduce the clinical feel of the service. Guests stay an average of two or three days, during which time they are left alone if wanted, and offered the chance to develop a recovery plan with the peer, or attend any of the daily groups. These optional groups are facilitated by peers and counsellors, and cover both recovery topics (e.g. goal-setting, low mood) and social activities. Given the proximity to Las Vegas, it may be no surprise that one group is a poker tournament. All groups take place with participants from the adjacent locked unit, and guests find themselves acting as peers for the locked unit in-patients – a beneficial opportunity to give something back and experience being valued. Mental health professionals provide input in the Living Room as needed, but none is based in the unit. Each guest is evaluated by a psychiatrist or nurse practitioner daily, and a treatment plan is developed by a counsellor or social worker.

A challenge has been how to respond when peer workers become unwell. The evolved practice is that they are, if wanted, admitted to the Living Room. The basis for this judgement is that in a recovery environment, everything is transparent – what is said to the person is consistent with what is recorded in notes.

A second challenge has been moving to non-use of force. Only two restraints or seclusions have ever been needed, and fewer than 1% of people are chemically sedated. One means of achieving this has been values-based, influenced by the presence of peers advocating non-coercive responses to conflict situations. A second route has been re-framing violent behaviour as a normal response to crisis – shouting, screaming and throwing things without damaging by-standers are all ways of coping with crisis, and not indicators of escalating hostility requiring intervention.

Further information: www.recoveryinnovations.org

Crisis is, though, about more than minimising the negative impact. The neglected aspect of crisis is that it can be a punctuation point in a person's life, through being a time either of acceptance or of developing a new trajectory in life. We turn now to how the positive benefits of crisis can be amplified.

Supporting identity in and through crisis

Relationships are of paramount importance during crisis[562]. Although a detached relationship may be the only type of connection possible with the person, the development of a partnership relation as soon as possible is central. How is this done? Peers can be particularly skilled at making this kind of connection, as we illustrate in our next case study of a peer-led in-patient service run by Wellink (www.wellink.org.nz) – an organisation with 35% peer employees.

Key recovery-promoting features are attention to environment, trying to keep the person in their life, and a balancing of the need for safety and the opportunity that being in crisis presents to learn from the past and to re-orient future plans.

Case study 15: Key We Way

Key We Way[a] is a four-bed peer-run residential alternative to an acute in-patient mental health unit. The service operates from a standard house overlooking a beautiful beach on Kapiti Coast, north-west of Wellington. No mental health professionals work in the service, which is instead staffed by 14 'recovery agents' – people with their own histories of using mental health services. Two recovery agents work in the home between 8 a.m. and midnight, and one from midnight to 8 a.m.

People are generally referred by the acute services co-ordinator or local Community Mental Health Team, although self-referral is also welcomed. Admission decisions are made by the local District Health Board (DHB), an arrangement which works because of the mature relationship between Wellink and the DHB.

What happens during an admission?
The average length of stay is three weeks. Residents do 'normal' healing things – walk on the beach, make things, cook, go for a drive, go on group outings, watch comedy on TV, do some gardening. The aim of the house is to be a place which is conducive to recovery. As part of this, family members are actively encouraged to visit and to stay for meals.

During their stay, the intention is that residents work actively on future-focussed plans with the recovery agents. Initially plans are focussed on short-term goals, such as staying safe. Over time, the focus shifts to the development of a **personal plan** – a creative process to facilitate the individual re-connecting with their personal dreams and aspirations. It may be written, or can be a collage, an audio recording, a mind-map, a portfolio of work, a song – anything that re-connects the person with their life. The aim is to move past a maintenance model to focus on process – the generation of hope, motivation and ultimately healing. After discharge, residents are offered an outreach programme for up to 6 weeks, which may involve further work on their personal plan.

Who does the service work with?
Key We Way works with both detained and non-detained patients. The proportion of compulsorily detained people is small, because each resident must consent to going there, and because some people consent to voluntary admission to Key We Way although they would need to be compulsorily admitted to the local statutory service. The intention is that the choice of where to be admitted rests with the person, although in reality it is normally the clinician who decides.

Key We Way seems to be most valuable for people who are having their first experience of in-patient mental health services. It provides highly visible role models of a potential positive future – 'here are people like me who are now working'. It is less suited for people who are not able to benefit from the peaceful environment (e.g. those who are loud and aggressive) or where absconding is an issue.

Case study 15: (*cont.*)

How is risk to self or others dealt with?
For each admitted resident there is initially daily contact with the clinical team, which reduces in frequency over time. All residents have a clinical risk management and care plan, developed by the statutory clinical service. Recovery agents support and supervise the taking of medication, but do not dispense. If someone refuses their medication this is reported to the clinician.

All staff are trained in conflict de-escalation. If the person's behaviour becomes unmanageable, the recovery agent will call the police (if life is threatened) or the local Crisis Assessment Team to make an emergency assessment.

How does the service compare with a professional-led in-patient unit?
There are similarities with good acute in-patient units. For example, the importance of supervision is emphasised by the recovery agents, and there is a willingness in supervision to discuss both personal and professional challenges of the role. This includes the extent to which self-disclosure is helpful – the line is drawn more towards the self-disclosing end of the spectrum than is common in professional-led services, but there is still a line. Similarly, there is an emphasis on accountability. The service is accountable to Wellink, which in turn is accountable to the commissioning DHB. This accountability is monitored by a general management structure within Wellink.

One notable difference is in terminology. For example, residents may have favourites among the staff whom they want to focus on, or may want more self-disclosure from the recovery agent than is helpful, or may evoke strong emotional responses in the recovery agent. These challenges would be framed clinically in terms of 'maintaining boundaries', but in Key We Way the challenge is framed as 'developing sustainable relationships'. In supervision this involves discussion of the same boundary issues that would feature in a statutory setting, but the implicit communication in the language is more strategic and less defensive.

A second difference is in role markers. Indicators of status (i.e. who are the recovery agents and who are the residents) are notably absent in dress, talk and behaviour. The disclosure of difficulties by the recovery agents is validated, as is the giving of support by the resident to the recovery agent. Advice is offered to residents not from a position of professional expertise, but from lived experience – 'I don't know if this will help you, but when I went through this I found it worked to. . .'.

Further information: www.wellink.org.nz

Note:
[a]The term 'Key We Way' is not a Māori word – it is a play on 'Kiwi' and also a pointer to the key being 'we'.

General strategies for supporting identity during crisis include:
- Keeping the person's normal life on the go: ensuring mail is collected, pets are fed, dependants cared for, bills paid, home secured, deliveries cancelled, etc.
- Maximising engagement from the person's support network, e.g. by abolishing visiting hours, and actively encouraging visitors and involving them in meals and other unit activities.
- Keeping life skills activated. If the person is able to cook for themselves, it is unhelpful for meals to be automatically provided. If the person enjoys reading or exercise (or any other form of personal medicine[521]), these are important to encourage.
- Reinforcing an identity as a person from the first contact, rather than starting with illness-focussed admissions procedures. Talking with the person about their life, what

they want from admission, what they hope to do after, etc. Amplifying the positive parts of the person's identity.

- Supporting the person, over time, to reflect on and make sense of their crisis. How did it arise? What is good and bad about it? What learning does it contain? What plans or goals or supports or skills will the person need in the future?
- Using time strategically. Individualising the support to the needs of the individual. This may involve giving the person space to regroup, or individual counselling to support recovery processes, or access to artistic media and therapies to allow the expression of experience. A recovery-focussed crisis service does not have a compulsory programme of activities.

The challenge is to intervene in ways which keep the person in their life, or minimise their removal from it. This may require structural change to ways services work. For example, the involvement of police in the compulsory detention of people who have committed no crime is stigmatising and, for some, shame-provoking. This point is made by a head teacher who experienced a psychotic breakdown[309]: 'Looking back I'm glad they made me accept treatment . . . but if I needed to go to hospital why did they call the police to take me and not an ambulance . . . I still can't face my neighbours' (p. 6).

In closing our discussion of crisis services, we mention two other structural aspects. First, there are several residential alternative models to traditional in-patient care[563], including short-stay crisis houses[564], Soteria or recovery houses[258], halfway hospitals[565] and peer-run in-patient services (see Case studies 13 and 14). There are also several non-residential alternatives, including day hospitals[566] and home treatment teams[567]. This last type of service involves increasing the level and type of support available to the person in a crisis through 24-hour intensive support, including medication, brief counselling, practical advice, information and other types of support for both the consumer and their informal carers. Unusually in comparison with the pattern of other service models, the findings from early evaluations[568] have been essentially replicated in later investigations[569;570]: home treatment is safe, effective, preferred by patients and suitable for up to 80% of people in crisis. What is less known is the extent to which they contribute to personal recovery. One home treatment team in New Zealand has actively embraced a recovery approach in its work[124]. People using this service identified helpful aspects: practical help; being around; being available to talk; providing advice; providing information about mental illness; and hooking up with other useful services. Recovery-promoting operating practices included availability, flexibility, treating people as individuals, the team working well together, support to the family, establishing of strong relationships with the consumer, giving hope and encouragement about recovery, going the extra mile, including consumers and family members in decisions, and dealing sensitively with issues around choice and control.

Second, since compulsion involves control, democratisation of this power and promoting community responsibility for deviance is one approach to reducing the potential for abuse of this power. This has led some commentators to call for increased involvement of non-statutory sector services in decision-making about compulsion in mental health services[26]. The extent to which this power is simply co-opted by other interest groups and whether there is sufficient community resource to take on this responsibility are questions which are amenable to evaluation.

We turn now to how to recognise, and evaluate the impact of, a recovery-focussed mental health service.

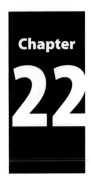

Recognising a recovery focus in mental health services

How can we recognise a recovery focus in mental health services? Which aspects of current practice should be amplified, and which discouraged? How should the effectiveness of mental health services be judged? This chapter addresses these questions.

A variety of quality indicators for a recovery-focussed mental health service are proposed in this chapter, along with an outcome evaluation strategy. These can be used as the focus of an audit cycle, especially using external[571] and user-led[186;572] approaches. Or they can be the focus of routine outcome assessment[545;573], an established healthcare technology[574]. The overall aim is to develop the culture of a learning organisation – giving the organisation the information (sometimes called practice-based evidence[575]) necessary to reflect on its performance against stated values, and the desire and empowerment to tailor behaviour towards these values.

Quality standards

There is as yet no accreditation process to identify a recovery focus in services. This is unfortunate, because it allows any service to incorporate the term recovery into its name, irrespective of its actual approach. In the future it will be of benefit when an accreditation process emerges, although this will be challenging: needing to consider staff values, engagement with community services, process issues such as hope promotion, and so forth: challenging but not impossible, as the fidelity measure for consumer-operated services[374] described in Box 12.1 showed.

Quality standards are emerging – see Case study 25. For example, the Pillars of Recovery Service Audit Tool (PoRSAT) identifies six pillars of service development: Leadership, Person-centred and empowering care, Hope-inspiring relationships, Access and inclusion, Education and Research/Evaluation[315]. The most widely used quality standards are the *Practice Guidelines for Recovery-Oriented Behavioral Health Care*, which cover eight domains[571;576]:

1. Primacy of participation
2. Promoting access and engagement
3. Ensuring continuity of care
4. Employing strengths-based assessment
5. Offering individualised recovery planning
6. Functioning as a recovery guide
7. Community mapping, development and inclusion
8. Identifying and addressing barriers to recovery.

Another approach is to investigate the consumer–clinician relationship. The Recovery-Promoting Relationships Scale is a 24-item consumer-rated measure about their experience of the relationship with their provider[577]. It includes items such as *My provider helps me recognize my strengths, My provider helps me find meaning in living with a psychiatric condition, My provider encourages me to take chances and try things, My provider sees me as a person and not just a diagnosis,* and *My provider believes in me.*

In the absence of universal quality standards, we now propose some litmus tests which indicate a focus on personal recovery.

Belief markers

Some beliefs in traditional and personal recovery-focussed services are compared in Table 22.1.

A recovery-focussed service has a balanced view about the impact of clinical models. It recognises that many consumers benefit from the traditional practices and values of mental health services. The problem is that not all consumers benefit, and some are harmed. So the orientation of the service is towards doing better over time. This creates a learning organisation culture, in which performance information is highly valued, and the twin characteristics of ambition and modesty are present.

Other beliefs become evident in behaviour. For example, if the consumer needs to 'game' to get their needs met (e.g. becoming abstinent before getting housing, or reporting no voices before being discharged), this may be because of unstated clinical assumptions that treatment needs to come before other types of help or support, or that illness-related needs should be met before meeting normal needs. The overarching behavioural marker is whether the person is treated as the professional would like to be treated. Housing provides an example. Some professionals would love to live with a group of other people from the same profession, and others would hate it. Few would be pleased if their request for housing was responded to with a requirement that they go on a course to learn to be a good tenant!

We turn now to the language of recovery.

Table 22.1 Beliefs in two types of mental health service

Belief in traditional mental health service	Belief in recovery-focussed mental health service
We already 'do' recovery	Recovery is a journey not a destination, and we are on the way, but have a long way to go
Recovery begins with recognising you have a mental illness	Recovery begins by reclaiming a sense of who you are
My job is to diagnose or formulate, then provide treatments or interventions for mental illness	My job is to support the person in their journey towards a more meaningful and enjoyable life
My primary approach to relating to consumers is as an expert	My primary approach to relating to consumers is as a coach or a mentor
I have a duty to intervene	I have some must-dos, but I employ several approaches to avoid my agendas dominating our work together
I decide when compulsory treatment is necessary	Approaches such as Advance Directives minimise the extent to which I decide when compulsion is necessary
Staff and consumers are fundamentally different – they have a mental illness, we do not	Staff and consumers are fundamentally similar – we are all trying to live a meaningful and enjoyable life
It is better not to be open if I have my own experience of mental health problems	Being open with other staff and clients about my own strengths and vulnerabilities is a positive asset

Discourse markers

There is no right way of talking about recovery. Language is constantly evolving, so any linguistic symbol (i.e. a word or phrase) attracts unintended meanings over time. For example, in New Zealand the term 'peer' is used for people who self-identify as having used mental health services, since the term 'service user' is seen by some as having negative connotations of being a ravenous consumer of resources. Similarly the term resilience is preferred to recovery by younger people, because it has fewer associations with illness.

To some extent, therefore, the language used is irrelevant. What matters is the core values, rather than the words an individual professional uses (which are influenced by profession, education, context, etc.). However, since language shapes how we see and construct the world, it is important to consider how language can encourage recovery, i.e. to use shorthands which foster rather than inhibit the recovery journey. Some general principles can be identified. For example, person-first language is helpful – talking about the person experiencing psychosis or the person with schizophrenia (or, even better, the person with a diagnosis of schizophrenia) rather than the schizophrenic or the schizophrenic patient serves to remind that diagnoses classify illnesses, not people[62]. Similarly, the avoidance of illness-saturated linguistic environments – in which the only visible part of the person is the mental illness part – is important, so language to describe strengths and aspirations is a necessary counter-balance to discourse around deficits and disabilities. In Table 22.2 some traditional clinical terms and more recovery-promoting alternatives are put forward. Because there is no single best language, the intention is not to identify right

Table 22.2 Discourse markers of a recovery-focussed mental health service

Clinical term	Problem	Potential alternative
Case management	*People are more than a case (of schizophrenia, depression etc.)*	Recovery support
Case presentation	*This creates an expectation that what needs presenting, and therefore what matters, is the illness part*	Recovery presentation
Has a diagnosis of. . .	*When used without any qualification this becomes reified – seen as a true thing instead of a professional construction*	Meets criteria for a diagnosis of. . .
Patient/ consumer/peer, etc.	*Puts the person and their experiences into a socially defined category, instead of encouraging self-definition*	Ask the person how they want to be referred to
Treatment-resistant	*Locates the reason for not benefiting as in the person AND pejorative AND normally a misleading synonym for medication-resistant*	Not benefiting from our work with him/her
The treatment aims are. . .	*Treatment should be secondary to recovery goals, rather than an end in itself*	The recovery processes being supported are. . .
Maintaining boundaries	*Has implications of a fortress mentality, and needing to defend against harm from 'the other'*	Creating sustainable relationships
Introducing as 'I am Dr Smith'	*Positions the professional as high social status and imposes a clinical frame of reference which constrains the resulting discourse*	'Please call me Sam or Dr Smith, as you prefer'
Maintenance, stabilisation	*Expecting no improvement is self-fulfilling AND pejorative*	Consolidating gains
Risk management	*Views all risks as to be avoided, so does not encourage personal growth*	Harmful risk and positive risk-taking

and wrong ways of talking. Rather, the aim is to make visible some embedded assumptions and to suggest one of many approaches to talking in ways which support recovery.

Other discourse markers which are harder to specify in concrete terms are being open to discussion of power and choice (and its limits), and having a meaningful concept in regular use of expert-by-experience.

Evaluating success

Assessing the outcome of mental health services is vital, for both external and internal reasons. Externally, the spending of tax-payers' money on mental health services rather than other demands can only be sustained long-term if there is evidence of value-for-money, and outcome evaluation provides the value data. Internally, a learning organisation requires regular feedback on its performance. How can we evaluate the impact of a mental health service in ways which promote a focus on recovery? The difficulty is summarised by Julie Repper and Rachel Perkins[4]:

> Traditional yardsticks of success – the alleviation of symptoms and discharge from services – are replaced by questions about whether people are able to do the things that give their lives meaning and purpose, irrespective of whether their problems continue and whether or not they continue to need help and support.
>
> (p. ix)

The challenge is to measure outcome in a way which is both aggregable and meaningful. Outcome data need to be aggregated across individuals in order to meet many of the information needs of modern society – at the team, service, programme, region and national planning levels. The problem from the consumer perspective with aggregation is loss of meaning (or granularity, as epidemiologists would put it). Collecting information primarily for aggregation purposes leads to a focus on quantitative rather than qualitative data and on average rather than individual ratings. Both of these features are experienced by many consumers as unhelpfully reductionist and associated with loss of individual identity.

Outcome evaluation should be based on a theoretical framework, and should measure what matters[578]. If not based on some form of theory, then it is incoherent. If not measuring what matters, then it becomes irrelevant. Having contributed to the evidence base on routine outcome assessment[545], I know very well that although these are easy statements to make, they are remarkably complex to implement[579]. Whilst noting the implementation challenges, we finish this chapter with a specific (untested) proposal for an outcome evaluation approach.

The Personal Recovery Framework outlined in Chapter 9 provides a theoretical basis for outcome assessment. It identifies two classes of outcome which matter (i.e. promote personal recovery): valued social roles which reinforce social identity, and individual goals which contribute to personal identity. Both classes of outcome have features which are relevant for outcome assessment.

Valued social roles include employee, partner, family member, friend, citizen, free (i.e. non-detained) person, etc. Their value is relatively invariant – most (but of course not all) people want a job, a relationship, contact with their family, some close friends, the ability to exercise citizenship rights such as voting, not to be held in hospital or prison, etc. Assessment tends to be quantitative and dichotomous (or at least on an ordinal scale, such as unemployed – voluntary work – part-time work – full-time work), and hence easy to aggregate with little loss of meaning. They can be measured using objective quality-of-life indicators. For example, the MHA Village uses ten observable outcome indicators:

1. Live in the most independent, least restrictive housing feasible in the local community
2. Engage in the highest level of work or productive activity appropriate to their abilities and experience
3. Create and maintain a support system consisting of friends, family and participation in community activities
4. Access an appropriate level of academic education or vocational training
5. Obtain an adequate income
6. Self-manage their illness and exert as much control as possible over both the day-to-day and long-term decisions which affect their lives
7. Access necessary physical health care and maintain the best possible physical health
8. Reduce or eliminate antisocial or criminal behaviour and thereby reduce or eliminate their contact with the criminal justice system
9. Reduce or eliminate the distress caused by their symptoms of mental illness
10. Reduce or eliminate the harmful effects of alcohol and substance abuse.

The primary advantage of this kind of outcome is that they are based on normal social values, and so avoid illness-focussed lowering of expectations (either by staff in an effort to be realistic or by patients with internalised stigmatising beliefs about what they can expect in life). Since most valued social roles occur outside the mental health system, they orient the actions of the service towards increasing integration and participation by the person into their social environment, rather than encouraging a decontextualised and service-focussed view of the person. Their primary disadvantage is their invariance – some people get along very well in life without friends, or a partner, or a job. Attempting to impose normal social roles has the potential to be oppressive. However, assessing outcome is intrinsically value-based. It is less oppressive to be concordant with a value of personhood – the person with mental illness is before all else a person[453] – than with a value of clinical imperatives being more important.

Unlike valued social roles, individual goals differ from person to person. There is simply no way around this. Any evaluation of this aspect using predefined categories necessarily loses some of that uniqueness. No standardised measure will have items such as *Swim with dolphins*, *Breed snakes*, *Ride a motorbike*, or any of the other idiosyncratic goals individuals set and attain on their recovery journey (these are all real-life examples of recovery goals). Any attempt to squeeze personal identity into predefined boxes can be justifiably criticised for its loss of meaning. This does not of course mean that personal goals should not be included in outcome evaluation – they remain central, despite the difficulties in assessing individual goal attainment. Rather, as Robert McNamara put it, 'The challenge is to make the important measurable, not the measurable important'[166].

There are developing technologies which allow for assessment of progress towards individualised goals. The most established approach is Goal Attainment Scaling, which involves the person identifying their own goals, along with markers of relative success or failure in attaining these goals[580]. The resulting data can be aggregated across individuals to give an indicator of the overall success of the service at helping people to reach personally valued goals. But the approach is time-consuming and complex. Another approach is to identify a list of standardised outcome measures covering a range of domains, and for the consumer to identify the most relevant outcome measure from the list[581]. This allows a degree of tailoring of outcome to each individual, without the complexity involved in Goal Attainment Scaling. Data can be easily aggregated, but using a predefined list of outcome measures reduces the extent to which assessment is individualised. The simplest approach is to periodically collect a dichotomous rating about whether each goal has been attained.

So an overall outcome evaluation strategy would measure two things: first, objective quality-of-life indicators, such as adequacy of housing, friendship, safety, employment, close relationships, etc.; second, progress towards personal goals. A mental health service which can show it is increasing the attainment of valued social roles and increasing the proportion of personally valued goals being met by people on its caseload is likely to be a recovery-focussed mental health service.

We have argued that recovery involves the development of valued social roles. This often involves the development of inter-dependency skills – we can't all be mechanics, but it helps to know how to access a mechanic if our car breaks down. It is to this wider world of social inclusion, or exclusion, which we now turn.

Chapter 23

Improving social inclusion

We have discussed the creation and fostering of hope, meaning and personal responsibility primarily at the level of the individual, with a particular focus on how these processes can be supported by mental health services. However, there is an interaction between hope and opportunity[4]. If no person is an island, then recovery cannot happen just within the individual. Access to and experience of valued social roles is the lifeblood of well-being for most people. And yet mental illness is associated with disconnection from these normal social experiences of community integration which are so central to supporting and buttressing the processes of recovery.

In this chapter, we argue that a focus on available resources in the environment creates more opportunity than a focus on environmental barriers. This is not to argue that if we ignore societal stigma and discrimination, the adverse impact of these factors will simply be nullified. Rather, just as we argued in Chapter 16 that an exclusive focus on the individual's deficits and dysfunction is unhelpful, it is recognising that individuals who are focussed on what they can do (the possible) rather than what they can't do (the impossible) are more likely to utilise available opportunities and to develop new opportunities.

Personal responsibility and social opportunity are the twin requirements for community integration. The individual needs to try to access the community, and the community needs to be accessible. These are not, of course, independent[330]: 'A central route to escaping this Catch-22 situation of needing to free oneself from the clutches of the illness in order to develop the capacities needed to free oneself from the clutches of the illness is for the person to reconstruct an effective sense of social agency in the midst of persistent symptoms and dysfunction' (p. 157). Social agency is the ability to view oneself as a person capable of choosing, initiating, doing and accomplishing things in the world. As described in Chapter 18, agency is central for self-management skills and for the attainment of valued social roles. The development of social agency is a key recovery process, and is difficult where the person experiences discrimination. The New Zealand blueprint for mental health services states[291]: 'One of the biggest barriers to recovery is discrimination. That is why stopping discrimination and championing respect, rights, and equality for people with mental illness is so important. It is as important as providing the best treatments or therapies' (p. 18).

To put this another way, Amartya Sen, who won the Nobel Prize for Economics in 1998, identifies the notion of substantial freedom, meaning that even where legally codified, freedom is effectively restrained when a lack of psychological, social and financial resources make it impossible to achieve goals and live a meaningful life[582]. In relation to mental health, Faith Dickerson asks some simple but important questions[583]:'How can one recover—in any sense of the term—in America in 2006 with a total monthly income of $500, or while homeless, or with no health insurance?' (p. 647). Creating pathways back into mainstream society has direct benefits for identity, self-managing the mental illness, and social role development[373]: 'The more you get out, the better you feel . . . It just opened my eyes that there are other things to think about beside mental illness . . . [that] I could go places and have fun' (p. 284).

Hopeful individuals can create opportunities. Changing environmental opportunities can engender hope. What does this person–environment interaction mean for mental health services? Comprehensive approaches to discrimination, including conceptual frameworks[86], impact[4,584] and remedial strategies[56,585], have been considered elsewhere. In this chapter we will identify the contribution of three groups who can improve social inclusion: mental health professionals, consumers and governments.

Mental health professionals can improve social inclusion

Mental health services have not always focussed on promoting non-patient roles. The sociologist Erving Goffman identified how characteristics of other total institutions (e.g. military, jails) applied in mental institutions[71], through processes such as institutional stripping – the systematic removal of identity markers from the person. The benign intent was to re-mould the individual into a more conforming or normal member of society, but this rehabilitative goal was found in practice to be outweighed for many individuals by the loss of a sense of self outside the institution. Institutionalisation leads to ex-military who can't survive in civvy street, recidivism by released convicts needing the security of prison, and mental patients for whom the hospital becomes their home.

We are now in the post-institution era of mental health, where this phenomenon is more clearly recognised. That said, there is an episodic nature to institutions – I was recently taken aback when teaching to be asked by a medical student, 'What's so bad about institutions?'. It was a reasonable question from someone who had never seen a back ward, as the warehouse wards used to be called. My first experience in the psychiatric system was doing voluntary work at school, and visiting a hospital (now closed). I walked in to see a man sitting masturbating in the day room. I was greeted by the staff, who walked me past him with a 'Never mind him – he's always doing that' comment. I was shown round, including the padded cell which contained a wild-eyed bound man, wriggling in a straitjacket. I don't need to ask the medical student's question, but new generations will.

The historical role of services in segregation, described in Chapter 7, means that the mental health system has been part of the problem. A new direction is needed if mental health services are to actively challenge the exclusion of people in the future, and instead to be part of the solution. What might this involve?

A central transition is to enlarge the focus of a clinician's role, to being about more than treating individual patients. Treatment is of course part of the job, but so too is supporting people to exercise their full citizenship rights. Overly focussing on doing things at the individual level creates ghettos of mental illness, in which special services, housing and employment for people with mental illness create a parallel mental health universe – a virtual institution[2] – in which exposure to everyday, non-mental-illness-defined experiences is almost entirely absent. To be part of the community involves exercising full rights of citizenship, and obtaining and maintaining social capital: 'people have a right to participate, as equal citizens, in all the opportunities available within the communities of their choice'[4] (p. x). It is insufficient to simply be geographically in the community in invisible ghettos of dedicated day services and accommodation. Segregation and social exclusion follow from an exclusive focus on individual treatment.

The contribution of mental health services to promoting social inclusion is not primarily about where mental health service buildings and resources are situated. Indeed, there are approaches that do not involve creating either real or virtual institutions. For example, the Fungrata Program in Bogota has no mental health centre – it works with homeless people with a mental illness by focussing on the development of natural supports and independence through work and rehabilitation[586].

Rather, the contribution of mental health services to social inclusion comes from how the service works. A central orientation of mental health services needs to be towards keeping people in their own lives, rather than transplanting them into mental health settings which inevitably reinforce an illness identity. Organising around this vision is difficult. For example, mental health services in England spend £123m per year on day services, yet a review of success in implementing a social inclusion agenda concluded that change is 'usually slow and difficult, with resistance being a common feature'[587] (p. 5). In particular, the review noted that 'User-run services appear to remain relatively uncommon, despite the prominence they are given in the commissioning guidance' (p. 4).

Keeping people in their lives does not mean casting them adrift: community integration should not mean community isolation. There is a role for specialist services, both as pathways into mainstream community activities and, for some people, as an end in themselves. The point is that the orientation needs to be towards creating a conveyor belt out of the mental health system and into a socially valued life. The implication is that workers in the mental health system 'need to move away from a perspective that considers "patients in our services" to one of serving people in their communities, enabling people to live the lives they wish to lead'[4]. This is underpinned by a fundamental re-orientation towards a view that[588]: 'the failure of a person to display competence is not due to deficits within the person but rather to the failure of the social systems to provide or create opportunities to be displayed or acquired' (p. 130). Employment provides a concrete example. It is a central part of recovery, not what happens after recovery. A key challenge is to avoid impoverished expectations[55]: 'Currently services aren't geared towards you getting access to education, training, or employment, unless you want to do the three Fs: filth, food, and filing. These are your choices, you can be a cleaner, you can be a waitress, or you can file stuff. I'm too bright for that!' (p. 10).

How do these low expectations arise? One reason is that a focus on clinical recovery involves cessation of normal expectations whilst the person gets back to normal: 'Let's think about work when you're feeling better'. This is one way in which a focus on clinical recovery can be toxic to personal recovery – it fails to recognise that work is something that for many people creates and maintains wellness, rather than something to do once well[56]: 'I always get this remark that I should take it easy, I shouldn't stress myself as if I'm a weakling, or maybe because of what has happened to me I can no longer do things that I used to do and I don't like that. I want to feel like everybody else' (p. 30).

A central insight of the recovery approach is that social agency and the attainment of valued social roles is not what happens *after* the person is better. Rather, it is for many people the vehicle of their recovery. This challenges many current practices. The person who wants to experience love is given social skills training. The person who wants a home must show they are abstinent from alcohol. The person who wants a pet must first prove they can be responsible. The person who wants to have some fun is put into a leisure group. The alternative, recovery-focussed orientation is to recognise that people learn from real experiences, and rise to real challenges. People experience love by being in social and work situations, and going on dates. People stay off alcohol because they prefer to keep their home. People rise to the challenge of looking after another being. People with mental illness have their own idea of fun, which is unlikely to be the same as everyone else's in the leisure group.

Another reason for low expectations is the chain of reasoning that work is stressful, and stress exacerbates symptoms which in people with a mental illness leads to hospitalisation, so work causes hospitalisation. Of course work is often stressful, but it has real benefits: pay, a social network (often of people with no mental illness), a non-illness role, etc. Just as a focus on deficit during assessment leads to a biased view of the person, a focus on the difficulties associated with work reduces access to the potential benefits. As ever, there is no invariant solution to this balance, other than recognising that it is a balance. For some people, being asked to meet the demands of employment is setting the person up to fail. But for many others, providing supportive pathways into real work is a central contribution to recovery. The challenge is to avoid a bias towards low expectations, by holding a values-based assumption that normal social roles such as employment should be available to all. Efforts then more easily become focussed towards making attainment of those roles possible, rather than towards encouraging realistic (i.e. low) expectations in patients.

A third reason for pessimism is reality. Whilst employment rates among the general population and among most disability groups rose in the UK between 2000 and 2005, they fell from 14% to 10% among people with moderate to severe mental illness[304]. Societal and professional pessimism about the ability of people with mental illness to work can be internalised by consumers[86]. This creates a vicious cycle, because internalised stigma prevents people from trying to obtain competitive employment[589].

Focussing on employment should not of course ignore the work-related difficulties which people with mental illness can experience due to the illness, rather than due to a negative societal response. Problems with concentration, personal organisation skills, hygiene, motivation and so forth can all be direct consequences which reduce work ability. A rehabilitation approach is important. This couples a positive expectation of success with a focus on developing relevant skills using evidence-based practices and providing support to bridge the gap between current capacity and goals. In practice, this means that individual-ised approaches to supporting the transition into work are needed, which focus on allowing the person to build up their work muscles over time.

A body of research into approaches to supporting people into employment is emerging[56]. The consistent message is that Individual Placement and Support (IPS) approaches which support the person to find and maintain mainstream employment are better than training the person in separate supported employment schemes in preparation for mainstream work. IPS is more effective – 50% get paid employment, compared with 20% in sheltered employment[590]. IPS also has indirect benefits, by directly challenging discriminatory recruitment and retention practices, and reducing the social distance between the general population and people with mental illness. Overall, the empirical finding is clear: the best preparation for work is work.

Mental health professionals can increase the access of service users to the valued social role of work by supporting the development of employment schemes[506]. The main evaluation of IPS initiatives has been in relation to people with long-term mental health problems, but the approach may be relevant early in an experience of mental illness. An initiative at ORYGEN Youth Health Service supports employment-seeking among young people.

Case study 16: IPS for young people

The Individual Placement and Support (IPS) initiative was aimed at young people experi-encing their first episode of psychosis. The goal is to support people into work before the formation of a stable and enduring illness identity. The support provided by the employment

Case study 16: (*cont.*)

worker during their six-month involvement includes use of an online careers guidance tool to clarify employment goals, CV preparation, cold-calling and visiting potential employers, and interview and post-placement support.

A central feature is that the gap between expressing willingness to work and starting work-related behaviours is brief. The employment worker is co-located with the service, and can be driving to potential employers with the young person on the same day as the person is referred by the case manager. For example, a woman who expressed an interest in screen-printing was taken to meet professional screen-printers, to identify the pathway into and nature of the career. This led to her signing on for a college course. A further type of support occurs post-recruitment, when the employment worker can be contacted by the employer if they have any concerns. Finally, the employment worker can discuss with the young person regarding whether and what to disclose. For example, they may discuss whether to get into the job, perform well, and then disclose about their mental illness after a few months, with or without support from their employment worker.

The integration of the employment worker with the mental health service avoids the inter-agency duplication of assessment and bureaucratic procedures which locally led to a two-month delay before job-seeking support was offered by mainstream employment support services.

The employment worker who was specifically focussed on supporting young people into mainstream work has been subjected to randomised controlled trial evaluation[a]. The only inclusion criterion for the trial was willingness to work – criteria such as 'readiness for work' or symptom status were specifically not used to select participants. Employment rates at the end of the trial were 10% in the control group who had access to the normal group programme (including vocationally oriented groups). By contrast, 65% of people in the intervention group were in work at the end of the study, having received additional input from the employment worker. Similarly, the end-of-trial proportions in either paid employment or vocational training were 30% in the control group and 85% in the intervention group.

Further information Eóin Killackey: eoin@unimelb.edu.au

Notes:
[a]Killackey E, Jackson H, McGorry PD. Vocational intervention in first-episode psychosis: individual placement and support v. treatment as usual. *British Journal of Psychiatry* 2008; 193:114–120.

One specific work opportunity is within mental health services. These are often large employers – the National Health Service in the UK is the largest employer in Europe. However, health services have a history of poor recruitment and retention approaches to attracting people with declared mental illness to work for them[4]. (Of course, many people working in these services have an undisclosed history of mental illness.) This is a wasted opportunity, and reinforces stigmatising us-and-them beliefs in the work-force. Actively encouraging applications from people who have used mental health services for all posts, and positively discriminating between applicants with the same skill level in favour of people with a history of mental illness are two relevant approaches. They directly challenge[56]: 'the common tendency in human service organisations to see workers as either healthy and strong and the donors of care, or as weak and vulnerable recipients' (p. 32).

If a single outcome measure had to be chosen to capture recovery, there would be a case to make that it should be employment status: not because of a value about economic productivity, but because work has so many associated benefits. This idea is captured in the notion of vocational recovery, defined as a level of vocational functioning after the onset of a mental illness above specified thresholds of stability and degree of workforce participation[591]. Developing an evidence base about vocational recovery is an important research focus. For example, a five-year longitudinal study involving 529 people in vocational recovery found 47% had continuous employment, 23% had interruptions each of less than six months during the five years, and 30% had fluctuating employment with interruptions of more than six months[592].

Moving beyond employment, a general approach to supporting recovery is to provide services outside the context of treatment. An alternative context is education. The social role of student is positively valued, and one in which diversity is more tolerated and valued. This is the approach taken in our next case study.

Case study 17: education for well-being

The Division of Recovery Services is part of the Center for Psychiatric Rehabilitation at Boston University. Since 1984 it has provided a service for people with psychiatric disabilities through an 'educational lens', based on adult learning principles.

People using the service are students rather than patients. The course is based on four non-negotiable, non-debatable values:
1. Hope – holding hope for the student until hope is internalised
2. Choice – working with rather than on the person
3. Self-determination – respect for personal decisions irrespective of the educator's opinion
4. Growth – the focus is on strengths, satisfaction, success and skills.

The resulting difference in relationship is profound – as one student contrasts it, 'In hospital they tend to limit our identity to an illness'.

Information about the service is disseminated through both clinical and community services, and people apply and register for courses. The attendance expectations (the term used in preference to 'rules') are made explicit, and currently 150 students are enrolled each year, with services provided by 26 educators (including over 50% consumer providers). There is a waiting list of 200 people. All courses are free to students, who receive a 'Recovery Scholarship' to the value of the course. This both normalises the educational process as costing money, gives students a sense of value and places students into the valued social role of scholarship recipient.

A wide range of courses are offered, including healthy lifestyle (Food education, Sexuality and intimacy, Supported physical activity), spiritual (Tai Chi, Mindful meditation, Laughter yoga), daily living skills (Computing, Personal organization, Stress hardiness) and mental illness specific (WRAP, Recovery workbook, Health management and recovery). For example, the Writing course involves students reading accounts of recovery, writing a response, writing their own story and then writing their 'future story' of where they will be in ten years time. The Community and Recovery course involves voluntary work. The Photovoice course involves people taking a photograph about an issue of importance to them in their recovery, learning to narrate it and then bringing the narrated picture to those who hold power over their lives to change their minds.

The service aims to promote role transition: from patient to student to peer provider teacher to mentor to colleague. A key focus is therefore on community integration, especially in relation to work. The *Training For The Future* programme involves full-time attendance at work-related (especially computing) courses for six months, followed by a six-month internship in local businesses.

Several principles have emerged from experience: autonomy (as opposed to paternalism); risk, success and failure (rather than compliance, compulsion and maintenance); disagreement is part of the growth process (so should not be pathologised or labelled); using

Case study 17: (*cont.*)

'readiness to change' as a means of developing motivation is more helpful than using perception of motivation to determine readiness for change; and 'dependency' is not a dirty word – people may need long-term support (despite the cultural value to the contrary).

Risk is dealt with using normal academic approaches, tailored to the needs of people with psychiatric disabilities: behavioural expectations are made explicit, university policies regarding smoking/drinking/violence are followed, and an information card records the student's emergency contact details along with elements from advance directives about their wishes for crisis response. Staff response to inappropriate behaviour is informed by frameworks from education, such as the LEAST approach: Leave it alone, Eyeball without confrontation, Attend to the problem (privately and directly), Strategise with the student about the skills and support needed to meet behavioural expectations, Take a break from the programme. No student has ever been permanently excluded.

Further information: Dori Hutchinson (dorih@bu.edu)

An important feature of this case study is that over 60% of the programme staff have their own lived experience of mental illness.

We end with concrete suggestions for how mental health professionals and teams can improve social inclusion.

Suggestion 1. Spend resources differently

A common experience of workers in the mental health system is frustration – a sense that these ideas about social inclusion, employment and social roles are all well and good, but impossible to implement within the existing constraints. The constraints differ from country to country (e.g. mental health policy, reimbursement arrangements, financing, workforce skills), but the implication is always the same – we can't do it here. At the heart of this issue is the question of what the job of mental health services is. We have argued that its primary task is *not* to provide treatment (with the implication that any other activity is a luxury), but to support personal recovery. Our next case study is an example of a system that decided to spend its available resources differently.

Case study 18: the MHA Village approach to employment

The Mental Health America (MHA) Village in Los Angeles works with people with mental illness who are homeless, deinstitutionalised and recently released from prison. Their goal is to 'help people create a life not defined by the illness' – and to replace the identity of patient with a more meaningful role. Their expectation is that altering day-to-day experiences leads to new roles, shifts in identity and, ultimately, changed behaviours and outcomes. Hence exposure to the experience of working is a central strategy.

The Village integrates its clinical support services with its employment services. This provides the opportunity for skills deficits and support needs to be met by a clinical staff while the employment service offers the realistic, 'normal' expectations of employees: that they show up for work, do what's asked of them, serve customers, and 'leave their mental illness at the door'. When is someone ready to use the employment service? When the person wants to work (i.e. a client's clinical state is not a primary criterion).

The features of any work environment capitalised on by the Village include non-disabled expectations, a focus on ability (to produce, serve, etc.), real work for which the client is needed, participation as part of a team rather than a target group, internal motivations to manage symptoms, tangible results and the opportunity to practise the role of a 'worker' repeatedly.

For people who are anxious about working, the Work-for-a-Day option offers the chance to work for one shift, with the immediate gratification of getting paid at the end of the shift. For people with little work experience, the Village runs in-house businesses including a café where people can work for up to nine months. Job seekers apply in writing, are interviewed, get hired and are paid standard wages. For people with criminal backgrounds or a weak work history, the Lease Labor option offers community employers the option of contracting with the Village (not the individual) to get the job done – the Village pays the worker the same day and bills the employer. For people who would feel more comfortable working with people they already know, group placements are found through a Village employment agency, which contracts with community employers (without disclosing about issues of mental illness). The agency provides quality assurance specialists who check on the person's progress and offer on-the-job support where necessary – a less stigmatising and disclosing approach than a 'job coach'. Other approaches include seasonal work, temporary labour (short-term community jobs where homelessness or proper identification is an issue) and, of course, competitive employment.

Even a failure at work is both normalising (most people have such experiences) and contributes to creating a life not defined by mental illness. The experience of working (even if the job only lasts a short time) contains seeds of growth. Village members learn which jobs they like or dislike, what behaviours work or don't work and which skills have yet to be mastered. It has proven far better for adults with mental illness to have tried and learned than to be denied the opportunity to fail and grow.

All of this probably sounds expensive. The Village describes it as a cost or allocation shifting. It is based on the view that 'you get what you pay for', a fiscal paradigm shift that requires an emphasis on spending money to promote wellness and recovery rather than promote stability and maintenance. This has practical financial consequences. The top three areas of expenditure are individualised case management (41%), work (25%) and community integration (12%)[a]. By contrast, the top three expenditures in the traditional clinical services were acute hospitalisation (28%), long-term care (23%) and out-patient therapy (23%). Since hospitalisations and living in institutional residence are markedly reduced for members attending the Village[b], the money saved is re-invested in work-supporting services. The evidence suggests that the reduction at the Village of costly hospitalisation rates and long-term care is a direct result of services that emphasise well-being.

Further information: www.mhavillage.org

Notes:
[a]Lewin-VHI I, Meisel J, Chandler D. *The Integrated Service Agency Model: A Summary Report to the California Department of Mental Health.* California: California Department of Mental Health; 1995.
[b]Chandler D, Meisel J, Hu T, McGowen M, Madison K. Client outcomes in a three-year controlled study of an integrated service agency model. *Psychiatric Services* 1996; 47:1337–1343.

Suggestion 2. Organise community-based events

One way in which the community can be influenced towards seeing mental illness as part of 'us' not 'them' (and consequently taking a level of ownership) is through exposure. For example, at the MHA Village there is an emphasis on activities which give back to the community. Staffing a water station for a marathon gave an opportunity for members and staff to dress up, have fun and literally give back to the local community. This has unexpected pay-offs – a 911 despatcher who had several times responded to emergency calls for police assistance to the Village was for the first time able to humanise the organisation which she had previously viewed as a problem group. A key role of mental health services is to create these positive community experiences. This both has benefits for consumers – giving back is an important human experience – and makes a positive impact on the community.

Suggestion 3. Educate employers about workplace accommodations

Workplace accommodations can involve People (focussing on interpersonal challenges), Places (focussing on where the work takes place), Things (focussing on equipment needed to do the job) or Activities (focussing on the work tasks). For people with physical disability, accommodation needs tend to relate to Places and Things. This is what employers are used to. In mental illness, People issues are often the central issue. Employers need educating about how these interpersonal needs can be tended to.

A key contribution from the clinician can be educating employers about their legal duties under relevant discrimination legislation and about reasonable workplace adjustments for people with mental illness, which might include[56]:

- addressing concentration problems by having a quieter work place with fewer distractions rather than an open-plan office
- the need to have some time away from other workers
- enhanced supervision to give feedback and guidance on job performance
- allowing the use of headphones to block out distracting noise (including hearing voices)
- flexibility in working hours, e.g. to attend clinical appointments or work when less impaired by medication
- mentor scheme for on-site orientation and support
- the need to talk to a supporter (e.g. a job coach) during a lunch break
- clear job description for people who find ambiguity and uncertainty difficult
- prior discussion about how leave due to illness will be managed, e.g. allowing the use of accrued paid and unpaid leave
- relocation of marginal job functions which are disturbing to the individual.

These accommodations often come down simply to good supervision: motivating the worker; providing clear and constructive feedback on role performance; and in general supporting the person to do a good job. Anticipating common problems experienced by people with mental illness moving into the workplace is also helpful, such as tensions around disclosure, needing to prove themselves more than other workers, and being reluctant to take sick days due to mental illness. Developing collaborative relationships with local employers is an important contribution which can be made by expert mental health professionals to increasing employment opportunities.

Suggestion 4. Use group skills in community settings

Most mental health services contain staff with a high level of skill in running groups in a mental health context. This does not promote social inclusion. Since the group is only for people who have a mental illness, this inadvertently reinforces an identity defined by the mental illness. Providing an in-house response to a need does not support a service orientation towards keeping the person in their life by supporting them to do things for themselves, or to harness their own existing natural supports, or to develop new natural supports. Finally, whilst community adult education services have had to make their services accessible to people with other forms of disability, the existence of special groups for people with mental illness allows mainstream discrimination to continue.

An alternative approach is for mental health staff with skills in running groups to approach local mainstream adult education services, and co-facilitate groups with adult education specialists in community settings. The groups would be on the same range of social and therapeutic topics as those currently run in mental health services, but would be open to anyone. The advantages of this approach are that the adult education service gains skills in accommodating to the needs of people with mental illness, the consumer experiences being referred to a mainstream group, and the group is genuinely community-based, involving participants with and without mental illness.

Suggestion 5. Amplify the voice of the consumer in society

Negative media portrayals of people with mental illness are pervasive[534;535]. Mental health professionals can directly address the absence of media stories involving people who have recovered from mental illness[593] by:

- Encouraging and training peer support specialists to be the spokesperson for a team
- Developing local bureaux of speakers who have recovered from mental illness[56] (see Case study 3)
- Refusing a media request to give a professional perspective without the guaranteed inclusion of a consumer perspective.

The role of consumers in improving social inclusion

A key approach to promoting social inclusion is to support the development of consumer activism. This has many potential benefits. It can be a pathway to recovery for the individual. It can provide a model of authentic partnership. It challenges social and professional beliefs about what recovery means – having someone talking about their own experiences of recovery is a powerful antidote to prejudicial beliefs about what is possible for people with mental illness[86].

This can be hard for mental health professionals. We are more used to seeing service users as the problem than as the solution. Yet the power of people with lived experience to impact on other consumers, professionals and society may be greater than that of professionals.

Ingrid Ozols is an example of a consumer-activist involved in employment. Ingrid's recovery journey has led her to the belief that getting well involves taking responsibility, and requires vigilance on her part. She has developed many supports: a doctor who acts as a temporary crutch (i.e. genuinely supportive but only in the short term – the goal being worked towards is always standing unsupported); medication (which 'lifts the fog' so she can see colours, think logically and get out of bed); a supportive partner and friends with normal (i.e. not over-compensating) expectations; and regular use of a coach who provides the occasional 'kick on the shins'. Ingrid identifies that she needed to get over the self-stigma of discussing her own experiences, and now uses her own story as the basis for a business.

Because it relies on the courage and strength of one person, this approach may not be generalisable. But it does point to the importance of mental health services looking out for potential consumer activists among people on the caseload.

Case study 19: Mental Health at Work

Mental Health at Work (mhatwork®) is a company started by Ingrid Ozols which works with workplaces to help promote mental healthiness in their workforce. The aim of mhatwork® is to increase retention and reduce claims against the corporation for mismanagement of

Case study 19: (cont.)

employees with stress and mental health problems and create a supportive environment. The business model is explicitly commercial – mhatwork® is not a 'worthy' activity or a not-for-profit organisation, but a commercial entity making a financial case for its services. Corporations, including some household names in Australia, employ the services of mhatwork® for financial not charitable reasons.

The company's emphasis is on promotion, prevention and early intervention, with the ultimate aim for the organisation to undergo a corporate culture change. To achieve this aim, mhatwork® consultants draw on their own lived experience of mental health problems (whether the experience has been direct or indirect) to model breaking the taboo about the topic. The goal is to teach employees and managers to become better at 'looking out for each other', through openness on the part of the employee and appropriate work-place accommodations on the part of the manager and employer. Methods used are varied:

- Individual consultation – for example, discussing with a manager how to work with employees in a way which is both emotionally supportive and meets legal and organisational responsibilities
- Workshops – 2–4-hour interactive workshops for 15–25 staff, based on adult learning principles. The content can cover topics such as recognising the signs and symptoms of potential mental health problems, how to manage and support them, values, balancing work and life, and building resilience to help plan ahead to avoid 'going crook'
- Educational materials – books, poster, pamphlets, e-learning resources
- Identifying and supporting local champions to provide peer support within the corporation.

Because of the emotional demands of self-disclosure, mental health support within mhatwork® is prioritised, including opportunities to debrief after each training session, and viewing peer support as normal rather than the exception.

Further information: www.mhatwork.com.au

A concern sometimes expressed about supporting consumer activism is whether people remain defined by their illness, rather than their personhood. A reasonable balance may be supporting people to use their own experiences because that's what they choose to do, rather than because that's all they are able to do. Many people who use their own history of using mental health services to develop a work role could clearly also prosper in other areas. However, there is no empirical evidence about what predicts whether becoming a consumer-activist is helpful or hindering of personal recovery. A consistent strategy is therefore to note the issue with the consumer and to support them to take responsibility for their own decisions.

The role of governments in improving social inclusion

Social inclusion can also be increased through interventions at local and national levels. A comprehensive range of interventions have been proposed by Graham Thornicroft[56;86], some of which are shown in Box 23.1.

Reducing stigmatising public attitudes will benefit people experiencing mental illness for the first time, since appropriate support-seeking in young people is hindered by low levels of information and negative images of mental illness[594]. It will also benefit people with ongoing difficulties, as a non-discriminating society is necessary if people with mental illness are to exercise their full rights of citizenship.

Box 23.1 Strategies to reduce discrimination

At the level of individuals and their families
- Develop new ways to offer diagnoses
- Actively provide factual information against popular myths
- Develop and rehearse accounts of mental illness experiences which do not alienate other people

At the local level
- Commission supported work schemes
- Increase the availability of psychological treatments
- Health and social care employers give recognition to 'expertise by experience' through positive support in recruitment and staff management practices
- Ensure people with mental illness and employers are properly informed of their rights and obligations
- Provide accurate data on mental illness recovery rates to mental health practitioners and service users and carers
- Support greater service user involvement in local speakers' bureaux

At the national level
- Promote a social model of disability which refers to human rights, social inclusion and citizenship
- Promote service user-defined outcomes
- Audit compliance with codes of good practice in providing insurance

The best way to reduce stigma is not to focus on mental illness as a medical disorder. International research consistently shows that biological or biogenetic attributions are associated with a perception of *higher* likelihood of impulsivity, unpredictability and dangerousness in the minds of the public[63]. This may be because the public equate biogenetic models with being deep and unchangeable, and therefore more 'other'. Nonetheless, mental health literacy campaigns often aim to communicate a message that mental illness is an illness like any other. One reason why this approach has been popular within mental health is suggested by Pat Bracken and Phil Thomas[26]: 'Psychiatrists have generally been keen to downplay the differences between their work and that of their medical colleagues . . . However, patients (and the public) are well aware that a diagnosis such as diabetes does not lead to compulsory detention in hospital, whereas the label schizophrenia is a major risk factor for this' (pp. 8–9).

Although some commentators call for a closer link between mental illness and chronic disease models[595], the epidemiological data on recovery rates reviewed in Chapter 3 suggest that such a linkage is not empirically justified. Broadly one third of people recover without any help from mental health services. This group, invisible to mental health services, become apparent in population surveys[596]. Even those who use mental health services can experience clinical recovery from severe mental illness. As Daniel Fisher (psychiatrist and co-director of the National Empowerment Center) put it[597]: 'I have recovered from schizophrenia. If that statement surprises you – if you think schizophrenia is a lifelong brain disease that cannot be escaped – you have been misled by a cultural misapprehension that needlessly imprisons millions under the label of mental illnesses.'

The more effective approach to reducing stigma is contact with people with a mental illness[585], where the person moderately disconfirms the negative stereotype. If they are consistent with the stereotype then it is reinforced, whereas if they are too different then they can be dismissed as an exception[598]. The contact needs to involve the same status and goals for the different groups, be collaborative rather than competitive and have senior managerial support[599].

Unfortunately, stigma is also found within mental health services. A good review of the available evidence about attitudes of mental health professionals is provided by Beate Schulze, who concludes[70]: 'In sum, findings indicate that, while mental health providers are well informed about mental illness, they nevertheless do not always hold positive opinions about the conditions and the people they treat.'

We have already identified working alongside peer support specialists and seeing people in recovery as well as in crisis as approaches to reducing stigmatising clinician beliefs. Another approach is to develop new ways of talking about constructs traditionally referred to as dichotomous and discontinuous (e.g. schizophrenia, insight, responsibility, capacity), perhaps with terms such as 'a touch of schizophrenia' and 'partial capacity'. Of course for some purposes it is necessary to use a binary classification, but since the experience of even apparently discontinuous phenomena such as psychotic symptoms proves to be much more common in the general population than previously thought[98;99;600], language emphasising difference is neither empirically supported nor helpful in relation to stigma.

Turning to attitudes of the wider public, stigmatising beliefs have practical consequences. For example, the Burdekin Inquiry in Australia identified widespread systemic discrimination in relation to mental illness, with under-funding especially in relation to accommodation, employment and crisis care[601]. What can be done about it?

In New Zealand, the inquiry by Judge Ken Mason in 1996 highlighted the negative way mental illness is viewed in society[602]. This led to an anti-stigma campaign, which is described in our next case study.

The aim in Section 3 has been to provide resources to crystallise and catalyse movement towards a recovery focus in mental health services. In Section 4, we identify some of the concerns this may raise, and concrete actions with which to start.

Case study 20: Like Minds, Like Mine campaign

Like Minds, Like Mine is a national anti-stigma campaign run by the New Zealand Ministry of Health. It has three levels of intended impact[a]:

1. Societal – a nation that values and includes all people with experience of mental illness
2. Organisational – all organisations have policies and practices to ensure people with experiences of mental illness are not discriminated against
3. Individual – people with experiences of mental illness have the same opportunities as everyone else to participate in society and in the everyday lives of their communities and whānau.

It supports three actions:

1. Providing opportunities for contact with people with experience of mental illness
2. Promoting rights and challenging organisations, communities and individuals not to discriminate
3. Delivering evidence-based education and training.

The most visible intervention is a rolling series of national television and radio advertisements. The content of the advertisements was deliberately non-clinical in its focus, and was influenced by the family orientation of Māori / Pacific Islander cultures, who make up 25% of the New Zealand population. In these traditions, mental ill-health is located in the family

Case study 20: (*cont.*)

rather than the individual, and so clinical models of understanding are less culturally conson-ant. The key focus in the adverts was on raising visibility of, and reducing social distance from, mental illness.

Adverts featured famous and non-celebrity New Zealanders who have experienced mental illness. They included first-person accounts of what the experience was like and what helped or didn't help, and family, friends and employers talking about the person as an individual (rather than as a mental patient). For example, rugby player John Kirwan talked with his friend Michael Jones[b]:

> KIRWAN: I was clinically depressed, but I like to call it freaking out, because depression is such a word that people say, 'Snap out of it.' . . . What gets you through? Love, family, communication's a big one. You've got to talk it through. It's terrible when you're in there. But it's no big deal, it's pretty normal.
>
> JONES: I personally noted, as a close mate, that I felt really guilty that I didn't recognise it . . . He went through something and he was prepared to face up to that demon, and that took guts and that took courage. You know, I'll always respect him and admire him and love him for that. (p. 195)

The tag-lines for the adverts are 'Don't judge a book by its cover', 'Are you prepared to judge?', 'Know me before you judge me' and 'The biggest barrier to recovery is discrimination'.

There have been many other initiatives. The programme is predominantly led, driven and delivered by people with experience of mental illness. In Capital and Coast District Health Board, the Mental Health Foundation of New Zealand (a national non-governmental organisa-tion) ran a series of workshops for local communities. A Māori-specific resource to address stigma and discrimination has been developed. Research into addressing internalised stigma is under way.

Evaluation has been central to the campaign. The proportion of positive media portrayals of mental illness rose from 5.7% in 1994 to 11.1% in 2004[c]. Tracking surveys of community attitudes to mental illness show improved public views about mental illness[d]. This has concrete benefits. In a survey of 266 people with experience of mental illness, more than half reported reduced stigma and discrimination from family, mental health services and the public[e].

The success of the campaign is shown by its extension to 2013.

Further information: www.likeminds.org.nz

Notes:

[a]Ministry of Health. *Like Minds, Like Mine National Plan 2007–2013: Programme to Counter Stigma and Discrimination Associated with Mental Illness*. Wellington: Ministry of Health; 2007.

[b]Mental Health Commission. *Te Haererenga mo te Whakaôranga 1996–2006. The Journey of Recovery for the New Zealand Mental Health Sector*. Wellington: Mental Health Commission; 2007.

[c]Mental Health Commission. *Discriminating Times? A re-survey of New Zealand print media reporting on mental health*. Wellington: Mental Health Commission; 2005.

[d]Vaughan G, Hansen C. 'Like Minds, Like Mine': a New Zealand project to counter the stigma and discrimination associated with mental illness. *Australasian Psychiatry* 2004; 12:113–117.

[e]Ball J. *'What's been happening?'. A summary of highlights, activity and progress on Like Minds, Like Mine 2003–2006*. Wellington: Quigley and Watts Ltd; 2006.

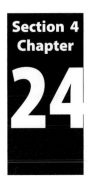

Section 4
Chapter

24

Challenges
Concerns held by clinicians

In this chapter some of the many potential questions and concerns raised by clinicians about recovery are identified and addressed. This and the next chapter (which relates to concerns held by consumers) are written as questions or objections with suggested responses. This format will facilitate their use when making the case for a focus on personal recovery.

To aid readability there is a deliberately minimal use of citations, balanced by references to earlier chapters where the relevant theme was explored in more depth. Some of the answers draw from published sources[603;604], and others are personal views.

Isn't the recovery movement simply antipsychiatry by another name?

No. The original antipsychiatry movement of the 1960s emerged from within psychiatry. The recovery movement has emerged from the individual and collective voice of people who have used mental health services (see Chapter 3). It has an overlap with antipsychiatry in some aims – such as a challenge to the right to impose an explanatory model on experience and an awareness of (and wariness about) professional power – but aims such as giving primacy to the priorities of the individual and the importance of high-quality mental health services are distinct. Indeed, although there has been a recent strengthening of the alignment[605], the antipsychiatry movement was criticised by early consumer activists as 'largely an intellectual exercise of academics'[606].

There's nothing new here – we do this already

It is certainly true that some of the values embedded in a recovery approach have featured previously in the history of mental health services, such as Tukes's moral treatment emphasising respect and dignity in nineteenth-century asylums, and the development of social psychiatry with its focus on the social context in the 1950s and 1960s. It is also true that many individual clinicians are highly skilled at supporting people to self-manage, develop support networks, develop a positive personal identity and work towards valued social roles.

However, systems have emergent properties. In Chapter 22 we considered some of the attitudinal, discourse and behavioural markers which characterise a focus on recovery. For services which exhibit those characteristics, the challenge may be communicating that practice to others. For services which do not yet exhibit those pro-recovery markers, it may be helpful to start with a recognition that there is a journey to make.

Recovery means cure – anything else is just twisting the meaning

I agree. The term is not ideal, partly because it places the discourse in an illness frame, and partly because the everyday meaning of recovery is indeed cure. As Roberts and Wolfson put it, 'In the context of a progressive dementia, for example, the victory over disease implied by "recovery" can seem a hollow example of society's need to sanitise the distress caused by events beyond our control'[466] (p.33). If we were starting again, a more neutral term such as a discovery approach or a forward-focussed approach would be preferable. But we are where we are. One positive suggestion would be to focus more on working within the Personal Recovery Framework and avoid sometimes polarised discussions about recovery as a concept.

However, the level of emotion often contained in this criticism suggests that it is not really about inexactitude of meaning, but more concerned with the underlying shift in values. As Oyebode put it, 'the involvement of governments in this endorsement of a peculiar departure in ordinary language demonstrates that we are here dealing with the politics of healthcare and not the clinical aspects'[607]. It does indeed. The real issue underpinning this objection may be a core disagreement with the whole recovery approach – an important, but different, concern.

People with mental illness lack capacity, so cannot take responsibility for their own lives

The embedded assumption that capacity is discontinuous, unidimensional and permanent is not true. It is true that a person with a mental illness may at particular times lack capacity to some degree in some areas of their life. In this, they are clearly similar to anyone else who has ever been drunk, excessively sleep-deprived, felt uncontrollable anger, or in any other way experienced a temporary loss of capacity. This understanding of capacity is much more useful, because it acknowledges that lack of capacity is possible, but assumes that the ability to express preferences and take some degree of personal responsibility is the norm rather than the exception. So the challenge is one of balancing the recognition that someone may have temporary decision-making incapacity whilst creating an orientation towards enhancing rather than diminishing an individual's ability to take personal responsibility. Even during crisis it is possible to minimise the loss of autonomy (see Chapter 21).

My job is to act in the patient's best interests, not on the basis of what they say they want

A focus on personal recovery is not consistent with this belief. History suggests that making decisions for people with mental illnesses has led to harm for many people (see Chapter 7). Also, such an approach is out of step with societal values: when people consult an expert, they expect to be given relevant information and then be the one who decides on action, either by stating their wishes or explicitly giving permission to the expert to decide. Why should it be any different for people with mental illness?

My job is to treat people

That is what many clinicians were trained for, and treatments are a major strength of mental health services. But we now recognise that an exclusive focus on treating illness is insufficient for some patients, and toxic for others (see Chapter 1). Focussing on promoting recovery involves placing more importance on well-being, on keeping the person in their life, and on the development of valued social roles and a positive identity (see Chapter 9). Clinical treatment skills are a vital contributor to this process for many people, but treatment is a means of meeting recovery goals, not an end in itself (see Chapter 18). The paradox is that working towards the individual's goals will lead to greater engagement in treatment, because it is then linked to a personally valued goal rather than because someone else thinks it is in the person's best interests. The job of a recovery-focussed clinician is to support recovery, not to provide treatment.

'You'd better wait until you're better before going back to work'

A key insight of a recovery approach is that it is unhelpful to put life on hold until the mental illness is successfully treated. Rather, it is better to put clinical effort and resources into helping the person to keep their life going, to retain existing social roles and to develop new roles. Work, as one of the primary means by which many of us define ourselves, is a vital early focus, and not something to consider at some point in the future.

How do I manage risk in a recovery-focussed service?

There is a political and professional reality that this is an expected function, so it is an important component of a recovery-focussed mental health service. Key strategies are distinguishing between harmful risks and positive risk-taking, having organisationally endorsed approaches to setting treatment goals to minimise harmful risks and recovery goals to maximise risk self-management, valuing the dignity of risk, and giving primacy as much as possible to recovery goals over treatment goals (Chapter 17). This involves reflective practice around how to minimise the clinical resources put into meeting treatment goals and maximise the clinical resources put into supporting recovery goals.

What is a recovery-focussed response to people who are a danger to themselves or others?

Key clinical strategies are: (i) skilled and collaborative assessment; (ii) promoting risk self-management by supporting the growth of personal responsibility; (iii) focus on the development of valued social roles, which buffer against acting on harmful impulses; (iv) use WRAP and early warning signs work to avert crises; (v) use advance directives to minimise loss of autonomy during crisis; and (vi) intervene with minimal compulsion where necessary (see Chapter 21).

What are the central values of recovery?

The core value is the primacy of personhood (see Chapter 15). As Bill Anthony put it, 'People with severe mental illnesses are people'[453]. This sounds prosaic, but is in fact transformational. It has implications for how clinicians relate to consumers (Chapter 13), seeing a person not an illness (Chapter 16), basic expectations of a good life for the person (Chapter 14), where responsibility for change lies (Chapter 18), needing the expertise of lived experience to do the clinical job (Chapter 12), and challenging stigmatising views held by clinicians and the public (Chapter 23).

Recovery will lead to a neglect of people with the most complex health and social needs

If the values of recovery are understood, there is no reason this should be so. Recovery is not about working mainly with people who are making progress and improving, or abandoning the most disabled. It is about using a different approach with exactly this most challenging group of people, to support them to lead the best life they can, *as they define it*. For some people, the gains will be very modest, and they will need long-term high levels of support. This, of course, should be available. Dependency is not a dirty word! The challenge, though, is to exhaust every avenue of support before reducing ambitions for the person.

Recovery is actively unhelpful for severely disabled people

The concern here is twofold. First, that setting up expectations of a better future will lead to hopes being dashed. However, we cannot judge who can recover, and therapeutic nihilism is self-fulfilling. Better surely to expect good things than to communicate impoverished expectations?

The second concern is that this will lead to people being abandoned[152]: 'Many individuals are so disabled with mental illness that they do not have the capacity to understand that they are ill. Giving such individuals the right to make decisions about their treatment is tantamount to abandonment' (p. 1464). This argument is particularly consonant with a perspective that mental illness is *essentially* a biological disorder[608]. We argued in Chapter 2 that this view of the person is unhelpful – mental illness is *essentially* a subjective experience, often of course expressed in a biological substrate. Similarly, recovery is not a thing you do once better, it is about winning small (and big) battles starting where you are. The challenge is supporting the person, whatever perceptions the observer has about their disability, to maximise what they can do, to work towards taking responsibility for their own lives, and to have hope for a better future. It is perhaps those people who are seen as most disabled, and written off as (literally) no-hopers, who have most to benefit from a recovery-focussed approach.

Diagnosis is a central protection for vulnerable people

This argument was first put forward by Anthony Clare[269] in his seminal book *Psychiatry in dissent* as a response to the antipsychiatry movement:

> What protects the dissident, the deviant, and the outsider from being labelled 'mentally ill' is not the psychiatrist who does not believe in psychiatric classifications. . .but rather the psychiatrist who acknowledges that people can suffer from serious mental disturbances, that the symptoms of these can be grouped and defined in such a way as to produce a reasonable degree of agreement to their validity and reliability, and that those people who do not show such symptoms cannot be classified as mentally ill, whatever society may say or do.
>
> (p. 156)

One can look at this in two ways. On the one hand, it is true that diagnostic taxonomies provide, if not protection, then at least the ability to argue that what is going on is not psychiatry. We mentioned in Chapter 7 the use of psychiatry for political purposes in the Soviet Union[278] and China[279]. On the other hand, there has not been a visible outcry from clinicians about other developments, such as the political construction in England of diagnoses such as dangerous and severe personality disorder, whose 'societal and legal convenience may appear substantially to exceed their clinical provenance'[609] (p. 344). Other issues with diagnosis were explored in Chapter 2.

The best balance point in promoting personal recovery is to view diagnosis as one highly developed and often useful tool, but only a means to an end, not an end in itself. The job of mental health services is not to diagnose and treat, but to support personal recovery. This may involve providing an explanatory model in which diagnosis features centrally. Or it may involve supporting the development of direct meaning in which diagnosis is peripheral. Or, most challengingly for current practice, recovery for some consumers may have nothing to do with (and be actively hindered by a clinical focus on) diagnosis.

People have a right to know their diagnosis

True, but misleading. If what is meant is simply that clinicians should share their understanding of what is going on with the consumer, then this is true as we emphasise in Chapter 16. Information should not be withheld when the individual asks for a clinical view. It is also the case that sometimes (as when the diagnosis is particularly stigmatising, such as schizophrenia) there is an argument that this should be shared slowly over time to allow integration and adjustment, but the goal should be openness and clear communication. The role of professional expertise and clinical judgement in the relationship is central.

However, it is misleading if the implicit assumption is that the diagnosis represents the privileged insight held by the clinician into what is really going on for the person, i.e. the person has the illness and it is the clinician's duty to let them know that they have it. This reification of diagnosis was challenged in Chapter 2, and it works against the tentativeness which is a central value for personal recovery. There is a world of difference between 'You have schizophrenia' and 'What you've described can be understood as being symptoms of schizophrenia'.

There aren't resources to offer treatments, so how can we be expected to do more tasks?

For over-worked, under-resourced clinicians this is a barrier to any change. Two suggestions are to spend differently and to 'code-share'. Spending the available resources to support recovery will be more effective than spending on the treatment of illness (See Case study 18). Code-sharing is the practice of an airline selling seats on a flight operated by another airline. Many must-do clinical activities can be done in a recovery-promoting way, to both feed the beast of professional or administrative requirements and to take advantage of the fact that the beast doesn't generally care what it is fed. So work differently, not more. Focus treatment planning towards recovery goals rather than treatment goals. Positively discriminate in favour of people with lived experience of mental illness in recruiting mental health staff. Harness the energy of consumers to run groups and develop community links. Train consumers to speak for the team to media. If placement reviews are the required mechanism to ensure taxpayers get value for money, then this has to be done – but by whom? Can some consumers in placements be supported to review the placement themselves? Can a consumer be trained in placement review as a means of developing job-related skills? If risk management plans are compulsory, then what stops it including a section on growth opportunities (i.e. risks needed for personal growth)?

We would do this if we weren't so over-run with trying to meet endless need with minimal resources

This realistic concern is important. It is unrealistic to expect hopeless and disempowered workers to promote recovery, or to expect clinicians to get to know someone if they have minimal interaction time and large amounts of paperwork, or to expect recovery-focussed services to be a way of saving money. A key function of leadership is to create an organisational context in which recovery-focussed work is possible, which will involve addressing these barriers to change.

What are the implications of recovery for the professions?

We don't know. Some potential positives are increased job satisfaction, less compulsory treatment (Chapter 21), seeing people moving on in their lives beyond what anyone thought possible (Chapter 18), and developing exciting new roles as promoters of well-being

(Chapter 14). There are potential negatives: professional role uncertainty (Chapter 13), leadership tensions (who should lead a clinical team?), values conflict where the professional identity emphasises nomothetic knowledge (Chapter 4) or deficit amelioration (Chapter 2), increased self-awareness about stigmatising beliefs (Chapter 12) and loss of status (e.g. in salary, or in relation to other specialities in the same profession).

Chapter 25

Concerns held by consumers

We consider here some of the concerns which I have heard raised by consumers about the recovery approach.

Recovery is a medical term

It does have medical overtones, although recovery in the sense in which it is used here has emerged from the stories of people who have experienced mental illness, rather than from clinicians. This is an example of where partnership is needed – if the clinical community seeks to understand and communicate this understanding of recovery back to the service user/survivor community from which it emerged, it is very likely to be framed as a professional initiative. What is needed is a mature service user–professional partnership, in which the values and practices of recovery are communicated to a service user audience primarily by other service users.

Interestingly, in New Zealand, which probably has the longest history of trying to develop recovery-focussed mental health services, there is a growing recognition of the need for consumer training in recovery – supporting individual service users to engage with mental health services in ways which support their own recovery.

There isn't one route to recovery, or one recovery model

Absolutely. Therefore it is more useful to talk about recovery as an approach, a set of values, or overarching guiding principles. As Repper and Perkins point out[4], this 'circumvents sterile arguments between competing intervention models (medication vs. therapy vs. employment vs. self-help vs. complementary therapy, etc.). All or none of these may contribute to the central overarching goal of growth and development'. This is why there is no mention in this book of *a* recovery model. Rather, a focus on personal recovery means incorporation of a set of values, and consequent working practices, into mental health services. That said, clinicians do think in terms of models. The Personal Recovery Framework presented in Chapter 9 seeks to bridge the gap, by being sufficiently individual to highlight the unique and idiosyncratic nature of recovery, whilst sufficiently general to be of use across mental health services.

Recovery is a cover for service cuts

Recovery has been used as a justification for cuts to services. A cost-reducing element of a recovery-focussed mental health system is the dismantling of mental illness ghettos, such as day-care services and daytime activities exclusively for people with a mental illness. A cost-generating element is the creation of pathways to social inclusion, including accessing normal mainstream community resources and opportunities to exercise full citizenship rights. Similarly, reducing dependency may lead to more people moving on from services (saving money), but working in an individualised way with each person is more time-consuming (costing money). The financial implications of a shift in values and practice towards personal recovery are unknown, but substantial cost savings are unlikely. Saving money by closing ghettoising services and increasing throughput without spending money on creating pathways into society and staff capacity to work alongside people as they struggle to re-engage in their lives should not be presented as a means of promoting recovery.

Taking away diagnostic labels will reduce access to services and benefits

Diagnosis is the means of access to many important forms of support, so in the short term diagnostic terms will remain important as gateways to health and social benefits and entitlements. A focus on personal recovery does not mean abandoning a diagnostic frame of reference. Rather, it means moving from diagnosis as a revealed truth to diagnosis as a working hypothesis to make sense of the individual's experience. Genuinely allowing individuals to determine their own meaning will involve open discussion about the merits of accepting or using a diagnostic label. For some people, the use of a diagnosis will fit their experiences and provide a helpful way forward. For others, they may not fully or at all understand their experiences within a diagnostic framework, but will accept the use of the diagnosis in order to access societal benefits. For others, they will decide that the use of a diagnostic label is personally unacceptable, even if this means not being able to access social benefits. The central principle is informed choice.

Recovery will be neutralised by professionals

There is a danger that the term becomes appropriated by professionals as a means of retaining the *status quo* and ensuring business as usual. The absence of any accreditation process for labelling a service as recovery-based creates the very real possibility that recovery teams will be established whose philosophy is based on clinical recovery, with primacy given to professional concerns about symptoms, risk, etc. Similarly, consumers often voice concern about the individualised nature of recovery becoming 'the recovery model' by the time it reaches professional level of discourse, suggesting a production-line mentality in which recovery is the next thing that professionals do to consumers.

This issue has been addressed in three ways. First, the difference between personal and clinical recovery was identified in Chapter 3. The aim of this book is to translate the consumer-developed idea of personal recovery into clinical practice, not to legitimise the professionally developed idea of clinical recovery. Second, the values and working practices needed in a mental health service focussed on personal recovery have been outlined in Chapters 15 to 21, and they are certainly not business-as-usual. Third, quality indicators for a recovery-focussed service have been proposed in Chapter 22, which make the embedded values transparent and amenable to debate.

Recovery is a consumer-developed concept being appropriated by professionals, when it's nothing to do with them

Underpinning this concern may be a view that the incorporation of the user-developed concept of recovery into mental health services necessarily involves a loss of its radical and oppositional edge, so there can be no real shifts in power and it will simply involve processing patients in a slightly different way: using modified language but with the same ultimate aim of controlling the individual. This criticism is difficult to address without agreeing with assumptions implicit in the concern. It is a central assumption in this book that mental health services have much to offer many, though not all, people with mental illness, and that whilst the mental health system has some damaging emergent properties, the vast majority of the individuals working in the system are altruistic, compassionate and skilled people. Supporting the consumer-developed idea of recovery will involve core shifts in the values and practices of mental health services. Persuading oppositional consumer activists – who view collaboration with services as 'supping with the devil'[610] – to move from a position of outsider to a position of partnership will be an indicator of the success of mental health services in embracing and operationalising personal recovery values.

All this talk about recovery ignores the human suffering caused by mental illness

A focus on personal recovery does not mean ignoring the all-too-real human suffering. It also does not involve being relentlessly up-beat in the face of this suffering. Acknowledging when life is hard is an authentic and helpful response for both the person with a mental illness and the professionals and non-professionals in their life. However, the development and consolidation of identity, the finding of hope, the creation of meaning and the grasping of personal responsibility all create ways forward from this suffering.

The recovery approach imposes a set of values on the individual

This concern can be held at two levels. First, the recovery literature is permeated by implicit notions of how people should be. The North American recovery literature 'projects traditional American values onto disabled people, such as rugged individualism, competition, personal achievement and self-sufficiency', and does not appreciate that for some people, 'independent living amounts to the loneliness of four walls in some rooming house'[119]. An emerging counterpoint is the New Zealand experience, which is influenced by non-American cultural views. Similarly, in this book the concept of identity (described in Chapter 9) has been deliberately positioned as neutral towards whether primacy should be given to the individual or the person-in-context.

A second level of this concern is as a tautology – any approach to working with other people contains implicit assumptions about values. Given that reality, it is helpful to make the values transparent, which at least makes them amenable to debate. This involves more explicit recognition of the values base held by practitioners, and its potential impact on clinical practice. As Bill Fulford put it, 'If . . . a psychiatrist cannot distance herself from the ideas about beneficial treatment endorsed by her profession, it is unlikely that they will appreciate the reasons behind their patients' preferences and concerns or will altogether fail to elicit these'[611] (pp. 706–707). Making values clear also allows services to be held accountable for living by them. For example, the closure of day centres or reduction in peer support services or imposing individual over communal living under the justification of increasing social inclusion can only be effectively challenged by holding the mental health system to account for the extent to which its services match its stated values.

I don't understand my experiences in a medical framework

A great advance offered by a recovery approach is that this is fine – the meaning of choice is the choice of meaning. A recovery-focussed mental health professional doesn't care what label someone puts on their experiences, or whether they accept they are ill. To an extent they even don't care about compliance with medication or treatment. Their starting point is what the person wants in their life. Their goal is to work collaboratively towards the consumer's goals, bringing their professional training as a resource to add to the person's expertise about their own experiences, values and goals. Because this means working differently to how many professionals were trained, consumers can help this process by communicating their goals as clearly as possible.

Taking responsibility is hard

Yes, it is. And so too is continuing to carry responsibility for one's life. Recovery is about values, and one value is that taking responsibility is an important underpinning for a good life. Clearly, some people at some points in their life cannot take full responsibility for themselves. One reason, amongst many, is mental illness. A recovery-focussed mental health service takes as little responsibility as possible away from the person, and actively supports the person to take back partial or full responsibility for their own life as soon as possible. This process can take time, as the person slowly builds confidence and skills at running their own life.

I may not meet expectations – recovery sets me up to fail

Failure is possible. Real success is not possible without the chance of failure, so people in recovery from mental illness can (and will) experience setbacks. Just like everyone else. The only way to avoid the chance of failing is to disengage from trying anything. The central recovery value is that engaging in life is better than trying to survive life. This is a value, not an objective truth. It is also not the only view – not everyone agrees with Tennyson that 'Tis better to have loved and lost than never to have loved at all'[612]. What is proposed here is that holding and communicating expectations of an engaged, meaningful and productive life is a *better* value for mental health services. The job of mental health professionals is then to be actively supporting the individual, both by helping the person to develop the skills and confidence to take on challenges, and where helpful to be a safety net for the person if things don't work out as planned.

I have nothing to recover to

The language of recovery may sound hollow to someone experiencing strong incentives to retain what status they have as a person with a mental illness, rather than trying to operate in a discriminating and suspicious society. So it is understandable that, initially at least, life as a patient may seem more attractive. But this simply points to the central challenge, which is finding the hope that meaning and purpose are possible, that an identity which is not defined by the mental illness can be developed, and that a valued life is attainable. This involves a move from an entitlement to an empowerment mind-set, which is difficult. Increasing the visibility of role models is a central contribution of mental health services to this process. Alongside this, part of the job of mental health professionals is improving social inclusion – working with communities to widen opportunities.

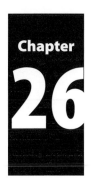

Chapter

26 Organisational transformation

In this concluding chapter, concrete actions are proposed for mental heath services which want to develop a recovery focus. Moving towards this focus will involve doing things differently, which is likely to include seven key actions.

Action one: lead the process

Leadership differs from management. Managers solve problems to make the organisation work more effectively or efficiently, and their basic orientation is towards control and administration. Leaders build the organisation's future, and their basic orientation is towards inspiring, influencing and guiding. Evolving towards a recovery focus starts, but does not end, with leadership. The first action is then to employ and legitimise leaders rather than managers in organisational positions of influence.

Bill Anthony identifies eight leadership principles[613], shown in Box 26.1.

Leaders understand that systems, like people, don't change easily. There is a need to introduce a level of survival anxiety – a sense that things cannot continue as they are. It often takes a jolt to the system to create change. For example, the Georgia Certified Peer Specialist Project began when the state government threatened to ask for a repayment of funds from the statutory mental health service after lobbying by local consumers about unsatisfactory outcomes and insufficient move-on[614]. It is now established with both state and federal funding[368]. Leaders recognise the stages of transforming systems[615]:

1. Establishing a sense of urgency
2. Forming a powerful guiding coalition
3. Creating a vision
4. Communicating the vision
5. Empowering others to act on the vision
6. Planning for and creating short-term wins
7. Consolidating improvements and producing still more change
8. Institutionalising new approaches

Key leadership strategies follow from this analysis.

Raise awareness

Measure and publicise empowerment levels among consumers. Support people to talk about their own recovery stories. Highlight anti-recovery practice. Audit treatment and care plans for the extent to which they promote self-determination and autonomy. Create token consumer roles on influential boards. Import charismatic recovery champions, either permanently into the workforce or temporarily as invited speakers at local events. Visit demonstration sites. Link in with existing networks (e.g. Coalition of Psychiatrists in Recovery – www.wpic.pitt.edu/AACP/CPR). Learn from others (e.g. www.calmend.org).

Box 26.1 Leadership principles

Principle 1: Leaders communicate a shared vision
Principle 2: Leaders centralise by mission and decentralise by operations
Principle 3: Leaders create an organisational culture that identifies and tries to live by key values
Principle 4: Leaders create an organisational structure and culture that empowers their employees and themselves
Principle 5: Leaders ensure that staff are trained in a human technology that can translate vision into reality
Principle 6: Leaders relate constructively to employees
Principle 7: Leaders access and use information to make change a constant ingredient of their organisation
Principle 8: Leaders build their organisation around exemplary performers

Create survival anxiety

Support existing consumer coalitions – their voice is often much stronger than clinicians' in calling for change. Support individual consumers wanting to complain. Develop advocacy services. Pilot pro-recovery ways of working. Locally publicise pro-recovery national policy. Encourage consumers to tell their stories in local and national media. Stock-take and publicise the level of valued social roles and rights (work, intimate relationships, housing, income). Increase disclosure in the workforce by including personal experience of mental illness as a desirable criterion in all job descriptions.

Develop new coalitions

Seek out local and national allies. Form local networks. Actively promote – literally if possible – recovery champions. Get to know influential opinion-formers and encourage pro-recovery values in them. Develop personal support networks to remain hopeful. Create a ground-swell about recovery by local learning sets, recovery meetings and team or programme-level commitments. Align with influential people who are highly negative in their views about recovery around a shared goal of making the lives of consumers better and ask for their help, rather than directly try to change the person into a recovery adherent. Remember that 'when you pit a bad system against a good performer, the system always wins'[616].

Have a plan

Act strategically and use the limited resource of your time and energy as productively as possible. Separate means and ends. Drop the term recovery if it provokes a knee-jerk negative response – find a more acceptable local term. Analyse organisational readiness to change[454;617]. Develop staff knowledge through teaching sessions (many short sessions, not one long session), policy, induction procedures, day-to-day discourse, educational materials, research presentations, conference attendance. Shape values through visits to exemplar sites, exposure to recovery narratives, consumer employees, supervision practices, management messages about the primary purpose of the organisation, workshops on values, bringing recovery heroes into the system as invited speakers or as employees. Increase skills through targeted skills workshops, supervised practice, leadership from opinion-formers, telling and supporting staff to change behaviour, new clinical processes. Embed change through a clear and visible mission, reviewing policy, amending record-keeping, using programme development consultancy expertise, asking all parts of the system (e.g. IT, human resources) to prepare recovery business plans – what they will do to support a recovery focus. Work around resistance rather than through it. Have goals about organisational transformation and celebrate success when they're met. Review the plan – as Winston Churchill put it, 'However beautiful the strategy, you should occasionally look at the results'. Learn from others[91;613;618].

Action two: articulate and use values

The second action is to make the organisational values explicit, and to collate and use evidence of consistency between these values and working practices. This involves difficult discussions about core values and identity. For example, some commentators propose that[619]: 'the medical/illness-based paradigm from which our mental health system has historically operated is perhaps the single-most overarching barrier impeding both consensus and implementation of person-centered planning' (p. 12). One component is the development of new clinical sayings. The Collaborative Recovery Model (CRM)[620], described in Case Studies 10 and 21, uses these:

1. Recovery is responsibility
2. Hope helps
3. There is evidence for alliance
4. Roll with resistance
5. Develop discrepancy
6. Avoid argumentation
7. Motivation is malleable
8. Champion capacity; disable deficit
9. Needs are negotiable
10. Goals should be meaningful, not just manageable
11. Review, Design, Assign [for homework tasks]

How is this translated into practice? Our next case study illustrates some of the benefits and challenges[621].

Case study 21: implementing the Collaborative Recovery Model

SNAP Gippsland Inc. began as a non-governmental housing initiative in 1992, and diversified into a focus on day programmes in 1996. It serves a rural population in south-east Victoria, and provides community-based support to people with mental illness. In 2003 the organisational commitment to recovery led to employment of a worker who had completed a one-year supervised training programme in the Collaborative Recovery Model (CRM). A condition of employment was that CRM be implemented in undiluted form. During the first three months employment, the CRM trainer led a top-to-bottom audit of the organisation's recovery focus. Following this review, a number of organisational change strategies have been implemented:

- Training staff in CRM, and then expecting the protocol to be used with at least one client, followed by more over time
- Developing supervision arrangements to promote reflective practice
- Developing personal mentorship arrangements
- The CRM trainer audits all paper-work, to maximise model fidelity
- Maintaining links with relevant academic centres, through monthly teleconferences and biannual visits. This enhances local credibility, and provides access to emerging practice developments

---

Case study 21: (*cont.*)

- Hosting a recovery-themed local conference with both internal and external speakers, to celebrate success, disseminate local stories of recovery, and promote a system-level identity as a recovery centre of excellence.

A central implementation step has been developing shared ownership: 'The whole organisation, from service-users to the Board of Management, must own and embrace the model in order to change the mindset and practice of the organisation as a whole' (p. 43). *For consumers, a developmental approach is needed*: 'Not all of my clients are happy to change to the CRM because they find it a bit scary. I'm working these clients up to it and slowly teaching them about the new program' (p. 48).

The reason these ideas have taken hold is because of their transformative potential. For example, Danielle is a woman with a history of multiple admissions, self-harm attempts and diagnoses (schizophrenia, depression, substance abuse) who was able to identify and implement a recovery goal of swimming with whales in Tonga. Or Ron, who reports 'One of the things about SNAP is that the people there can help you, but you have to do the work. I'm proud because I have accomplished things. I'm more open. The petals are open' (p. 59).

The service is now working with the idea of exit interviews with clients, to seek to understand their experience of using the service. This requires consideration of power issues (the person may come back, so may not feel they can be honest), who should do the interview (e.g. a consumer-advocate) and what to ask.

Key challenges have been:
- High turnover of SNAP workers, due to staff being unwilling or unable to move with the organisation: 'taking ownership of the recovery model represents a change in identity for the organisation' (p. 56)
- Employment of consumer-employees, who have not been able to separate their own recovery journey from that of the client they're talking with, leading to advice-giving on the basis of what worked for them. This has been exacerbated by a rhetoric about the consumer having the most expertise about recovery, which has now been refined to the consumer having the most expertise about their own recovery journey
- Difficulties in embedding ownership, shown by a high burden resting on the chief executive officer and the CRM trainer with consequent concerns about sustainability.

Further information: www.snap.org.au

Action three: maximise pro-recovery orientation among workers

Consumer narratives emphasise the importance of personal characteristics of the worker, in addition to technical competency. Desirable qualities include being kind, tenacious, tolerant, positive, warm, compassionate, optimistic and hopeful. The importance of being able to relate to people with mental illness as a person rather than an illness is central. Yet mental health services have traditionally emphasised technical competency, professional group and accreditations, rather than personal qualities. This has practical implications: core professional training is one barrier to a focus on personal recovery[622]:

> An analysis of the training standards and curricula for psychiatrists, comprehensive nurses, diploma level social workers and mental health support workers showed that there are some gaps in the recognition of recovery competencies . . . There was little or no reference in most of these documents to:

- a recovery approach
- the different understandings of mental health and mental illness
- supporting the personal resourcefulness of service users

(p. 1)

This is beginning to change, with the development of recovery competencies. In New Zealand there is a recognition of the scale of the task[292]: 'The recovery-based competencies . . . signal a fundamental change to all aspects of the education of mental health workers. They require that some new material be taught. But they also require that some existing material be taught differently' (p. 2). The ten New Zealand recovery competencies[622] are shown in Box 26.2.

As another example, a review of the capabilities needed by a modern mental health workforce in England identified gaps in professional training in relation to: user and carer involvement; mental health promotion; values and evidence-based practice; working with families; multidisciplinary working; and working with diversity. This led to the development of ten Essential Shared Capabilities as a foundation for all workers in the mental health system[623], shown in Box 26.3.

What both these approaches have in common is that they relate to *how* staff work with patients. The third action is therefore to increase the pro-recovery orientation of workers in the system, through both recruitment strategies and workforce development.

How can people with pro-recovery views be identified during recruitment? Being explicit about organisational values in the information about the post allows potential applicants to self-select. Interview questions such as 'Why do you suppose people with psychiatric disabilities want to work?' give a chance for applicants to demonstrate their values. Involving consumers and carers in the recruitment process gives some information about how interviewees relate to people they will work with. The Boston University Center for Psychiatric Rehabilitation requires basic knowledge, attitudes and skills in relation to recovery to be shown during selection[454]:

Box 26.2 New Zealand recovery competencies

A competent mental health worker . . .
1. understands recovery principles and experiences in the Aotearoa/NZ and international contexts
2. recognises and supports the personal resourcefulness of people with mental illness
3. understands and accommodates the diverse views on mental illness, treatments, services and recovery
4. has the self-awareness and skills to communicate respectfully and develop good relationships with service users
5. understands and actively protects service users' rights
6. understands discrimination and social exclusion, its impact on service users and how to reduce it
7. acknowledges the different cultures of Aotearoa/NZ and knows how to provide a service in partnership with them
8. has comprehensive knowledge of community services and resources and actively supports service users to use them
9. has knowledge of the service user movement and is able to support their participation in services
10. has knowledge of family/Whānau perspectives and is able to support their participation in services.

Box 26.3 The ten Essential Shared Capabilities in England

1. Working in partnership
2. Respecting diversity
3. Practising ethically
4. Challenging inequality
5. Promoting recovery
6. Identifying people's needs and strengths
7. Providing service-user-centred care
8. Making a difference
9. Promoting safety and positive risk-taking
10. Personal development and learning

Basic knowledge includes knowing the current research with respect to recovery and recovery outcomes as well as, for example, research related to the role of prejudice and discrimination as obstacles to recovery. Basic attitudes include the extent to which the four key values *[person orientation, person involvement, self-determination, growth potential]* are incorporated into a candidate's way of thinking about individuals with disabilities or psychiatric histories . . . Basic skills include skills such as the skill of engaging an individual in a partnership, inspiring hopefulness, connecting with that individual in a personal way, as well as supporting and facilitating the individual's recovery journey.

(pp. 153–154)

For the existing workforce, stage-based training is needed. For workers in the precontemplative phase, approaches include learning about recovery (using websites with recovery-focussed resources – see Appendix), reading the accounts of recovered consumers[55;106–108;118], understanding how recovery happens in stages[123;137;318], exposure to people in recovery, and training on national policy. For those in the contemplative phase, staff development approaches include identifying personal values and practices[309], developing communication skills through reading information written for consumers about recovery[28;296;624;625] and visiting demonstration sites.

Like several others, this action is not possible without support to legitimise doing things differently. The more powerful the support is, the better. Radical transformation at the national level is occurring in some countries, notably New Zealand and Italy. In New Zealand, the shift towards non-governmental organisation involvement in *providing* services emerged from a system-level crisis, and has required radical shifts in core assumptions.

In Italy, system transformation has involved a focus on laws rather than policies. The advantage of a legal framework is that laws are subject to judicial oversight, and in contrast to policies they cannot be easily sabotaged by unenthusiastic clinicians or managers, or by resource arguments. See www.triestesalutementale.it for more information.

Case study 22: implementing pro-recovery policy

After 67 consecutive inquiries, it became clear that the mental health system in New Zealand was unable to improve acute care services through internal change. In 1996, Judge Ken Mason produced a report into mental health services[602]. Unlike the previous inquiries, the Mason Report led to innovative developments. It made a small number of recommendations:

Case study 22: (*cont.*)

1. A national anti-stigma campaign
This was described earlier in Case study 20.

2. A coordinating Mental Health Commission
The Commission has overseen the strategic development of mental health services, and its directors come from both mental health professional and consumer backgrounds. It has published many practical resources, including the recovery competencies for mental health workers[292], a systematic review of the evidence about consumer-led services[293] and recovery-focussed research on consumer narratives[107], media reporting[294] and in-patient[295], home treatment[124], forensic[126] and early psychosis[125] services. Two publications to highlight are a consumer-written guide for service users to get the most from mental health services[296], and a celebration of recovery-focussed mental health workers[297]. Both contribute to the mature and genuinely collaborative relationship needed for mental health services to promote recovery. All are available at www.mhc.govt.nz.

3. A funding stream which came to be known as Blueprint funding
The Blueprint was published in 1998[291], and stated:

> Recovery is a journey as much as a destination. It is different for everyone . . . Recovery is happening when people can live well in the presence or absence of their mental illness and the many losses that come in its wake, such as isolation, poverty, unemployment, and discrimination . . . Historically, mental health services have failed to use a recovery approach. Recovery could never take place in an environment where people were isolated from their communities, where power was used to coerce people and deny them choices, and where people with mental illness were expected to never get better. Some people have experienced recovery without using mental health services. Others have experienced recovery in spite of them. But most will do much better if services are designed and delivered to facilitate their recovery.
>
> (pp. 1–2)

This statement involves a commitment to a recovery-focussed future (which is now common in international policy) and a recognition of past failings (which is unique to New Zealand). This latter aspect may be the reason why the policy commitment to recovery has become deeply embedded in practice. An important engine of innovation has been Blueprint funding – the partial redistribution of public funds for acute care outside the statutory sector. For example, this led to the development of peer-led and peer support services, including the in-patient unit described in Case study 15. This creates flexibility in services, and means there's more than one model – and hence more than one real choice.

Looking back on the impact of his report, Mason commented that 'A huge advantage of our inquiry was that we weren't required to look at issues of guilt, as so many inquiries are. What we had to determine was whether there were deficiencies within the system . . . and how could they best be resolved'[91] (*p. 5*).

There are ongoing challenges. It has been difficult to make the development of recovery a whole-system approach. For example, a lot of resourcing has been focussed on in-patient services, which are arguably not the best start point because the primary goal is often safety, and the expectations of disempowering coercion are highest. Other system transformation challenges have been:
1. Embedded attitudes amongst professionals
2. The change in the power relationships experienced by both clinicians and the families of service users
3. The development of better exit strategies – how to move people on from the mental health system

Case study 22: (*cont.*)

4. The shortage of access to adequate housing and employment
5. Keeping people's lives afloat during admission. On admission people often aren't asked whether they have children, other dependants or pets, and they don't volunteer this information for fear they'll be taken away. The challenge is keeping employers in the loop, and more generally keeping life on the go whilst the person is ill.

The next phase in the evolution of services will be to link the recovery concept with the Māori concept of Whānau Ora – wider population-level understandings, such as resilience. Although older consumer activists prefer the term recovery (as it has produced a partial power shift), younger people prefer the less stigmatising term resilience – everyone needs resilience, but only ill people need to recover. This also links with the culturally embedded construct of resilience, which is needed by both the individual and the group to survive. It is therefore applicable to the whole population, and a necessary and normal component of individual and cultural well-being.

Further information: www.mhc.govt.nz

Action four: develop specific pro-recovery skills in the workforce

The next action is to develop three specific skills. The first is to train staff to assess capabilities as well as disabilities, and support the use of this skill through ongoing training and supervision. This skill is a necessary counterbalance to the deficit bias we discussed in Chapter 2. How is this done? In Case study 13 we described a service based on the Strengths Model[72]. We now describe how the service change was made.

Case study 23: implementing the Strengths Model

Since 2004, workers in the St Vincent's Hospital system had been grappling to define the model for adult rehabilitation and continuing care services. Several models were considered in relation to:

1. evidence base
2. fit with existing service structures, language and practical constraints
3. existence of experienced clinicians who had implemented the model and were willing to share their experiences
4. being person-centred, based on consumer goals, with consumer-held records
5. fitting with local values of the hospital: Compassion, Justice, Human Dignity, Excellence and Unity.

Existing expertise in the Strengths Model[72] was identified in Timaru Mental Health Services in New Zealand, which has been implementing the model since 2001. Staff from Timaru shared training materials freely, and were happy to discuss its implementation via videoconference. The decision was made in 2005 to adopt the Strengths Model at St Vincent's.

Implementation began with a visit by a multidisciplinary group of clinicians and managers from St Vincent's to Timaru. The programme comprised a five-day training workshop (as given to local Timaru staff), implementation planning and train-the-trainers work. The advantages of going to the expert service were that each stakeholder had more chance to address their own questions.

Managers wanted to know whether the service was sufficiently similar for comparison to be meaningful, whether it could be implemented locally, whether the model would build on what was already in place rather than devaluing existing skills and whether the investment of time and effort was worthwhile. Managers saw the inpatient unit, met consumers, followed the use of documentation and talked with the local trainers and senior clinicians.

Clinicians were struck by the positive engagement approaches which were possible even with consumers who rejected illness labels or the need for treatment, the emphasis on learning and changing for both consumers and staff, the recognition of the self-fulfilling nature of a focus on problem and deficit, and the expectation that interventions are not planned or implemented without the approval of the consumer, except in the specific context of the Mental Health Act. The emphasis on the community as a supporter of recovery, rather than an obstacle to recovery, was congruent with assertive outreach approaches. The relationship between the clinician and the consumer correlated positively with good outcomes.

Following this visit, a series of two-day and shorter training courses have been run at St Vincent's. Training initially involved a local St Vincent's trainer and visiting Timaru trainers, using Timaru-developed training programmes. A training team has now incorporated local examples from both staff and consumers into the programmes, leading to greater local ownership and visibility of the model. Training is now provided exclusively by St Vincent's staff, with consultation support from Timaru.

The ongoing mentoring relationship has been experienced positively by Timaru staff, who identify the following benefits:
- affirmation of the Timaru service as being valued by others
- reassurance that local issues were similar to those faced by St Vincent's
- recognising that training in itself is insufficient, and having to make concrete the key elements needed for successful transition to the new model: developing a motivated group of key people, securing management buy-in, revising policy, conducting regular audits
- positive reinforcement of giving an open and welcoming response to enquiries from external services
- enhanced credibility with the local District Health Board

Overall this approach to system transformation has been positively valued by both sides. A term used is that the services are 'travelling together', indicating both value being placed on the current arrangements and a learning and development orientation towards the future.

Further information: Bridget Hamilton (Bridget.hamilton@svmh.org.au)

The second specific skill is identifying and planning action towards recovery goals. This involves clinical processes and working practices which orient mental health services more towards recovery goals, and views treatment goals as necessary but not the primary purpose of the organisation. A range of approaches were identified in Chapter 17. Audit strategies can include the proportion of care plans which are focussed on recovery rather than treatment goals, the proportion which harness approach rather than avoidance motivation, and the extent to which attention (e.g. in clinical meetings) and resources (e.g. money, workforce skills) are focussed on recovery goals rather than on treatment goals.

The third specific staff skill is recognising the central importance of developing personal meaning. This involves links with mutual self-help groups, training for staff in the distinction between supporting meaning and promoting insight, and using written and verbal communication which validates the individual's perspective.

Action five: make role models visible

The fifth action involves services working in ways which make people in recovery more visible, to both consumers and staff. Potential initiatives include training in telling one's story (Case study 3), running events celebrating success (Case study 12), developing a consumer speakers' bureau and providing consumer-led staff training.

The development of peer support specialist roles in teams and employment of people in recovery from mental illness throughout the system is crucial. However, it is unlikely to be sustainable before the earlier actions. This involves ring-fencing dedicated posts for people with their own experience of mental illness throughout the system, and ensuring there is access to initial training and ongoing support for people in this role. The transformative potential of this single action is high, as shown in our next case study.

Case study 24: Recovery Innovations

META Services is a mental health service based in Phoenix, Arizona. In 1999 the organisation's chief executive, Gene Johnson, attended a national workshop in which service recipients talked about feeling continually discounted, disempowered and disrespected[604]. The discomfort created by this experience kick-started a process of organisational transformation, from being a traditional service provider to one where 139 (54%) of its 256 staff are peers. Peer-operated services now account for $4m of its $12m annual revenue[614]. This transformation was done in stages[630]:

1. Revising the mission statement: 'Our mission is to create opportunities and environments that empower people to recover, to succeed in accomplishing their goals, and to reconnect to themselves, others, and meaning and purpose in life'.

2. Recruiting people with lived experience of mental illness ('peers') to the management team and into full-time (36%) and part-time (72%) posts at all levels in the organisation. These new peer recruits were carriers of a recovery culture into the organisation.

3. Achieving early wins, such as the elimination over a two-year period of seclusion and restraint from services.

4. Moving from a therapeutic to an educational model. This was central because 'we wanted our Centre to be about reinforcing and developing people's strengths, rather than adding to the attention placed on what was "wrong" with them'[631]. Most training is prepared and delivered by peer specialists, such as WRAP[632] and many college credited and non-credited courses, tailored to contain a recovery focus. In 2006/07, 5660 people received 98 900 hours of education in 6730 classes.

5. A key innovation has been the Peer Employment Training Program, which is a 20-module, 80-hour training course to prepare people to work as peer support specialists. Entry requirements are lived experience, having a high school diploma, having completed a WRAP and wanting to attend and find a job. The course covers both general work skills and the role of the peer support worker (e.g. telling your personal story, being with people in challenging situations). Post-training options include an 80-hour internship, support from a job placement service, and 90-day employment follow-up services. In-class transformation is common: over 95% of participants graduate, and 89% of peer support specialists were working at one-year follow-up[631]. The peer training is accredited, earning college credits which allow peers to work towards an associate arts degree. Ongoing support and supervision is provided for peer specialists, to avoid washout of their unique contribution. By June 2008, 796 peer specialists had been trained, of whom 76% have obtained employment. The training model is being adopted in other States and internationally (e.g. Scotland (see Case study 4), New Zealand).

Case study 24: (*cont.*)

6. Growing flexibly and opportunistically, by retaining the recovery values whilst responding to market need. For example, partnering with a local college to offer a wider range of educational options, developing a wellness centre, and creating innovative alternatives for people in crisis (see Case study 14).

7. Evaluation is central, since money identified as being saved on admission rates (reduced by 56%[631]) has been used to develop new peer support worker roles, including: recovery educators and coaches in case management teams; crisis specialists in the Living Room; peer advocates in in-patient services; and peer recovery teams as an alternative to case management teams.

The driving force within the organisation has been placing value on lived experience. Since most of the workforce now have experience of mental illness in their lives or those close to them, the 'them–us' distinction is broken down; as one worker noted, 'it [mental illness] is all around us'. The 'them–us' distinction is further reduced by requiring peer and non-peer staff to go through recovery training together, which culminates in a 'telling your story' day in which participants describe a personal recovery experience. Sometimes this creates discomfort, when the organisation is confronted with its own professional biases and stigmatising beliefs and practices. The process of organisational 'recovery' has involved increasing the extent to which workers experience the five recovery pathways (choice, hope, empowerment, spirituality and recovery environment). The processes of organisational recovery parallel personal recovery in several ways: shifting from an entitlement to an empowerment culture; focus groups to understand the needs of staff rather than a sole focus on organisational imperatives; leadership training to enhance self-direction and self-management skills; supporting managers to 'get out of the way' of the worker's desire to do a good job, e.g. through the use of coaching (recoveryopportunity.com) rather than a prescriptive management style. Gene Johnson characterises the resulting changes as 'a profound, deep, intense, and penetrating alteration in the status quo'.

Further information: www.recoveryinnovations.org

Action six: evaluate success in relation to social roles and goal attainment

This action involves orienting the service towards supporting the attainment of valued social roles and personally valued goals by the individual. Once this orientation is in place, pro-recovery behaviours are increased by using these outcomes as key performance indicators by which organisational and individual worker performance is appraised. Our next case study describes one approach to identifying and evaluating recovery standards.

Case study 25: Recovery Devon

The county of Devon in England has a population of 850 000. Following a conference in 2003 with Mary-Ellen Copeland as an invited speaker, a recovery-focussed partnership of service users, carers and staff has developed, initially intentionally outside, but with informal support from, statutory sector services. Partnership activities included providing WRAP training[351] to over 300 staff and service users, establishing a quarterly newsletter and web-site (www.recoverydevon.co.uk), and developing intentional peer support training[360]. In 2006 a second conference was held, consolidating a 'recovery way of working' – again with inspirational invited speakers (Frank Bristol, David Gonzales, Shery Mead), a quota of an equal split of service user/carers and professionals, and name badges with first names only.

Case study 25: *(cont.)*

Since 2006 the Devon and Torbay local implementation team has provided the focus for a broad mental health and well-being network (growing out of this partnership), comprising commissioners and providers of mental health services from the statutory, voluntary and independent sectors. There is less need to refer to 'service users, carers and professionals' because (for some network members) this has become the meaning of these units – the them–us distinction has in places disappeared.

The voluntary and independent sectors have been an engine of innovation. For example, the Community Care Trust (www.community-care-trust.co.uk) is an independent provider operating in-patient and community-based services which focus on supporting recovery by:

- Inviting consumers to stay at the service when well, to get to know them and hence be holders of hope for them when in crisis
- Inviting consumers to bring a guest for a night or two when coming to the service in crisis, to make the admission experience safer
- Focussing on the development in its workforce of important qualities (e.g. authenticity, integrity, presence) in addition to skills
- Using coaching skills as the preferred method of interaction
- Signing up to holding others to account and being held to account in all matters, e.g. requiring all staff to complete WRAP, using a recovery approach to sickness self-management and disciplinary procedures
- Living the value of 'there is no other', so anyone using the service simultaneously becomes a resource for the service.

Informed by these innovations in other network members, the statutory mental health provider (www.devonpartnership.nhs.uk) has also identified an aim of 'putting recovery at the heart of everything we do'. Their service is being re-structured, with the design of each function being set by a professional expert group and endorsed by a clinical cabinet of senior clinicians, with accountability to a programme board. Change is being supported through the use of team coaches – 20 people are employed to work across 57 teams, supporting the teams to work better (e.g. through amplifying negotiation and conflict-resolution skills, supporting good leadership, encouraging reflective practice). Leadership buy-in has been increased by all the Trust executives attending WRAP training. Using these in-system approaches has maximised ownership of the change process.

Ten core standards for all commissioned mental health and social care services in Devon and Torbay have been agreed:

1. The recovery approach – all staff have relevant knowledge and skills
2. Recovery outcome evaluation – all services have a regular cycle of measuring recovery outcomes
3. Coherent and effective service configuration – services are constructed on recovery principles and delivered by teams that are managed and led so as to be coherent and effective contributors
4. Network partnership relationships – relationships are characterised by good communication, clarity, consistency and respect
5. Staff and service performance – all practitioners, teams and services are subject to regular performance review
6. The experience of networks – there is excellent 'customer care', receptive to personal preferences and diverse needs
7. Satisfaction – from those who use the services, their families and providers of related services. The general public have confidence in the services provided to their communities

Case study 25: (*cont.*)

8. Social inclusion – all services demonstrate practices which are supportive of people living ordinary lives in ordinary settings, especially in relation to accommodation, occupation, education, personal relationships, money and participation in community life

9. Building mental well-being – all service users and providers are supported to maintain well-being and build resilience

10. Challenging stigma and discrimination – all services are able to engage and effectively respond to issues of prejudice, stigma and discrimination.

The long-term aim is to 'design in' recovery into services by commissioning on the basis of these standards. Approaches to measuring success for each criterion (e.g. using DREEM[633]) are being investigated in 16 pilot sites.

Further information: www.recoverydevon.co.uk

Action seven: amplify the power of consumers

This final action involves ceding power, and occurs at the end rather than the beginning of organisational transformation. People with their own experience of mental illness are an under-used resource for organisational and societal change. Supporting consumer activism to challenge anti-recovery assumptions and obstacles in the mental health system and wider society is a hallmark of a recovery-focussed service[404]:

> When such obstacles are encountered on an individual's pathway to recovery, it is the job of the guide to work in collaboration with the client to identify the roadblock and to find routes under, around, over, or through it. This might mean encouraging the client to challenge the 'rules' by becoming active in the agency's or the system's various decision-making bodies . . . or becoming active yourself.
>
> (p. 497)

One approach is to engage with people outside the clinical context. An example is the trialogue initiative in German-speaking Europe, described in our final case study.

Case study 26: Trialogues

An innovative approach to changing community and clinical attitudes to mental illness is the Trialogue initiative[634], also known as Psychosis Seminars[635]. These have been held in German-speaking countries since 1990. A Trialogue group involves users, carers and mental health workers meeting regularly in an open discussion forum on neutral territory, away from any therapeutic, familial or institutional context. The aim of these meetings is to learn from each other, by discussing the experiences and consequences of mental health problems and mental illness and different ways of responding. Patients who attend are more likely to be critical of current services, and one important motivation to attend is to be actively involved and initiating change in the way mental health care is practised. Family members tend to feel under-supported by services, or live with a consumer who does not willingly accept any treatment. Their motivation is to increase their knowledge about the illness and to share their feelings and learning points with others. Professionals who attend tend to be more senior and are motivated by a desire to reflect on their own practice and learn about psychosis processes.

The groups also lead to initiation of activities, such as serving on quality control boards and a trialogic day in the training of police officers about interacting with people with mental illness. Over 130 regular Trialogue groups are now attended by approximately 5000 people. Trialogues are inexpensive, widely seen as beneficial, and have developed concepts and terminology which differ from a biomedical model of mental illness (which is still widely prevalent in the mental health system). Specifically, they provide an opportunity to interact outside role stereotypes, and a learning forum for working together on an equal basis – as 'experts by experience' and as 'experts by training'.

Further information: michaela.amering@meduniwien.ac.at

We have identified seven key actions for organisations wanting to develop a focus on personal recovery. We end by looking ahead.

The future

Developing a focus on recovery will be resisted by parts of the mental health system. Personal resistance will arise because of the risk to job security (can I do what is being asked?) and role security (do I want to do what is asked?). Failure is likely with any change – Samsung's motto is 'fail often to succeed often' – and the need to expose oneself is anxiety-provoking for the individual and the organisation. A recovery approach challenges fundamental assumptions about the purpose of mental health services[333]:

> The new paradigm also changes the nature of solutions and remedies from 'fixing'
> individuals or correcting their deficits to removing barriers and creating access
> through accommodation and promotion of wellness and well-being . . .
> Simultaneously, the source of intervention moves from predominantly mental health
> professionals and clinical/rehabilitation service providers to that of fully incorporating
> social capital development, mainstream health providers, natural supports and
> peer / consumer advocacy, information and support services. Most important, the role
> of the person with a psychiatric disability shifts from being the focus of an
> intervention to one of a customer, empowered peer, and decision maker.
>
> (p. 18)

This clearly involves more than the incorporation of new ways of working into mental health services. Working in ways which support recovery will, for example, require a different professional identity[619]:

> A dramatic paradigm shift which fundamentally alters the ways in which professionals,
> individuals, families, and the community behave and interact is necessary . . . We must
> work together to move away from 'medical necessity' toward 'human need,' away from
> managing illness to promoting recovery, away from deficit-oriented to strengths-based,
> and away from symptom relief to personally-defined quality of life. Perhaps most
> critical is the fundamental shift in power involved in realigning systems to promote
> person and/or family-centered planning—the shift away from prioritizing 'expert'
> knowledge over respect for individual autonomy and self-determination
>
> (p. 4)

There are already signs of active professional resistance to this direction of travel[626]. Evolving towards a recovery vision may prove impossible without fundamental transformation – a paradigm shift. Although challenging at the time, changes in paradigm are a healthy sign. Kuhn proposed that 'Successive transition from one paradigm to another via revolution is the usual developmental pattern of mature science'[627] (p. 12). This book has argued that the process of recovery is far more wide-reaching and long-lasting than getting rid of symptoms, restoring social functioning, avoiding relapse and the other preoccupations of the current paradigm. Therefore, arguing for a focus on personal recovery *is* arguing for a paradigm shift, in which:

- previous preoccupations (e.g. risk, symptoms, hospitalisations) become seen as a subset or special case of the new paradigm
- what was previously of peripheral interest (i.e. the patient's perspective) becomes central
- the intellectual challenge emerges from outside the dominant scientific paradigm (the understanding of recovery emerges from people who have experienced mental illness, not from mental health professionals).

A reversal of some traditional clinical assumptions is at the heart of a recovery approach. Mental illness is a part of the person, rather than the person being a mental patient. Having valued social roles improves symptoms and reduces hospitalisation, rather than treatment being needed before the person is ready to take on responsibilities and life roles. The recovery goals come from the patient and the support to meet these goals comes from the clinician among others, rather than treatment goals being developed which require compliance from the patient. Assessment focusses more on the strengths, preferences and skills of the person than on what they cannot do. The normal human needs of work, love and play *do* apply – they are the ends to which treatment may or may not contribute. People with mental illness are fundamentally normal, i.e. like everyone else in their aspirations and needs. They will over time make good decisions about their lives if they have the opportunity, support and encouragement, rather than being people who will in general make bad decisions so professionals need to take responsibility for them.

The Personal Recovery Framework of Chapter 9 provides one way of understanding the processes involved in the central recovery task of reclaiming identity. It is superordinate to clinical models of mental illness, which provide explanatory models for the 'Mental illness part' of the framework. It is in this sense depicting a paradigm shift, in which the previously dominant clinical models become seen as a special case in the new paradigm. This is more than a change in rhetoric. As John McKnight put it[628]: 'Revolutions begin when people who are defined as problems gain the power to redefine the problem' (p. 16). A genuine shift in power is involved, with the priorities of the consumer moving to a position of central importance. If power remains held within the mental health system, then recovery will simply be the latest thing to do to patients. As Bracken and Thomas put it[26]:

> Insofar as citizenship is inextricably tied to democracy and human rights, it is not within the 'gift' of professionals. It is, perhaps, just as paternalistic for mental health professionals to say to service users 'Look! Here is citizenship. Take it! It is good for you. It will liberate you' as it is for them to say. 'Look! Here is Prozac. Take it. It will make you feel better.'

> (p. 254)

This book has tried to translate the consumer-developed idea of recovery into the clinical world. This aim is a stepping-stone to a more distant goal of there being no 'other'. Some of the steps along the way have already been taken, with service users having an increasingly audible voice, and a recognition of the need for user involvement. The next step may be the change from involvement (clinicians choosing to involve service users in decision-making) to partnership (needing the person to be involved). This will involve the deep transformation of coming to see the person with mental illness as part of the solution, not part of the problem. In parallel, it will involve an acknowledgement that the mental health system has been part of the problem: an acknowledgement which is necessary before the system can truly become part of the solution.

The implications for both consumers and professionals of embarking on a recovery journey are profound. It most obviously has the potential to empower and transform consumers. However, the change does not stop there. A recovery approach also has the potential to liberate professionals from unmeetable expectations: diagnose this person; treat this illness; cure this patient; manage risk effectively; keep the public safe; exclude deviance from society. We close with the words of Brazilian political activist Paulo Freire[629]:

> This, then, is the great humanistic and historical task of the oppressed: to liberate themselves and their oppressors as well . . . Only power that stems from weakness of the oppressed will be sufficiently strong to free both.
>
> (p. 26)

The recovery agenda will be complete when there are simply groups and communities and networks in which there is no caseload because there is no service user – there are only people.

Appendix: Electronic resources to support recovery

Organisation	Web address
General recovery resources	
Mental Health Commission	www.mhc.govt.nz
Boston University Center for Psychiatric Research	www.bu.edu/cpr
Ohio Department of Mental Health	www.mhrecovery.com
National Empowerment Center	www.power2u.org
Queensland Alliance	www.qldalliance.org.au/resources/recovery.chtml
Scottish Recovery Network	www.scottishrecovery.net
Recovery Devon	www.recoverydevon.co.uk/
Yale Program for Recovery and Community Health	www.yale.edu/prch
Specific recovery-focussed approaches	
Intentional care	www.intentionalcare.org
Tidal Model	www.clan-unity.co.uk
Intentional Peer Support	www.mentalhealthpeers.com
Wellness Recovery Action Planning (WRAP)	www.mentalhealthrecovery.com
The Village	www.mhavillage.org
Hearing Voices Network	www.hearing-voices.org
Promoting resilience	www.resilnet.uiuc.edu
Stigma initiatives/consumer narratives	
Mental Health Media	www.mhmedia.com
Time to change	www.time-to-change.org.uk
Like Minds, Like Mine	www.likeminds.org.nz
See me	www.seemescotland.org
Narratives Research Project	www.scottishrecovery.net
Mental health stigma	www.mentalhealthstigma.com
National Mental Health Awareness Campaign	www.nostigma.org
StigmaBusters	www.nami.org
Positive Psychology resources	
Australian coalition	www.positivepsychologyaustralia.org
Centre for Applied Positive Psychology	www.cappeu.org
Positive Psychology Center	www.ppc.sas.upenn.edu
Centre for Confidence and Well-being	www.centreforconfidence.co.uk
Values in Action Inventory of strengths	www.viastrengths.org

Organisation	Web address
Critical/oppositional sites[a]	
Successful schizophrenia	www.successfulschizophrenia.org
Critical Psychiatry	www.critpsynet.freeuk.com
Stop shrinks	www.stopshrinks.org
Psychiatric drug facts	www.breggin.com
Coming Off Psychiatric Medication	www.comingoff.com
Psychiatry Anti-Psychiatry	antipsychiatry.wetpaint.com
The Icarus project	www.theicarusproject.net
Freedom Center	www.freedom-center.org
Shoshanna's Psychiatric Survivor's Guide	www.harborside.com/~equinox
Mad not bad	www.madnotbad.co.uk

Notes:
[a]A goal of this book is to be a constructive messenger, and so some of the more oppositional literature referred to has been sanitised in its presentation. This section lists web sites which are more overtly challenging to the status quo. One view would be that polemic and 'one-sided' perspectives such as these have no place in an academic book. However, I suspect that my experience as a clinician of feeling misunderstood and misrepresented when reading these articles, and consequently feeling hurt and angry, mirrors the feelings some consumers get when in contact with mental health services.

Reference list

1. Anthony WA. Recovery from mental illness: the guiding vision of the mental health system in the 1990s. *Innovations and Research* 1993; **2**:17–24.
2. Priebe S, Turner T. Reinstitutionalisation in mental health care. *BMJ* 2003; **326**:175–176.
3. Mencken HL. *The Divine Afflatus. A Mencken Chrestomathy.* 1949.
4. Repper J, Perkins R. *Social Inclusion and Recovery.* London: Baillière Tindall; 2003.
5. Crossley ML, Crossley N. 'Patient' voices, social movements and the habitus; how psychiatric survivors 'speak out'. *Social Science and Medicine* 2001; **52**:1477–1489.
6. Baker M, Menken M. Time to abandon the term mental illness. *BMJ* 2001; **322**:937.
7. Murray R. Phenomenology and life course approach to psychosis: symptoms, outcome, and cultural variation. *Psychiatric Research Report* 2006; **22**(3):13.
8. Roth A, Fonagy P. *What Works for Whom?* New York: Guildford Press; 1997.
9. Read J, Mosher L, Bentall RP (eds). *Models of Madness: Psychological, Social and Biological Approaches to Schizophrenia.* Hove: Brunner-Routledge; 2004.
10. Boyle M. *Schizophrenia: A Scientific Delusion?* London: Routledge; 1990.
11. Kingdon D, Kinoshita K, Naeem F, Swelam M, Hansen L, Vincent S et al. Schizophrenia can and should be renamed. *BMJ* 2007; **334**:221–222.
12. Oak, D. Let's Stop Saying "Mental Illness". http://www.mindfreedom.org/kb/mental-health-abuse/psychiatric-labels/not-mentally-ill [2007, cited 2008 Jan. 2].
13. Kingdon D. Down with schizophrenia. *New Scientist* 2007; **2625**:22.
14. Bentall RP. *Madness Explained. Psychosis and Human Nature.* London: Penguin; 2003.
15. Gelder M, Lopez-Ibor J, Andreasen N, Geddes J (eds). *New Oxford Textbook of Psychiatry,* 2nd edn. Oxford: Oxford University Press; 2008.
16. Thornicroft G, Szmukler G (eds). *Textbook of Community Psychiatry.* Oxford: Oxford University Press; 2001.
17. Kanner AM. Is major depression a neurologic disorder with psychiatric symptoms? *Epilepsy & Behaviour* 2004; **5**(5):636–644.
18. Tyrer P, Steinberg D. *Models for Mental Disorder: Conceptual Models in Psychiatry.* Chichester: Wiley; 2005.
19. Chodoff P. The medicalization of the human condition. *Psychiatric Services* 2002; **53**:627–628.
20. Svensson T. *On the Notion of Mental Illness: Problematizing the Medical-model Conception of Certain Abnormal Behaviour and Mental Afflictions.* Brookfield VT: Avebury; 1995.
21. Roberts G, Davenport S, Holloway F, Tattan T. *Enabling Recovery. The Principles and Practice of Rehabilitation Psychiatry.* London: Gaskell; 2006.
22. Whitwell D. *Recovery Beyond Psychiatry.* London: Free Association Books; 2005.
23. Wade DT, Halligan PW. Do biomedical models of illness make for good healthcare systems? *BMJ* 2004; **329**:1398–1401.
24. Jaspers K (Trans.), Hoenig J, Hamilton MW. *General Psychopathology.* Manchester: Manchester University Press; 1963.
25. Mortimer A. Phenomenology: its place in schizophrenia research. *British Journal of Psychiatry* 1992; **161**:293–297.
26. Bracken P, Thomas P. *Postpsychiatry. Mental Health in a Postmodern World.* Oxford: Oxford University Press; 2005.
27. Johnstone L. *Users and Abusers of Psychiatry: A Critical Look at Psychiatric Practice.* 2nd edn. London: Routledge; 2000.
28. Heyes S, Tate S. *Art of Recovery.* Yeovil: Speak Up Somerset; 2005.

29. Allan C. Roads to freedom. *Guardian* 2007;**5**.

30. Engel GL. The need for a new medical model: a challenge to biomedical science. *Science* 1977; **196**:129–136.

31. Kiesler D. *Beyond the Disease Model of Mental Disorder.* Westport CT: Praeger Publishers; 2000.

32. Nuechterlein K, Dawson ME. A heuristic vulnerability-stress model of schizophrenia. *Schizophrenia Bulletin* 1984; **10**:300–312.

33. Barrett RJ. *The Psychiatric Team and the Social Definition of Schizophrenia: An Anthropological Study of Person and Illness.* London: Cambridge University Press; 1996.

34. Coker E. Narrative strategies in medical discourse: constructing the psychiatric "case" in a non-western setting. *Social Science and Medicine* 2003; **57**(5):905–916.

35. Johnstone L. *People with problems, not patients with illness.* Presentation at *'Schizophrenia: A new way of thinking'.* Liverpool: 2007.

36. Borrell-Carrió F, Suchman AL, Epstein RM. The biopsychosocial model 25 years later: principles, practice, and scientific inquiry. *Annals of Family Medicine* 2004; **2**(6):576–582.

37. Loveland D, Randall KW, Corrigan PW. Research methods for exploring and assessing recovery. In: Ralph RO, Corrigan PW, eds. *Recovery in Mental Illness. Broadening our Understanding of Wellness.* Washington DC: American Psychological Association; 2005. 19–59.

38. Andreasen N. *The Broken Brain: The Biological Revolution in Psychiatry.* New York: Harper & Row; 1984.

39. Double D. The limits of psychiatry. *BMJ* 2002; **324**:900–904.

40. Laing R.D. *The Divided Self: A Study of Sanity and Madness.* London: Tavistock; 1960.

41. Moncrieff J. *The Myth of the Chemical Cure. A Critique of Psychiatric Drug Treatment.* London: Palgrave Macmillan; 2007.

42. Romme M, Escher S. *Making Sense of Voices – A guide for professionals who work with voice hearers.* London: Mind Publications; 2000.

43. Szasz T. *The Myth of Mental Illness.* New York: Harper and Row; 1961.

44. Fava GA, Sonino N. The biopsychosocial model thirty years later. *Psychotherapy and Psychosomatics* 2008; **77**:1–2.

45. Goodwin D, Guze S. *Psychiatric Diagnosis.* 5th edn. Oxford: Oxford University Press; 1996.

46. Pawson R, Tilley N. *Realistic Evaluation.* London: Sage; 1997.

47. Harré R. *The Philosophies of Science.* Oxford: Oxford University Press; 1972.

48. Kendler KS. Explanatory models for psychiatric illness. *American Journal of Psychiatry* 2008; **165**:695–702.

49. American Psychiatric Association. DSM-IV-TR. Frequently asked questions about DSM. http://www.dsmivtr org/2-1faqs cfm [2008, cited 2008 Mar. 20].

50. Moser C, Kleinplatz PJ. DSM-IV-TR and the paraphilias: an argument for removal. *Journal of Psychology and Human Sexuality* 2005; **17**:91–109.

51. Fink M, Taylor MA. Issues for DSM-V: the medical diagnostic model. *American Journal of Psychiatry* 2008; **165**:799.

52. Summerfield D. Depression: epidemic or pseudo-epidemic. *Journal of the Royal Society of Medicine* 2006; **99**:161–162.

53. Moynihan R, Heath I, Henry D. Selling sickness: the pharmaceutical industry and disease mongering. *BMJ* 2002; **324**:886–891.

54. Kutchins H, Kirk S. *Making Us Crazy. DSM: The Psychiatric Bible and The Creation of Mental Disorders.* London: Constable; 1999.

55. Scottish Recovery Network. *Journeys of Recovery. Stories of hope and recovery from long term mental health problems.* Glasgow: Scottish Recovery Network; 2006.

56. Thornicroft G. *Actions Speak Louder . . . Tackling Discrimination Against People with Mental Illness.* London: Mental Health Foundation; 2006.

57. Wright BA, Lopez SJ. Widening the diagnostic focus. A case for including human strengths and environmental resources. In: Snyder CR, Lopez SJ, eds. *Handbook of Positive Psychology.* New York: Oxford University Press; 2002. 26–44.

58. Tajfel H (ed). *Differentiation Between Social Groups: Studies in the Social Psychology of Intergroup Relations.* London: Academic Press; 1978.

59. Brewer MB. The social self: on being the same and different at the same time. *Personality and Social Psychology Bulletin* 1991; **17**:475–482.

60. Cohen CE. Person categories and social perception: testing some boundaries of the processing effects of prior knowledge. *Journal of Personality and Social Psychology* 1981; **40**:441–452.

61. American Psychiatric Association. *Diagnostic and Statistical Manual of Mental Disorders*, 4th edn. Washington DC: American Psychiatric Association; 1994.

62. Davidson L, Flanagan EH. "Schizophrenics," "borderlines," and the lingering legacy of misplaced concreteness: an examination of the persistent misconception that the DSM classifies people instead of disorders. *Psychiatry* 2007; **70**:100–112.

63. Read J, Haslam N, Sayce L, Davies E. Prejudice and schizophrenia: a review of the 'mental illness is an illness like any other' approach. *Acta Psychiatrica Scandinavica* 2006; **114**:303–318.

64. Thomas P, Bracken P. Critical psychiatry in practice. *Advances in Psychiatric Treatment* 2004; **10**:361–370.

65. Wright BA. Attitudes and the fundamental negative bias. In: Yuker HE, ed. *Attitudes Towards Persons with Disabilities.* New York: Springer; 1991. 3–21.

66. Masten AS, Reed M-GJ. Resilience in development. In: Snyder CR, Lopez SJ, eds. *Handbook of Positive Psychology.* New York: Oxford University Press; 2002. 74–88.

67. Chadwick PK. *Schizophrenia: The Positive Perspective.* London: Routledge; 1997.

68. Strauss JS. Subjective experiences of schizophrenia: toward a new dynamic psychiatry-II. *Schizophrenia Bulletin* 1989; **15**:179–187.

69. Chadwick PK. The artist's diagnostic and statistical manual of mental disorders (DSM V). *Journal of Critical Psychology, Counselling and Psychotherapy* 2003; **3**:45–47.

70. Schulze B. Stigma and mental health professionals: a review of the evidence on an intricate relationship. *International Review of Psychiatry* 2007; **19**:137–155.

71. Goffman E. *Asylums: Essays on the Social Situation of Mental Patients and Other Inmates.* Harmondsworth: Penguin; 1968.

72. Rapp C, Goscha RJ. *The Strengths Model: Case Management With People With Psychiatric Disabilities*, 2nd edn. New York: Oxford University Press; 2006.

73. Rogers A, Pilgrim D, Lacey R. *Experiencing Psychiatry: Users' Views of Services.* London: Macmillan; 1993.

74. Slade M, Luke G, Knowles L. *Developing recovery-focused mental health services: evaluation of a training pilot. Clinical Psychology Forum* 2009; **193**: 10–15.

75. Pressman J. *Last resort: Psychosurgery and the Limits of Medicine.* Cambridge: Cambridge University Press; 1998.

76. Perkins R. My three psychiatric careers. In: Barker P, Davidson B, Campbell P, eds. *From the Ashes of Experience.* London: Whurr Publications; 1999.

77. Kelly GA. *The Psychology of Personal Constructs.* Vol. **1**. New York: W.W. Norton; 1955.

78. Barone DF, Maddux JE, Snyder CR. *Social Cognitive Psychology: History and Current Domains.* New York: Plenum; 1997.

79. Maddux JE. Stopping the "madness". Positive psychology and the deconstruction of the illness ideology and the DSM. In: Snyder CR, Lopez JS, eds. *Handbook of Positive Psychology.* New York: Oxford; 2002. 13–24.

80. Johnstone L, Dallos R (eds). *Formulation in Psychology and Psychotherapy: Making Sense of People's Problems.* London: Routledge; 2006.

81. Ryle A. *Cognitive Analytical Therapy, Developments in Theory and Practice.* London: Wiley; 1995.

82. Pilgrim D. *Psychotherapy and Political Evasions. Psychotherapy and its Discontents.* Oxford: Oxford University Press; 1992.

83. Roberts G. Understanding madness. In: Roberts G, Davenport S, Holloway F, Tattan T, eds. *Enabling Recovery. The Principles and Practice of Rehabilitation Psychiatry.* London: Gaskell; 2006. 93–111.

84. Sayce L. *From Psychiatric Patient to Citizen. Overcoming Discrimination and Social Exclusion.* London: Macmillan; 2000.

85. Perkins R. I have a vision... *Open Mind* 2000; **104**:6.

86. Thornicroft G. *Shunned: Discrimination against People with Mental Illness.* Oxford: Oxford University Press; 2005.

87. Spaniol L, Gagne C, Koehler M. Recovery from serious mental illness: what it is and how to assist people in their recovery. *Continuum* 1997; **4**:3–15.

88. Boardman J. Work, employment and psychiatric disability. *Advances in Psychiatric Treatment* 2003; **9**:327–334.

89. Peterson D. *I Haven't Told Them, They Haven't Asked. The Employment Experiences of People with Experience of Mental Illness.* Auckland: Mental Health Foundation of New Zealand; 2007.

90. Curtis T, Dellar R, Leslie E. *Mad Pride: A Celebration of Mad Culture.* London: Chipmunkapublishing; 2000.

91. Mental Health Commission. *Te Haererenga mo te Whakaôranga 1996–2006. The Journey of Recovery for the New Zealand Mental Health Sector.* Wellington: Mental Health Commission; 2007.

92. Kessler RC, McGonagle KA, Zhao S, Nelson CB, Hughes M, Eshleman S et al. Lifetime and 12-month prevalence of DSM-III-R psychiatric disorders in the United States. Results from the National Comorbidity Survey. *Archives of General Psychiatry* 1994; **51**:8–19.

93. Jacobi F, Wittchen H-U, Hölting C, Höfler M, Pfister H, Müller N et al. Prevalence, co-morbidity and correlates of mental disorders in the general population: results from the German Health Interview and Examination Survey (GHS). *Psychological Medicine* 2004; **34**:597–611.

94. Oakley Browne MA, Wells JE, Scott KM, McGee MA, New Zealand Mental Health Survey Research Team. Lifetime prevalence and projected lifetime risk of DSM-IV disorders in Te Rau Hinengaro: the New Zealand Mental Health Survey. *Australian and New Zealand Journal of Psychiatry* 2006; **40**:865–874.

95. Kendler KS, Gallagher TJ, Abelson JM, Kessler RC. Lifetime prevalence, demographic risk factors, and diagnostic validity of nonaffective psychosis as assessed in a US community sample. The National Comorbidity Survey. *Archives of General Psychiatry* 1996; **53**:1022–1031.

96. Poulton R, Caspi A, Moffitt TE, Cannon M, Murray R, HonaLee Harrington BS. Children's self-reported psychotic symptoms and adult schizophreniform disorder: a 15-year longitudinal study. *Archives of General Psychiatry* 2000; **57**:1053–1058.

97. Scott J, Chant D, Andrews G, McGrath J. Psychotic-like experiences in the general population: the correlates of CIDI psychosis screen items in an Australian sample. *Psychological Medicine* 2006; **36**:231–238.

98. Johns LC, van Os J. The continuity of psychotic experiences in the general population. *Clinical Psychology Review* 2001; **21**:1125–1141.

99. Peters E, Day S, McKenna J, Orbach G. Delusional ideation in religious and psychotic populations. *British Journal of Clinical Psychology* 1999; **38**:83–96.

100. Preti A, Bonventre E, Ledda V, Petretto DR, Masala C. Hallucinatory experiences, delusional thought proneness, and psychological distress in a nonclinical population. *Journal of Nervous and Mental Disease* 2007; **195**:484–491.

101. Varghese D, Scott J, McGrath J. Correlates of delusion-like experiences in a non-psychotic community sample. *Australian and New Zealand Journal of Psychiatry* 2008; **42**:505–508.

102. Millham A, Easton S. Prevalence of auditory hallucinations in nurses in mental health. *Journal of Psychiatric and Mental Health Nursing* 1994; **5**:95–99.

103. Post F. Creativity and psychopathology: a study of 291 world-famous men. *British Journal of Psychiatry* 1994; **165**:22–34.

104. Post F. Verbal creativity, depression and alcoholism: an investigation of one hundred American and British writers. *British Journal of Psychiatry* 1996; **168**:545–555.

105. Lawrence PN. *Impressive Depressives. 75 historical cases of manic depression from seven centuries.* London: Manic Depressive Fellowship; 1998.

106. Barker PJ, Davidson B, Campbell P (eds). *From the Ashes of Experience.* London: Whurr Publications; 1999.

107. Lapsley H, Nikora LW, Black R. *Kia Mauri Tau! Narratives of Recovery from Disabling Mental Health Problems.* Wellington: Mental Health Commission; 2002.

108. McIntosh Z. *From Goldfish Bowl to Ocean: personal accounts of mental illness and beyond.* London: Chipmunkapublishing; 2005.

109. Jamison KR. *An Unquiet Mind: a memoir of moods and madness.* New York: The Free Press; 1995.

110. Alexander D. A death-rebirth experience. In: Spaniol L, Koehler M, eds. *The Experience of Recovery.* Boston: Center for Psychiatric Rehabilitation; 1994. 36–39.

111. Torgalsbøen AK. Full recovery from schizophrenia: the prognostic role of premorbid adjustment, symptoms at first admission, precipitating events and gender. *Psychiatry Research* 1999; **88**:143–152.

112. Libermann RP, Kopelowicz A. Recovery from schizophrenia: a challenge for the 21st Century. *International Review of Psychiatry* 2002; **14**:242–255.

113. Harding CM, Brooks G, Ashikage T, Strauss JS, Brier A. The Vermont longitudinal study of persons with severe mental illness II: long-term outcome of subjects who retrospectively met DSM-III criteria for schizophrenia. *American Journal of Psychiatry* 1987; **144**:727–735.

114. Hopper K, Harrison G, Janca A, Sartorius N. *Recovery From Schizophrenia: An International Perspective. A Report From the WHO Collaborative Project, the International Study of Schizophrenia.* Oxford: Oxford University Press; 2007.

115. Warner R. Review of "Recovery From Schizophrenia: An International Perspective. A Report From the WHO Collaborative Project, the International Study of Schizophrenia". *American Journal of Psychiatry* 2007; **164**:1444–1445.

116. Coleman R. *Recovery - an Alien Concept.* Hansell; 1999.

117. Ralph RO, Corrigan PW (eds). *Recovery in Mental Illness. Broadening our Understanding of Wellness.* Washington DC: American Psychological Association; 2005.

118. Ridgway P. Restorying psychiatric disability: learning from first person narratives. *Psychiatric Rehabilitation Journal* 2001; **24**(4):335–343.

119. Deegan P. Recovery: the lived experience of rehabilitation. *Psychosocial Rehabilitation Journal* 1988; **11**:11–19.

120. Fisher DV. Health care reform based on an empowerment model of recovery by people with psychiatric disabilities. *Hospital and Community Psychiatry* 1994; **45**:913–915.

121. Davidson L, Strauss J. Sense of self in recovery from severe mental illness. *British Journal of Medical Psychology* 1992; **65**:131–145.

122. O'Hagan M. Two accounts of mental distress. In: Read J, Reynolds J, eds. *Speaking our Minds.* London: Macmillan; 1996.

123. Andresen R, Oades L, Caputi P. The experience of recovery from schizophrenia: towards an empirically-validated stage model. *Australian and New Zealand Journal of Psychiatry* 2003; **37**:586–594.

124. Goldsack S, Reet M, Lapsley H, Gingell M. *Experiencing a Recovery-Oriented Acute Mental Health Service: Home Based Treatment from the Perspectives of Services Users, their Families and Mental Health Professionals.* Wellington: Mental Health Commission; 2005.

125. Barnett H, Lapsley H. *Journeys of Despair, Journeys of Hope. Young Adults Talk About Severe Mental Distress, Mental Health Services and Recovery*. Wellington: Mental Health Commission; 2006.

126. Mental Health Commission. *Three forensic service users and their families talk about recovery*. Wellington: Mental Health Commission; 2000.

127. Scottish Recovery Network. *Routes to recovery. Collected wisdom from the SRN Narrative Research Project*. Glasgow: Scottish Recovery Network; 2007.

128. Davidson L, Sells D, Sangster S, O'Connell M. Qualitative studies of recovery: what can we learn from the person? In: Ralph RO, Corrigan PW, eds. *Recovery in Mental Illness. Broadening our Understanding of Wellness*. Washington DC: American Psychological Association; 2005. 147–170.

129. Spaniol L, Koehler M (eds). *The Experience of Recovery*. Boston, MA: Center for Psychiatric Rehabilitation; 1994.

130. Spaniol L, Wewiorski N, Gagne C, Anthony W. The process of recovery from schizophrenia. *International Review of Psychiatry* 2002; **14**:327–336.

131. Ralph RO. Recovery. *Psychiatric Rehabilitation Skills* 2000; **4**:480–517.

132. Davidson L, Schmutte T, Dinzeo T, Andres-Hyman R. Remission and recovery in schizophrenia: practitioner and patient perspectives. *Schizophrenia Bulletin* 2008; **34**(1):5–8.

133. Secker J, Membrey H, Grove B, Seebohm P. Recovering from illness or recovering your life? Implications of clinical versus social models of recovery from mental health problems for employment support services. *Disability & Society* 2002; **17**(4):403–418.

134. Bellack A. Scientific and consumer models of recovery in schizophrenia: concordance, contrasts, and implications. *Schizophrenia Bulletin* 2006; **32**:432–442.

135. Schrank B, Slade M. Recovery in psychiatry. *Psychiatric Bulletin* 2007; **31**:321–325.

136. South London and Maudsley NHS Foundation Trust. *Social Inclusion, Rehabilitation and Recovery Strategy 2007–2010*. London: South London and Maudsley NHS Foundation Trust; 2007.

137. Ralph RO. Verbal definitions and visual models of recovery: focus on the recovery model. In: Ralph RO, Corrigan PW, eds. *Recovery in Mental Illness. Broadening our Understanding of Wellness*. Washington DC: American Psychological Association; 2005. 131–145.

138. Resnick SG, Fontana A, Lehman A, Rosenheck RA. An empirical conceptualization of the recovery orientation. *Schizophrenia Research* 2005; **75**:119–128.

139. Care Services Improvement Partnership, Royal College of Psychiatrists, Social Care Institute for Excellence. *A common purpose: Recovery in future mental health services*. Leeds: CSIP; 2007.

140. Higgins ET. *Approach/avoidance Orientations and Operations*. New York: Columbia University; 1990.

141. Leete E. A consumer perspective on psychosocial treatment. *Psychosocial Rehabilitation Journal* 1988; **12**:45–52.

142. National Institute for Clinical Excellence. *Schizophrenia. Core interventions in the treatment and management of schizophrenia in primary and secondary care*. London: NICE; 2002.

143. May R. Making sense of psychotic experience and working towards recovery. In: Gleeson JFM, McGorry PD, eds. *Psychological Interventions in Early Psychosis*. Chichester: John Wiley & Sons; 2004. 246–260.

144. Menninger K. Hope. *American Journal of Psychiatry* 1959; **116**(12):481–491.

145. Deegan P. Spirit breaking: when the helping professions hurt. *Humanistic Psychology* 1990; **18**(3):301–313.

146. Rinaldi M. *Insufficient Concern*. London: Merton Mind; 2000.

147. Berrios GE. Delusions as 'wrong beliefs': a conceptual history. *British Journal of Psychiatry* 1991; **159**(Suppl. 14):s6–s13.

148. Topor A. *Managing the Contradictions. Recovery from Severe Mental Disorders. Stockholm Studies of Social Work 18*. Stockholm: Stockholm University Press; 2001.

149. McGorry PD. The concept of recovery and secondary prevention in psychotic disorders. *Australian and New Zealand Journal of Psychiatry* 1992; **26**:3–17.

150. Tait L, Birchwood M, Trower P. Predicting engagement with services for psychosis: insight, symptoms and recovery style. *British Journal of Psychiatry* 2003; **182**:123–128.

151. Morgan K. *Insight and psychosis: an investigation of social, psychological and biological factors (PhD Thesis).* London: King's College London; 2003.

152. Frese FJ, Stanley J, Kress K, Vogel-Scibilia S. Integrating evidence-based practices and the recovery model. *Psychiatric Services* 2001; **52**:1462–1468.

153. Fisher D, Ahern L. Evidence-based practices and recovery. *Psychiatric Services* 2002; **53**:633–634.

154. Dijksterhuis EJ (Trans.) Dikshoorn C. *The Mechanization of the World-picture.* Oxford: Oxford University Press; 1961.

155. Bacon F (ed. Fowler T). *Novum Organum Scientarium.* Oxford: Oxford University Press; 1620.

156. Geddes J, Harrison P. Closing the gap between research and practice. *British Journal of Psychiatry* 1997; **171**:220–225.

157. Greenhalgh J. How to read a paper: getting your bearings. *British Medical Journal* 1997; **315**:243–246.

158. Department of Health, Department of Mental Health National Service Framework. London: The Stationery Office; 1999.

159. Bolton D. Knowledge in the human sciences. In: Priebe S, Slade M, eds. *Evidence in Mental Health Care.* Hove: Brunner-Routledge; 2002.

160. Wittgenstein L (Trans. Ogden CK). *Tractatus Logico-Philosophicus.* Routledge & Kegan Paul; 1922.

161. Rand A. *Introduction to Objectivist Epistemology.* New York: Meridian; 1979.

162. Kraepelin E (Trans. Barclay RM, ed. Robertson GM). *Dementia Præcox and Paraphrenia.* Edinburgh: E. & S. Livingstone; 1919.

163. Bleuler E. Dementia praecox oder die grüppe der schizophrenien. In: Aschaffenburg A, ed. *Hanbuch der psychiatrie.* Leipzig: Deuticke; 1911.

164. Arieti S. *Interpretation of Schizophrenia.* 2nd edn. New York: Basic Books; 1974.

165. American Psychiatric Association. *Practice Guideline for the Treatment of Patients With Schizophrenia,* 2nd edn. 2004.

166. Slade M, Priebe S (eds). *Choosing Methods in Mental Health Research.* Hove: Routledge; 2006.

167. Oakley A, Strange V, Bonell C, Allen E, Stephenson J. Process evaluation in randomised controlled trials of complex interventions. *BMJ* 2006; **332**:413–416.

168. Shill MA, Lumley MA. The Psychological Mindedness Scale: factor structure, convergent validity and gender in a non-psychiatric sample. *Psychology and Psychotherapy: Theory, Research and Practice* 2002; **75**(2):131–150.

169. Garety P, Fowler D, Kuipers E, Freeman D, Dunn G, Bebbington P et al. London-East Anglia randomised controlled trial of cognitive-behavioural therapy for psychosis. II: Predictors of outcome. *British Journal of Psychiatry* 1997; **171**:420–426.

170. Rosen F. *Classical Utilitarianism from Hume to Mill.* Hove: Routledge; 2003.

171. Thro M. Apollo vs Dionysius: The only theme your students will ever need in writing about literature. *VCCA Journal* 1996; **10**(2):11–18.

172. Fonagy P, Roth A, Higgitt A. The outcome of psychodynamic psychotherapy for psychological disorders. *Clinical Neuroscience Research* 2005; **5–6**:367–377.

173. Schön D. *Educating the Reflective Practitioner.* New York: Jossey-Bass; 1987.

174. Schön D. *The Reflective Practitioner.* New York: Basis Books; 1983.

175. Eraut M. Schön shock: a case for reframing reflection-in-action. *Teachers and Teaching: Theory and Practice* 1995; **1**(1):9–22.

176. Grimmett P, Erikson G (eds). *Reflection in Teacher Education.* New York: Teacher's College Press; 1988.

177. Hamilton B, Roper C. Troubling 'insight': power and possibilities in mental health care. *Journal of Psychiatric and Mental Health Nursing* 2006; **13**:416–422.

178. Pilgrim D, Rogers A. The troubled relationship between psychiatry and sociology. *International Journal of Social Psychiatry* 2002; **51**:228–241.

179. Murphy N, Canales M. A critical analysis of compliance. *Nursing Inquiry* 2001; **8**:173–181.

180. Benson A, Secker J, Balfe E, Lipsedge M, Robinson S, Walker J. Discourses of blame: accounting for aggression and violence on an acute mental health inpatient unit. *Social Science and Medicine* 2003; **57**:917–926.

181. Boyle M. *Schizophrenia, a Scientific Delusion?* 2nd edn. London: Routledge; 2002.

182. Speed E. Patients, consumers and survivors: a case study of mental health service user discourses. *Social Science and Medicine* 2006; **62**:28–38.

183. Galbraith JK. *American Capitalism: The Concept of Countervailing Power.* New York: Houghton Mifflin; 1952.

184. Foucault M. Two lectures. In: (Trans.) Marshall GC, Marshall L, Soper K, eds. *Power / Knowledge: Selected Interviews and Other Writings 1972–1977.* New York: Pantheon Books; 1980. 78–108.

185. Othmer E, Othmer SC. *The Clinical Interview Using DSM-IV-TR,* 3rd edn. Washington DC: American Psychiatric Publishing; 2002.

186. Faulkner A, Layzell S. *Strategies for Living. A report of user-led research into people's strategies for living with mental distress.* London: Mental Health Foundation; 2000.

187. Harvey D. Class relations, social justice and the politics of difference. In: Keith M, Pile S, eds. *Place and the Politics of Identity.* London: Routledge; 1993. 41–66.

188. Whitley R. Cultural competence, evidence-based medicine, and evidence-based practices. *Psychiatric Services* 2007; **58**:1588–1590.

189. Flexner S, Flexner D. *Wise Words and Wives' Tales: The Origins, Meanings and Time-Honored Wisdom of Proverbs and Folk Sayings Olde and New.* New York: Avon Books; 1993.

190. Edgeworth M. *Harry and Lucy Concluded: Being the last part of early lessons.* London: R. Hunter; 1825.

191. Meaney MJ. Nature, nurture, and the disunity of knowledge. *Annals of the New York Academy of Sciences* 2004; **935**:50–61.

192. Piaget J. *Logique et Connaissance Scientifique. Encyclopédie de la Pléiade.* Paris: Gallimard; 1967.

193. Mahoney MJ. Constructivism and positive psychology. In: Snyder CR, Lopez SJ, eds. *Handbook of Positive Psychology.* New York: Oxford University Press; 2002. 745–750.

194. Mahoney MJ. *Constructive Psychotherapy: The Heart of Positive Practice.* New York: Guilford; 2000.

195. Randall KW, Salem DA. Mutual-help groups and recovery: the influence of settings on participants' experience of recovery. In: Ralph RO, Corrigan PW, eds. *Recovery in Mental Illness. Broadening our Understanding of Wellness.* Washington DC: American Psychological Association; 2005. 173–205.

196. Grypdonck MHF. Qualitative health research in the era of evidence-based practice. *Qualitative Health Research* 2006; **16**:1371–1385.

197. Foucault M. *Language, Counter-Memory, Practice.* Ithaca NY: Cornell University Press; 1977.

198. Bloch S, Green SA. An ethical framework for psychiatry. *British Journal of Psychiatry* 2006; **188**:7–12.

199. Fulford KWM, Thornton T, Graham G. *Oxford Textbook of Philosophy and Psychiatry.* Oxford: Oxford University Press; 2006.

200. Szmukler G, Appelbaum P. Treatment pressures, leverage, coercion, and compulsion in mental health care. *Journal of Mental Health* 2008; **17**:233–244.

201. Mind. *Ward Watch.* Mind's campaign to improve hospital conditions for mental health patients. London: Mind; 2004.

202. Gert B, Culver CM, Clouser KD. *Bioethics: A Systematic Approach.* 2nd edn. New York: Oxford University Press; 2006.

203. Chamberlin J. Citizenship rights and psychiatric disability. *Psychiatric Rehabilitation Journal* 1998; **21**:405–408.

204. *Mental Capacity Act*. 2005.

205. Wirtz V, Cribb A, Barber N. Patient-doctor decision-making about treatment within the consultation - A critical analysis of models. *Social Science and Medicine* 2006; **62**:116–124.

206. Beauchamp T, Childress J. *Principles of Biomedical Ethics*, 5th edn. Oxford: Oxford University Press; 2001.

207. Mosher L, Burti L. *Community Mental Health: A Practical Guide*. New York: W.W. Norton; 1994.

208. Healthcare Commission. *Adult survey of users of mental health services*. London: Healthcare Commission; 2005.

209. Healthcare Commission. *Talking about Medicines*. London: Healthcare Commission; 2007.

210. Mental Health Foundation. *Up and Running? Exercise therapy and the treatment of mild or moderate depression in primary care*. London: Mental Health Foundation; 2005.

211. National Institute for Clinical Excellence. *Depression. Management of depression in primary and secondary care*. London: National Institute for Clinical Excellence; 2004.

212. Joy I, Miller I. *Don't Mind Me. Adults with Mental Health Problems: a Guide for Donors and Funders*. London: New Philanthropy Capital; 2006.

213. Office of the Deputy Prime Minister. *Mental Health and Social Exclusion*. London: Social Exclusion Unit; 2004.

214. Herxheimer A. Relationships between the pharmaceutical industry and patients organisations. *British Medical Journal* 2003; **326**:1208–1210.

215. Moynihan R, Henry D. The fight against disease mongering: generating knowledge for action. *PLoS Medicine* 2006; **3**(4):e191.

216. Healy D. The latest mania: selling bipolar disorder. *PLoS Medicine* 2006; **3**(4):e185.

217. Phillips CB. Medicine goes to school: teachers as sickness brokers for ADHD. *PLoS Medicine* 2006; **3**(4):e182.

218. Horwitz AV. *Creating Mental Illness*. Chicago: University of Chicago Press; 2002.

219. Young A. *The Harmony of Illusions: Inventing Post-traumatic Stress Disorder*. Princeton, NJ: Princeton University Press; 1995.

220. Boseley S. *Just say no to drug ads. Guardian* 2001;17.

221. Lancet. Europe on the brink of direct-to-consumer drug advertising. *Lancet* 2002; 359: 1709.

222. Bodenheimer T. Uneasy alliance - clinical investigators and the pharmaceutical industry. *New England Journal of Medicine* 2000; **342**:1539–1544.

223. Maynard A. Economic Issues. In: Rowland N, Goss S, eds. *Evidence-based Counselling and Psychological Therapies*. London: Routledge; 2000. 44–56.

224. Bekelman EJ, Li Y, Gross CP. Scope and impact of financial conflicts of interest in biomedical research. *JAMA* 2003; **289**:454–465.

225. Krimsky S, Rothenberg LS, Stott P, Kyle G. Scientific journals and their authors' financial interests: a pilot study. *Psychotherapy and Psychosomatics* 1998; **67**:194–201.

226. Lexchin J, Bero LA, Djulbegovic B, Clark O. Pharmaceutical industry sponsorship and research outcome and quality: systematic review. *BMJ* 2003; **326**:1167–1176.

227. Whitaker R. *Mad In America: Bad Science, Bad Medicine, and the Enduring Mistreatment of the Mentally Ill*. Perseus Publishing; 2002.

228. Moncrieff J. *Is Psychiatry for Sale?* London: Maudsley Discussion Paper; 2003.

229. Melander H, Ahlqvist-Rastad J, Meijer G, Beerman B. Evidence b(i)ased medicine–selective reporting from studies sponsored by pharmaceutical industry: review of studies in new drug applications. *BMJ* 2003; **326**:1171–1175.

230. Duggan L, Fenton M, Dardennes RM, et al. *Olanzapine for schizophrenia (Cochrane review)*. Oxford: Update Software; 1999.

231. Duggan L, Fenton M, Rathbone R, Dardennes RM, El-Dosoky A, Indran S. Olanzapine for schizophrenia. *Cochrane Database of Systematic Reviews* 2005;(2):CD001359.

232. Wahlbeck K, Tuunaaineen A, Gilbody SM, Adams CE. Influence of methodology on outcomes of randomised clozapine trials. *Pharmacopsychiatry* 2000; **33**:54–59.

233. Safer DJ. Design and reporting modifications in industry sponsored comparative psychopharmacology trials. *Journal of Nervous and Mental Disease* 2002; **190**:583–592.

234. Turner EH, Matthews AM, Linardatos E, Tell RA, Rosenthal R. Selective publication and antidepressant trials and its influence on apparent efficacy. *New England Journal of Medicine* 2008; **358**:252–260.

235. Kirsch I, Deacon BJ, Huedo-Medina TB, Scoboria A, Moore TJ, Johnson BT. Initial severity and antidepressant benefits: a meta-analysis of data submitted to the Food and Drug Administration. *PLoS Medicine* 2008; **5**(2):e45.

236. Lenzer J. Bush plans to screen whole US population for mental illness. *British Medical Journal* 2004; **328**:1458.

237. Abraham J. Making regulation responsive to commercial interests: streamlining drug industry watchdogs. *British Medical Journal* 2002; **325**:1164–1167.

238. Lièvre M. Alosetron for irritable bowel syndrome. Some patients may pay a high price for the FDA's decision to put the drug back on the market. *British Medical Journal* 2002; **325**:555–556.

239. Read J. Schizophrenia, drug companies and the internet. *Social Science and Medicine* 2008; **66**:99–109.

240. Choudry NK, Stelfox HT, Detsky AS. Relationships between authors of clinical practice guidelines and the pharmaceutical industry. *Journal of the American Medical Association* 2002; **287**:612–617.

241. Ioannidis JPA. Effectiveness of antidepressants: an evidence myth constructed from a thousand randomized trials? *Philosophy, Ethics, and Humanities in Medicine* 2008; **3**:14.

242. Tsapakis EM, Soldani F, Tondo L, Baldessarini RJ. Efficacy of antidepressants in juvenile depression: meta-analysis. *British Journal of Psychiatry* 2008; **193**:10–17.

243. Angell M. *The Truth About the Drug Companies. How they Deceive Us and What to Do About It.* New York: Random House; 2004.

244. Moynihan R. Who pays for the pizza? Redefining the relationships between doctors and drug companies. 1: Entanglement. *British Medical Journal* 2003; **326**:1189–1192.

245. Khan A, Khan SR, Leventhal RM, Brown WA. Symptom reduction and suicide risk among patients treated with placebo in antipsychotic clinical trials: an analysis of the Food and Drug Administration database. *American Journal of Psychiatry* 2001; **158**:1449–1454.

246. Khan A, Warner HA, Brown WA. Symptom reduction and suicide risk in patients treated with placebo in antidepressant clinical trials. *Archives of General Psychiatry* 2000; **57**:311–317.

247. Lewis S, Lieberman J. CATIE and CUtLASS: can we handle the truth? *British Journal of Psychiatry* 2008; **192**:161–163.

248. Sharfstein SS. Big pharma and American psychiatry: the good, the bad and the ugly. *Psychiatric News* 2005; **40**:3.

249. Paton C, Barnes T, Cavanagh M-R, Taylor D, Lelliott P. High-dose and combination antipsychotic prescribing in adult acute wards in the UK: the challenges posed by p.r.n. prescribing. *British Journal of Psychiatry* 2008; **192**:435–439.

250. Tauscher-Wisniewski S, Zipursky RB. The role of maintenance pharmacotherapy in achieving recovery from a first episode of schizophrenia. *International Review of Psychiatry* 2002; **14**:284–292.

251. Cramer JA, Rosenthal R. Compliance with medication regimens for mental and physical disorder. *Psychiatric Services* 1998; **49**:196–201.

252. Blackwell B. From compliance to alliance: a quarter century of research. *Netherlands Journal of Medicine* 1996; **48**:140–149.

253. Day JC, Bentall RP, Roberts C, Randall F, Rogers A, Cattell D et al. Attitudes towards antipsychotic medication. The impact of clinical variables and relationships with health professionals. *Archives of General Psychiatry* 2005; **62**:717–724.

254. Pyne JM, McSweeney J, Kane HS, Harvey S, Bragg L, Fischer E. Agreement between patients with schizophrenia and providers on factors of antipsychotic medication adherence. *Psychiatric Services* 2006; **57**:1170–1178.

255. Fenton WS, Blyler CR, Heinssen RK. Determinants of medication compliance in schizophrenia. *Schizophrenia Bulletin* 1997; **23**:637–651.

256. Lehtinen V, Aaltonen J, Koffert T, Räkkölainen V, Syvälahti E. Two-year outcome in first-episode psychosis treated according to an integrated model. Is immediate neuroleptisation always needed? *European Psychiatry* 2000; **15**:312–320.

257. Moncrieff J. Does antipsychotic withdrawal provoke psychosis? Review of the literature on rapid onset psychosis (supersensitivity psychosis) and withdrawal-related relapse. *Acta Psychiatrica Scandinavica* 2006; **114**:3–13.

258. Bola J, Mosher L. Treatment of acute psychosis without neuroleptics: two-year outcomes from the Soteria Project. *Journal of Nervous and Mental Disease* 2003; **191**:219–229.

259. Fenton W, Hoch J, Mosher L, Dixon L. Cost and cost-effectiveness of hospital vs. residential crisis care for patients who have serious mental illness. *Archives of General Psychiatry* 2002; **59**:357–364.

260. Porter R. *A Social History of Madness: Stories of the Insane*. London: Weidenfeld and Nicolson; 1987.

261. Scull A. *Museums of Madness*. Harmondsworth: Penguin; 1979.

262. Tuke S. Reprinted (1996) with an introduction by K. Jones. *Description of The Retreat*. London: Process Press; 1813.

263. Sargant W, Slater E. *An Introduction to Physical Methods of Treatment in Psychiatry*, 1st edn. Edinburgh: E & S Livingstone; 1944.

264. Ackner B, Harris A, Oldham AJ. Insulin treatment of schizophrenia; a controlled study. *Lancet* 1957; **272**:355–357.

265. Lerner BH. Last-ditch medical therapy - revisiting lobotomy. *New England Journal of Medicine* 2005; **353**:119–121.

266. Lind J. *A Treatise of the Scurvy in Three Parts. Containing an inquiry into the Nature, Causes and Cure of that Disease, together with a Critical and Chronological View of what has been published on the subject*. London: A. Millar; 1753.

267. Lambert TJ. Switching antipsychotic therapy: what to expect and clinical strategies for improving therapeutic outcomes. *Journal of Clinical Psychiatry* 2007; 68 suppl. **6**:10–13.

268. British Psychological Society Division of Clinical Psychology. *Recent advances in understanding mental illness and psychotic experiences*. Leicester: British Psychological Society; 2000.

269. Clare AW. *Psychiatry in Dissent: Controversial Issues in Thought and Practice*. London: Tavistock; 1976.

270. Sullivan PF. The genetics of schizophrenia. *PLoS Medicine* 2005; **2**(7):e212 0614–0618.

271. Sanders AR, Duan J, Levinson DF, et al. No significant association of 14 candidate genes with schizophrenia in a large European ancestry sample: implications for psychiatric genetics. *American Journal of Psychiatry* 2008; **165**:497–506.

272. Mulligan K. Caring for patients' graves helps hospitals reconcile with living. *Psychiatric Services* 2001; **36**:10.

273. Querido A. The shaping of community mental health care. *British Journal of Psychiatry* 1966; **114**:293–302.

274. Lazare A. *On Apology*. New York: Oxford University Press; 2004.

275. Satyanand A. Te Âiotanga. *Report of the Confidential Forum for Former In-patients of Psychiatric Hospitals*. Wellington: Department of Internal Affairs; 2007.

276. Ellard J. The history and present status of moral insanity. *Australian and New Zealand Journal of Psychiatry* 1988; **22**(4):383–389.

277. Faustman WO. Aversive control of maladaptive behavior: past developments and future trends. *Psychology* 1976; **13**:53–60.

278. Bloch S, Reddaway P. *Soviet Psychiatric Abuse: The Shadow over World Psychiatry*. London: Victor Gollancz; 1984.

279. Human Rights Watch and Geneva Initiative on Psychiatry. *Dangerous Minds: Political Psychiatry in China Today and Its Origin in the Mao Era*. New York: Human Rights Watch; 2002.

280. Stone AA. Investigating psychiatric abuses. *Psychiatric Times* 2002; **19**.

281. Compagni A, Adams N, Daniels A. *International Pathways to Mental Health System Transformation: Strategies and Challenges*. California: California Institute for Mental Health; 2007.

282. New Freedom Commission on Mental Health. *Achieving the Promise: Transforming Mental Health Care in America. Final report*. Rockville, MD: U.S. Department of Health and Human Services; 2003.

283. American Psychiatric Association. *Position Statement on the Use of the Concept of Recovery*. Washington DC: American Psychiatric Association; 2005.

284. Australian Health Ministers. *National Mental Health Plan 2003–2008*. Canberra: Australian Government; 2003.

285. Queensland Health. *Sharing Responsibility for Recovery: creating and sustaining recovery oriented systems of care for mental health*. Brisbane: Queensland Government; 2005.

286. South Australian Social Inclusion Board. *Stepping Up: A Social Inclusion Action Plan for Mental Health Reform 2007–2012*. Government of South Australia: Adelaide; 2007.

287. ACT Government. *ACT Mental Health Strategy & Action Plan 2003–2008*. Canberra: ACT Health; 2004.

288. Department of Health and Human Services. *Strategic Plan 2006–2011 partners. . .towards recovery*. Tasmania: Mental Health Service; 2006.

289. Department of Human Services. *New Directions for Victoria's Mental Health Services*. Melbourne: Victorian Government; 2002.

290. Department of Health. *A Recovery Vision For Rehabilitation. Psychiatric Rehabilitation Policy And Strategic Framework*. Perth: Government of Western Australia; 2004.

291. Mental Health Commission. *Blueprint for Mental Health Services in New Zealand*. Wellington: Mental Health Commission; 1998.

292. Mental Health Commission. *Recovery Competencies. Teaching Resource Kit*. Wellington: Mental Health Commission; 2001.

293. Doughty C, Tse S. *The effectiveness of service user-run or service user-led mental health services for people with mental illness: A systematic literature review*. Wellington: Mental Health Commission; 2005.

294. Mental Health Commission. *Discriminating Times? A re-survey of New Zealand print media reporting on mental health*. Wellington: Mental Health Commission; 2005.

295. O'Hagan M. *The Acute Crisis. Towards a recovery plan for acute mental health services in New Zealand*. Wellington: Mental Health Commission; 2006.

296. Mental Health Commission. *Oranga Ngākau. Getting the most out of mental health services. A recovery resource for service users*. Wellington: Mental Health Commission; 2003.

297. Mental Health Commission. *awhi, tautoko, aroba. Celebrating recovery-focused mental health workers*. Wellington: Mental Health Commission; 2001.

298. Scottish Executive. *Delivering for mental health*. Edinburgh: Scottish Executive; 2006.

299. *Delivering for Mental Health: The Scottish Recovery Indicator*. Edinburgh: 2007.

300. Scottish Recovery Network. *The role and potential development of peer support services*. Glasgow: Scottish Recovery Network; 2005.

301. Department of Health. *The Journey to Recovery - The Government's vision for mental health care.* London: Department of Health; 2001.

302. Department of Health. *The Expert Patient: A new approach to chronic disease management for the 21st century.* London: Department of Health; 2001.

303. Department of Health. *Supporting people with long-term conditions to self-care: A guide to developing local strategies and good practice.* London: Department of Health; 2006.

304. Cabinet Office. *Reaching Out: An Action Plan on Social Inclusion.* London: Cabinet Office; 2006.

305. Department of Health. *Creating a patient-led NHS.* London: Department of Health; 2005.

306. College of Occupational Therapists. *Recovering ordinary lives: The strategy for occupational therapy in mental health services 2007–2017.* London: College of Occupational Therapists; 2006.

307. Department of Health. *From values to action: The chief nursing officer's review of mental health nursing.* London: HMSO; 2006.

308. Department of Health. *Self-assessment toolkit. From values to action: The Chief Nursing Officer's review of mental health nursing.* London: Department of Health; 2006.

309. Woodbridge K, Fulford KWM. *Whose values? A workbook for values-based practice in mental health care.* London: Sainsbury Centre for Mental Health; 2004.

310. Department of Health. *The Ten Essential Shared Capabilities - A Framework for the whole of the Mental Health Workforce.* London: Department of Health; 2004.

311. Care Services Improvement Partnership. *ESC Recovery Training. A 2-day training programme for the mental health workforce.* Care Services Improvement Partnership; 2006.

312. Care Services Improvement Partnership. *Consultation on guidance on 'Finding a shared vision of how people's mental health problems should be understood'.* Essex: Care Services Improvement Partnership; 2007.

313. Department of Health. *From segregation to inclusion: Commissioning guidance on day services for people with mental health problems.* London: National Social Inclusion Programme; 2006.

314. Mental Health Commission. *A Vision for a Recovery Model in Irish Mental Health Services.* Dublin: Mental Health Commission; 2005.

315. Higgins A. *A recovery approach within the Irish Mental Health Services. A framework for development.* Dublin: Mental Health Commission; 2008.

316. Kirby M. Mental health in Canada: out of the shadows forever. *Canadian Medical Association Journal* 2008; **178**:1320–1322.

317. Amering M, Schmolke M. *Recovery. Das Ende der Unheilbarkeit.* Bonn: Psychiatrie-Verlag; 2007.

318. National Institute for Mental Health in England. *Emerging Best Practices in Mental Health Recovery.* London: NIMHE; 2004.

319. Baxter EA, Diehl S. Emotional stages: consumers and family members recovering from the trauma of mental illness. *Psychiatric Rehabilitation Journal* 1998; **21**:349–355.

320. Young SL, Ensing DS. Exploring recovery from the perspective of people with psychiatric disabilities. *Psychiatric Rehabilitation Journal* 1999; **22**:219–231.

321. Pettie D, Triolo AM. Illness as evolution: the search for identity and meaning in the recovery process. *Psychiatric Rehabilitation Journal* 1999; **22**:255–262.

322. Townsend W, Boyd S, Griffin G, Hicks PL. *Emerging Best Practices in Mental Health Recovery.* Columbus, OH: Ohio Department of Health; 1999.

323. Cohen P, Cohen J. The clinician's illusion. *Archives of General Psychiatry* 1984; **41**:1178–1182.

324. Leary MR, Tangney JP. *Handbook of Self and Identity.* New York: Guilford Press; 2003.

325. Flood J. *Archaeology of the Dreamtime: The Story of Prehistoric Australia and its People.* Sydney: Collins; 1991.

326. Cross T, Earle K, Echo-Hawk-Solie H, Manness K. Cultural strengths and challenges in implementing a system of care model in American Indian communities. *Systems of Care: Promising Practices in Children's Mental Health, 2000 series*, Vol. 1. Washington DC: Center for Effective Collaboration and Practice, American Institutes for Research; 2000. 8–14.

327. Goffman E. *Stigma: Notes on the Management of Spoiled Identity.* London: Prentice-Hall; 1963.

328. Breakwell G. *Coping with Threatened Identities*. London: Methuen; 1986.

329. Estroff SE. Self, identity, and subjective experiences of schizophrenia. In search of the subject. *Schizophrenia Bulletin* 1989; **15**:189–196.

330. Davidson L, Shahar G, Lawless MS, Sells D, Tondora J. Play, pleasure and other positive life events: "non-specific" factors in recovery from mental illness? *Psychiatry* 2006; **69**:151–163.

331. Kupersanin E. Psychosis fails to block psychiatrist's career path. *Psychiatric News* 2002; **37**:5.

332. Walsh D. A journey towards recovery: from the inside out. *Psychiatric Rehabilitation Journal* 1996; **20**:85–90.

333. Onken SJ, Craig CM, Ridgway P, Ralph RO, Cook JA. An analysis of the definitions and elements of recovery: a review of the literature. *Psychiatric Rehabilitation Journal* 2007; **31**:9–22.

334. Deegan P. *A letter to my friend who is giving up*. Cromwell, CT: Connecticut Association of Rehabilitation Facilities; 1989.

335. Erikson E. *Identity: Youth and Crisis*. New York: W.W. Norton; 1968.

336. Viney LL. A sociophenomenological approach to life-span development complements Erikson's sociodynamic approach. *Human Development* 1987; **30**:125–136.

337. Cox LM, Lyddon WJ. Constructivist conceptions of self: a discussion of emerging identity constructs. *Journal of Constructivist Psychology* 1997; **10**:201–209.

338. Markus H, Nurius P. Possible selves. *American Psychologist* 1986; **41**(9):954–969.

339. Boyatzis RE, Groenen PJF. The ideal self as the driver of intentional change. *Journal of Management Development* 2006; **25**(7):624–642.

340. Dunkel CS, Anthis KS. The role of possible selves in identity formation: a short term longitudinal study. *Journal of Adolescence* 2001; **24**:765–776.

341. Marcia JE. Development and validation of ego-identity status. *Journal of Personality and Social Psychology* 1966; **3**(5):551–558.

342. Resnick SG, Rosenheck RA. Recovery and positive psychology: parallel themes and potential synergies. *Psychiatric Services* 2006; **57**(1):120–122.

343. Chamberlin J. *Confessions of a non-compliant patient*. National Empowerment Center Newsletter 1997; Summer/Fall:9–10.

344. Vincent SS. *Using findings from qualitative research to teach mental health professionals about the experience of recovery from psychiatric disability*. Presentation at Harvard University Graduate School of Education 4th Annual Student Research Conference, Cambridge, MA: 1999.

345. Pargament KI. *Spiritually Integrated Psychotherapy*. New York: Guilford; 2007.

346. Davidson L. *Living Outside Mental Illness: Qualitative Studies of Recovery in Schizophrenia*. New York: New York University Press; 2003.

347. Pargament KI. The psychology of religion *and* spirituality? Yes and no. *International Journal for the Psychology of Religion* 1999; **9**:3–16.

348. Pargament KI, Mahoney A. Spirituality. Discovering and conserving the sacred. In: Snyder CR, Lopez SJ, eds. *Handbook of Positive Psychology*. New York: Oxford University Press; 2002. 646–659.

349. Pargament KI. *The Psychology of Religion and Coping: Theory, Research, Practice*. New York: Guilford; 1997.

350. Averill JR. Spirituality: from the mundane to the meaningful - and back. *Journal of Theoretical and Philosophical Psychology* 1999; **18**:101–126.

351. Copeland ME. *Wellness Recovery Action Plan*. Brattleboro: VT: Peach Press; 1999.

352. Russinova Z, Blanch A. Supported spirituality: a new frontier in the recovery-oriented mental health system. *Psychiatric Rehabilitation Journal* 2007; **30**:247–249.

353. Frith C. *Cognitive Neuropsychology of Schizophrenia*. Hove: Erlbaum; 1992.

354. Henquet C, Krabbendam L, Spauwen J, Kaplan C, Lieb R, Wittchen H-U et al. Prospective cohort study of cannabis use, predisposition for psychosis, and psychotic symptoms in young people. *BMJ* 2005; **330**:11.

355. Bebbington P, Kuipers L. The predictive utility of expressed emotion in schizophrenia: an aggregate analysis. *Psychological Medicine* 1994; **24**:707–718.

356. Slade M, Pinfold V, Rapaport J, Bellringer S, Banerjee S, Kuipers E et al. Best practice when service users do not consent to sharing information with carers: national multi-method study. *British Journal of Psychiatry* 2007; **190**:148–155.

357. Slade M, Loftus L, Phelan M, Thornicroft G, Wykes T. *The Camberwell Assessment of Need.* London: Gaskell; 1999.

358. Phelan M, Slade M, Thornicroft G, Dunn G, Holloway F, Wykes T et al. The Camberwell Assessment of Need: the validity and reliability of an instrument to assess the needs of people with severe mental illness. *British Journal of Psychiatry* 1995; **167**:589–595.

359. Clay S, Schell B, Corrigan P, Ralph R (eds). *On Our Own, Together. Peer Programs for People with Mental Illness.* Nashville, TN: Vanderbilt University Press; 2005.

360. Mead S, Mead. *Intentional Peer Support: an alternative approach.* Plainfield, NH: Shery Mead Consulting; 2005.

361. Kirkpatrick H, Landeen J, Byrne C et al. Hope and schizophrenia. Clinicians identifying hope-instilling strategies. *Journal of Psychosocial Nursing and Mental Health Services* 1995; **33**:15–19.

362. Chamberlin J. *On Our Own: Patient-Controlled Alternatives to the Mental Health System.* New York: Hawthorn; 1978.

363. Maton KI, Salem DA. Organizational characteristics of empowering community settings: a multiple case study approach. *American Journal of Community Psychology* 1995; **23**:631–657.

364. Rappaport J. Narrative studies, personal stories, and identity transformation in the mutual help context. *Journal of Applied Behavioral Science* 1993; **29**:239–256.

365. Meehan T, Bergen H, Coveney C, Thornton R. Development and evaluation of a training program in peer support for former consumers. *International Journal of Mental Health Nursing* 2002; **11**:34–39.

366. Craig T, Doherty I, Jamieson-Craig R, Boocock A, Attafua G. The consumer-employee as a member of a Mental Health Outreach Team. *Journal of Mental Health* 2004; **13**:59–69.

367. Corrigan P, Mueser KT, Bond GR, Drake RE, Solomon P. *Principles and Practice of Psychiatric Rehabilitation: an empirical approach.* New York: Guilford Press; 2008.

368. Division of Mental Health DDaAD. Georgia's Consumer-Driven Road to Recovery. *A Mental Health Consumer's Guide for Participation In and Development Of Medicaid Reimbursable Peer Support Services.* Georgia: Office of Consumer Relations; 2003.

369. Wells D. The experience of role strain from the perspective of consumers / employees in mental health settings. In: Mental Health Commission, ed. *Book of Collected Articles. A Companion to Mental Health Recovery Competencies Teaching Resource Kit.* Wellington: Mental Health Commission; 1999.

370. Chinman MJ, Rosenheck RA, Lam JA, Davidson L. Comparing consumer and nonconsumer provided case management services for homeless persons with serious mental illness. *Journal of Nervous and Mental Disease* 2000; **188**:446–453.

371. White W. *Sponsor, Recovery Coach, Addiction Counselor: The Importance of Role Clarity and Role Integrity.* Philadelphia PA: Philadelphia Department of Behavioral Health and Mental Retardation Services; 2006.

372. Granfield R, Cloud W. *Coming Clean: Overcoming Addiction without Treatment.* New York: New York University Press; 1999.

373. Davidson L, Haglund KE, Stayner DA, Rakfeldt J, Chinman ML. "It was just realising that life isn't one big horror": A qualitative study of supported socialization. *Psychiatric Rehabilitation Journal* 2001; **24**:275–292.

374. Johnsen M, Teague GB, Herr EM. Common ingredients as a fidelity measure for peer-run programs. In: Clay S, Schell B, Corrigan P, Ralph R, eds. *On Our Own, Together. Peer Programs for People with Mental Illness.* Nashville, TN: Vanderbilt University Press; 2005. 213–238.

375. Solomon P. Peer support / peer provided services. Underlying processes, benefits and critical ingredients. *Psychiatric Rehabilitation Journal* 2004; **27**:392–401.

376. Campbell J. The historical and philosophical development of peer-run programs. In: Clay S, Schell B, Corrigan P, Ralph R, eds. *On Our Own, Together. Peer Programs for People with Mental Illness*. Nashville, TN: Vanderbilt University Press; 2005. 17–66.

377. Davidson L, Chinman MJ, Kloos B, Weingarten R, Stayner D, Tebes JK. Peer support among individuals with severe mental illness: a review of the evidence. *Clinical Psychology - Science and Practice* 1999; **6**:165–187.

378. Simpson EL, House AO. Involving users in the delivery and evaluation of mental health services: systematic review. *BMJ* 2002; **325**:1265.

379. Crawford MJ, Rutter D, Manley C, Weaver T, Bhui K, Fulop T et al. Systematic review of involving patients in the planning and development of health care. *British Medical Journal* 2002; **325**:1263–1267.

380. Rogers ES, Teague GB, Lichenstein C, Campbell J, Lyass A, Chen R et al. Effects of participation in consumer-operated service programs on both personal and organizationally mediated empowerment: results of multisite study. *Journal of Rehabilitation Research & Development* 2007; **44**:785–800.

381. Dumont JM, Jones K. Findings from a consumer/survivor defined alternative to psychiatric hospitalization. *Outlook* 2002; Spring:4–6.

382. Van Tosh L, Del Vecchio P. *Consumer Operated Self-help Programs: A Technical Report*. Rockville, MD: US Center for Mental Health Services; 2000.

383. Forquer S, Knight E. Managed care: Recovery enhancer or inhibitor. *Psychiatric Services* 2001; **52**:25–26.

384. Galanter M. Zealous self-help groups as adjuncts to psychiatric treatment: a study of Recovery, Inc. *American Journal of Psychiatry* 1988; **145**:1248–1253.

385. Powell TJ, Yeaton W, Hill EM, Silk KR. Predictors of psychosocial outcomes for patients with mood disorders: the effects of self-help group participation. *Psychiatric Rehabilitation Journal* 2001; **25**:3–11.

386. Yanos PT, Primavera LH, Knight EL. Consumer-run service participation, recovery of social functioning, and the mediating role of psychological factors. *Psychiatric Services* 2001; **52**:493–500.

387. Chamberlin J, Rogers ES, Ellison ML. Self-help programs: a description of their characteristics and their members. *Psychiatric Rehabilitation Journal* 1996; **19**:33–42.

388. Gelso CJ, Kelley FA, Fuertes JN, Marmarosh C, Holmes SE, Costa C et al. Measuring the real relationship in psychotherapy: initial validation of the therapist form. *Journal of Counseling Psychology* 2005; **52**(4):640–649.

389. Greenson RR. *The Technique and Practice of Psychoanalysis*. New York: International Universities Press; 1967.

390. Mental Health Commission. *Te Hononga 2015. Connecting for greater well-being*. Wellington: Mental Health Commission; 2007.

391. Kovel J. *The Radical Spirit. Essays on Psychoanalysis and Society*. London: Free Association Books; 1988.

392. Ingleby D (ed). *Critical Psychiatry: The Politics of Mental Health*. Harmondsworth: Penguin; 1981.

393. Roper C (ed). *Sight Unseen: Conversations Between Service Receivers*. Melbourne: Centre for Psychiatric Nursing Research and Practice; 2003.

394. Slade M, Leese M, Cahill S, Thornicroft G, Kuipers E. Patient-rated mental health needs and quality of life improvement. *British Journal of Psychiatry* 2005; **187**:256–261.

395. Crane-Ross D, Lutz WJ, Roth D. Consumer and case manager perspectives of service empowerment: relationship to mental health recovery. *Journal of Behavioral Health Services & Research* 2006; **33**:142–155.

396. Priebe S, Gruyters T. The role of the helping alliance in psychiatric community care: a prospective study. *Journal of Nervous and Mental Disease* 1993; **181**:552–557.

397. Beauford JE, McNiel DE, Binder RL. Utility of the initial therapeutic alliance in evaluating psychiatric patients' risk of violence. *American Journal of Psychiatry* 1997; **154**:1272–1276.

398. Zuroff DC, Blatt SJ, Sotsky SM, Krupnick JL, Martin DL, Sanislow CA et al. Relation of therapeutic alliance and perfectionism to outcome in brief outpatient treatment of depression. *Journal of Consulting and Clinical Psychology* 2000; **68**:114–224.

399. Svensson B, Hansson L. Therapeutic alliance in cognitive therapy for schizophrenic and other long-term mentally ill patients: development and relationship to outcome in an in-patient treatment programme. *Acta Psychiatrica Scandinavica* 1999; **99**:281–287.

400. Topor A, Borg M, Mezzina R, Sells D, Marin I, Davidson L. Others: the role of family, friends, and professionals in the recovery process. *American Journal of Psychiatric Rehabilitation* 2006; **9**:17–37.

401. Borg M, Kristiansen K. Recovery-oriented professionals: helping relationships in mental health services. *Journal of Mental Health* 2004; **13**:493–505.

402. Topor A. *Breaking the rules - the professionals contribution to recovery* (Conference presentation). University of Hertfordshire: 18–19 September; 2007.

403. Curtis L, Hodge M. Old standards, new dilemmas: ethics and boundaries in community support services. *Psychosocial Rehabilitation Journal* 1994; **18**:13–33.

404. Davidson L, Tondora J, Staeheli M, O'Connell M, Frey J, Chinman MJ. Recovery guides: an emerging model of community-based care for adults with psychiatric disabilities. In: Lightburn A, Sessions P, eds. *Community Based Clinical Practice*. Oxford: Oxford University Press; 2003. 476–501.

405. Green LS, Oades L, Grant AM. Cognitive-behavioural, solution-focused life coaching: enhancing goal striving, well-being and hope. *Journal of Positive Psychology* 2006; **1**(3):142–149.

406. Seligman M, Csikszentmihalyi M. Positive psychology: an introduction. *American Psychologist* 2000; **55**:5–14.

407. Seligman M. *Authentic Happiness: Using the new positive psychology to realize your potential for lasting fulfillment*. New York: Free Press; 2002.

408. Jayawickreme J, Pawelski J, Seligman M. *Positive Psychology and Nussbaum's Capabilities Approach*. Conference presentation: Subjective Measures of Well-Being and the Science of Happiness: Historical origins and philosophical foundations. Birmingham AL: 2008.

409. Snyder CR, Lopez JS. *Handbook of Positive Psychology*. New York: Oxford University Press; 2002.

410. Keyes CLM, Haidt J (eds). *Flourishing: Positive psychology and the life well lived*. Washington DC: American Psychological Association; 2003.

411. Peterson C. *A Primer in Positive Psychology*. New York: Oxford University Press; 2006.

412. Compton W. *An Introduction to Positive Psychology*. Belmont CA: Thomson-Wadsworth; 2005.

413. Linley PA, Joseph S. *Positive Psychology in Practice*. Hoboken NJ: John Wiley; 2004.

414. World Health Organization. *Promoting Mental Health. Concepts, Emerging Evidence, Practice*. Geneva: World Health Organization; 2004.

415. Ryff CD, Keyes CLM. The structure of psychological well-being revisited. *Journal of Personality and Social Psychology* 1995; **69**:719–727.

416. Frisch MB, Cornell J, Villanueva M, Retzlaff PJ. Clinical validation of the Quality of Life Inventory: a measure of life satisfaction for use in treatment planning and outcome assessment. *Psychological Assessment* 1992; **4**:92–101.

417. Keyes CLM. Mental illness and/or mental health? Investigating axioms of the complete state model of health. *Journal of Consulting and Clinical Psychology* 2005; **73**:539–548.

418. Keyes CLM, Lopez SJ. Toward a science of mental health. In: Snyder CR, Lopez SJ, eds. *Handbook of Positive Psychology*. New York: Oxford University Press; 2002. 45–59.

419. Keyes CLM. Promoting and protecting mental health as flourishing. A complementary strategy for improving national mental health. *American Psychologist* 2007; **62**:95–108.

420. Keyes CLM. Social well-being. *Social Psychology Quarterly* 1998; **61**:121–140.

421. Keyes CLM. Mental health in adolescence: is America's youth flourishing? *American Journal of Orthopsychiatry* 2006; **76**(3):395–402.

422. Seligman M. The effectiveness of psychotherapy: the Consumer Reports study. *American Psychologist* 1995; **50**:965–974.

423. Shahar G, Davidson L. Depressive symptoms erode self-esteem in severe mental illness: a three-wave, cross-lagged study. *Journal of Consulting and Clinical Psychology* 2003; **71**:890–900.

424. Cook JA, Jonikas J. Self-determination among mental health consumers/survivors: using lessons from the past to guide the future. *Journal of Disability Policy Studies* 2002; **13**:87–95.

425. Russinova Z. Providers' hope-inspiring competence as a factor optimizing psychiatric rehabilitation outcomes. *Journal of Rehabilitation* 1999; Oct–Dec:50–57.

426. Snyder CR. *Handbook of Hope*. San Diego: Academic Press; 2000.

427. Coutu DL. How resilience works. *Harvard Business Review* 2002; May:46–55.

428. Klausner E, Snyder CR, Cheavens J. A hope-based group treatment for depressed older outpatients. In: Williamsone GM, Parmalee PA, Shaffer DR, eds. *Physical Illness and Depression in Older Adults: A Handbook of Theory, Research and Practice*. New York: Plenum; 2000. 295–310.

429. Irving LM, Snyder CR, Cheavens J, Gravel L, Hanke J, Hilberg P et al. The relationships between hope and outcomes at the pretreatment, beginning, and later phases of psychotherapy. *Journal of Psychotherapy Integration* 2004; **14**(4):419–443.

430. Snyder CR, Feldman DB, Taylor JD, Schroeder LL, Adams V. The roles of helpful thinking in preventing problems and enhancing strengths. *Applied and Preventive Psychology* 2000; **15**:262–295.

431. Snyder CR, Pulvers K. Dr Seuss, the coping machine, and "Oh, the places you will go.". In: Snyder CR, ed. *Coping with Stress: Effective People and Places*. New York: Oxford University Press; 2001. 3–19.

432. Michael ST. Hope conquers fear: Overcoming anxiety and panic attacks. In: Snyder CR, ed. *Handbook of Hope: Theory, Measures and Applications*. San Diego, CA: Academic Press; 2000. 355–378.

433. Sarason BR, Sarason IG, Pierce GR (eds). *Social Support: An Interactional View*. New York: Wiley; 1990.

434. Nakamura J, Csikszentmihalyi M. *The Concept of Flow. Handbook of Positive Psychology*. New York: Oxford University Press; 2002. 89–105.

435. Layard R. *Happiness. Lessons from a new science*. London: Penguin; 2005.

436. Sheldon KM, Williams G, Joiner T. *Self-Determination Theory in the Clinic: Motivating Physical and Mental Health*. New Haven: Yale University Press; 2003.

437. Sheldon KM, Kasser T, Smith K, Share T. Personal goals and psychological growth: testing an intervention to enhance goal attainment and personality integration. *Journal of Personality* 2002; **70**:5–31.

438. Crowe T, Deane F, Oades LG, Caputi P, Morland KG. Effectiveness of a collaborative recovery training program in Australia in promoting positive views about recovery. *Psychiatric Services* 2006; **57**(10):1497–1500.

439. Shapiro DH. *Meditation: Self-regulation Strategy and Altered States of Consciousness*. New York: Aldine; 1980.

440. Davidson R, Kabat-Zinn J, Schumacher J, Rosenkranz M, Muller D, Santorelli S et al. Alterations in brain and immune function produced by mindfulness meditation. *Psychosomatic Medicine* 2003; **65**:564–570.

441. Thich Nhat Hanh. *Anger: Buddhist Wisdom for Cooling the Flames*. London: Rider; 2001.

442. Segal Z, Teasdale J, Williams M. *Mindfulness-Based Cognitive Therapy for Depression*. New York: Guilford Press; 2002.

443. Elbert T, Pantev C, Wienbruch C, Rockstroh B, Taub E. Increased cortical representation of the fingers of the left hand in string players. *Science* 1995; **270**:305–307.

444. Harris A, Thoresen CE. Extending the influence of positive psychology interventions into health care settings: lessons from self-efficacy and forgiveness. *Journal of Positive Psychology* 2006; **1**:27–36.

445. Shapiro SL, Schwartz GER, Santerre C. Meditation and positive psychology. In: Snyder CR, Lopez SJ, eds. *Handbook of Positive Psychology*. New York: Oxford University Press; 2002. 632–645.

446. Niederhoffer KG, Pennebaker JW. Sharing one's story. On the benefits of writing or talking about emotional experience. In: Snyder CR, Lopez SJ, eds. *Handbook of Positive Psychology*. New York: Oxford University Press; 2002. 573–583.

447. Baumeister RF, Vohs KD. The pursuit of meaningfulness in life. In: Snyder CR, Lopez SJ, eds. *Handbook of Positive Psychology*. New York: Oxford University Press; 2002. 608–618.

448. Bauer JJ, McAdams DP, Pals JL. Narrative identity and eudaimonic well-being. *Journal of Happiness Studies* 2008; **9**:81–104.

449. Smyth JM. Written emotional expression: effect sizes, outcome types, and moderating variables. *Journal of Consulting and Clinical Psychology* 1998; **66**:174–184.

450. Christensen AJ, Smith TW. Cynical hostility and cardiovascular reactivity during self-disclosure. *Psychosomatic Medicine* 1993; **55**:193–202.

451. Paez D, Velasco C, Gonzalez JL. Expressive writing and the role of alexithymia as a dispositional deficit in self-disclosure and psychological health. *Journal of Personality and Social Psychology* 1999; **77**:630–641.

452. Seligman M, Rashid T, Parks AC. Positive psychotherapy. *American Psychologist* 2006; **61** (8):774–788.

453. Anthony W. The principle of personhood: the field's transcendent principle. *Psychiatric Rehabilitation Journal* 2004; **27**:205.

454. Farkas M, Gagne C, Anthony W, Chamberlin J. Implementing recovery oriented evidence based programs: identifying the critical dimensions. *Community Mental Health Journal* 2005; **41**:141–158.

455. Anthony W. Value based practices. *Psychiatric Rehabilitation Journal* 2005; **28**:205–206.

456. Farkas M. The vision of recovery today: what it is and what it means for services. *World Psychiatry* 2007; **6**:4–10.

457. Greenhalgh T, Hurwitz B. Narrative based medicine. Why study narrative? *BMJ* 1999; **318**:48–50.

458. Greenhalgh T. *Narrative Based Medicine*. London: BMJ Books; 1998.

459. Roberts G. Narrative and severe mental illness: what place do stories have in an evidence-based world? *Advances in Psychiatric Treatment* 2000; **6**:432–441.

460. Lodge D. *Consciousness and the Novel*. Secker & Warburg; 2002.

461. Roberts G. *Briefing paper on the setting of standards and measurement of outcomes for the Mental Health and Wellbeing Networks of Devon and Torbay*. Devon: Recovery and Independent Living Professional Advisory Group (R&IL PAG). Advisory Paper No: 2; 2008.

462. Deegan P. *Best practice*. www.senseinternet.com.au/fintry/bestpractice.htm: 1988.

463. Royal College of Psychiatrists. *Fair deal for mental health*. London: Royal College of Psychiatrists; 2008.

464. Allott P, Loganathan L, Fulford KWM. Discovering hope for recovery: a review of a selection of recovery literature, implications for practice and systems change. *Canadian Journal of Community Mental Health* 2002; **21**(2):13–34.

465. Roberts G, Wolfson P. The rediscovery of recovery: open to all. *Advances in Psychiatric Treatment* 2004; **10**:37–49.

466. Roberts G, Wolfson P. New directions in rehabilitation: learning from the recovery movement. In: Roberts G, Davenport S, Holloway F, Tattan T, eds. *Enabling Recovery. The Principles and Practice of Rehabilitation Psychiatry*. London: Gaskell; 2006. 18–37.

467. Farkas M, Gagne C, Anthony W. *Recovery and Rehabilitation: A Paradigm for the New Millennium*. Boston, MA: Center for Psychiatric Rehabilitation; 1999.

468. Baumeister RF. *Meanings of Life*. New York: Guilford; 1991.

469. Emmons RA. Motives and goals. In: Hogan R, Johnson JA, eds. *Handbook of Personality Psychology*. San Diego, CA: Academic Press; 1997. 485–512.

470. Jacobson N, Curtis L. Recovery as policy in mental health services: Strategies emerging from the states. *Psychiatric Rehabilitation Journal* 2000; **23**:333–341.

471. Bateson G. *Steps to an Ecology of Mind*. St Albans: Paladin; 1973.

472. Stastny P, Lehmann P (eds). *Alternatives Beyond Psychiatry*. Shrewsbury: Peter Lehmann Publishing; 2007.

473. Deegan P. Recovering our sense of value after being labelled mentally ill. *Journal of Psychosocial Nursing and Mental Health Services* 1993; **31**:7–11.

474. Deegan P. Recovery as a journey of the heart. *Psychosocial Rehabilitation Journal* 1996; **19**:91–97.

475. Byrne S, Birchwood M, Trower P, Meaden A. *A Casebook of Cognitive Behaviour Therapy for Command Hallucinations*. Routledge: Hove; 2005.

476. Lazarus RS, Folkman S. *Stress, Appraisal and Coping*. New York: Springer; 1984.

477. Amirkhan JH. A factor analytically derived measure of coping: the Coping Strategy Indicator. *Journal of Personality and Social Psychology* 1990; **5**:1066–1074.

478. Folkman S, Lazarus RS. If it changes it must be a process: study of emotion and coping during three stages of a college examination. *Journal of Personality and Social Psychology* 1985; **48**:150–170.

479. Mikulincer M. *Human Learned Helplessness: A Coping Perspective*. Springer; 1994.

480. Pakenham KI, Rinaldis M. The role of illness, resources, appraisal, and coping strategies in adjustment to HIV/AIDS: the direct and buffering effects. *Journal of Behavioral Medicine* 2001; **24**:259–279.

481. Horowitz MJ. Psychological responses to serious life events. In: Hamilton V, Warbuton DM, eds. *Human Stress and Cognition: An information-processing approach*. Toronto: Wiley; 1979. 235–263.

482. Peterson C, Seligman M. *Character Strengths and Virtues*. New York: Oxford University Press; 2004.

483. Watson D, Clark LA. *The PANAS-X: Manual for the Positive and Negative Affect Schedule – Expanded Form*. Iowa City: University of Iowa; 1994.

484. Hawkins D, Stayner D. *Recovery Foundations Practice Change* (Conference presentation). Herts: "From here to recovery", September 19; 2007.

485. Cooperrider D, Whitney D. *A Positive Revolution in Change: Appreciative Inquiry*. Taos, NM: Corporation for Positive Change; 1999.

486. Henry J. Positive psychology and the development of well-being. In: Haworth J, Hart G, eds. *Well-being: Individual, Community and Societal Perspectives*. Basingstoke: Palgrave Macmillan; 2007. 25–40.

487. Park N, Peterson C, Seligman M. Character strengths in fifty-four nations and the fifty US states. *Journal of Positive Psychology* 2006; **1**(3):118–129.

488. Marin I, Mezzina R, Borg M, Topor A, Lawless MS, Sells D et al. The person's role in recovery. *American Journal of Psychiatric Rehabilitation* 2005; **8**:223–242.

489. Davidson L, O'Connell M, Tondora J, Evans AC. Recovery in serious mental illness: a new wine or just a new bottle? *Professional Psychology: Research and Practice* 2005; **36**(5):480–487.

490. Sanderson H, Smull M. *Essential Lifestyle Planning for Everyone*. London: Helen Sanderson Associates; 2005.

491. Adams N, Grieder DM. *Treatment Planning for Person-Centered Care.* Burlington, MA: Elsevier; 2005.

492. Spaniol L, Koehler M, Hutchinson DS. *The Recovery Workbook: Practical Coping and Empowerment Strategies for People with Psychiatric Disability.* Boston, MA: Center for Psychiatric Rehabilitation; 1994.

493. Coleman R, Baker P, Taylor K. *Working to Recovery. Victim to Victor III.* Gloucester: Handsell Publishing; 2000.

494. Ridgway P, McDiarmid D, Davidson L, Bayes J, Ratzlaff S. *Pathways to Recovery: A Strengths Recovery Self-Help Workbook.* Lawrence, KS: University of Kansas School of Social Welfare; 2002.

495. Mead S, Copeland M. What recovery means to us: consumers' perspectives. *Community Mental Health Journal* 2000; **36**:315–328.

496. Gingerich S, Mueser KT. Illness management and recovery. In: Drake RE, Merrens MR, Lynde DW, eds. *Evidence-Based Mental Health Practice: a Textbook.* New York: Norton; 2005.

497. Griffiths KM, Christensen H, Jorm AF, Evans K, Groves C. Effect of web-based depression literacy and cognitive-behavioural therapy interventions on stigmatising attitudes to depression: randomised controlled trial. *British Journal of Psychiatry* 2004; **185**:342–349.

498. Barlow JH, Ellard DR, Hainsworth JM, Jones FR, Fisher A. A review of self-management interventions for panic disorders, phobias and obsessive-compulsive disorders. *Acta Psychiatrica Scandinavica* 2005; **111**:272–285.

499. Stevens S, Sin J. Implementing a self-management model of relapse prevention for psychosis into routine clinical practice. *Journal of Psychiatric and Mental Health Nursing* 2005; **12**:495–501.

500. Warner R, Huxley P, Berg T. An evaluation of the impact of clubhouse membership on quality of life and treatment utilization. *International Journal of Social Psychiatry* 1999; **45**:310–320.

501. Davidson L, Stayner D, Lambert S, Smith P, Sledge W. Phenomenological and participatory research on schizophrenia: recovering the person in theory and practice. *Journal of Social Issues* 1997; **53**:767–784.

502. Sayce L, Perkins R. Recovery: beyond mere survival. *Psychiatric Bulletin* 2000; **24**:74.

503. Henderson C, Flood C, Leese M, Thornicroft G, Sutherby K, Szmukler G. Effect of joint crisis plans on use of compulsory treatment in psychiatry: single blind randomised controlled trial. *BMJ* 2004; **329**:136–140.

504. Tarrier N. Cognitive behaviour therapy for schizophrenia – a review of development, evidence and implementation. *Psychotherapy and Psychosomatics* 2005; **74**:136–144.

505. Allen MH, Carpenter D, Sheets JL, Miccio S, Ross R. What do consumers say they want and need during a psychiatric emergency. *Journal of Psychiatric Practice* 2003; **9**:39–58.

506. Becker DR, Drake RE. *A Working Life for People with Severe Mental Illness.* Oxford: Oxford University Press; 2003.

507. Thornicroft G, Rose D, Huxley P, Dale G, Wykes T. What are the research priorities of mental health service users? *Journal of Mental Health* 2002; **11**:1–5.

508. Bower SA, Bower GH. *Asserting Yourself. A Practical Guide for Positive Change.* Cambridge, MA: Da Capo Press; 2004.

509. Carver CS, Scheier MF, Weintraub JK. Assessing coping strategies: a theoretically based approach. *Journal of Personality and Social Psychology* 1989; **56**:267–283.

510. Barham P, Hayward R. In sickness and in health: dilemmas of the person with severe mental illness. *Psychiatry* 1998; **61**:163–170.

511. Corin E. The thickness of being: intentional worlds, strategies of identity, and experience among schizophrenics. *Psychiatry* 1998; **61**:133–146.

512. Miller WR, Rollnick S. *Motivational Interviewing: Preparing people to change (addictive behavior).* New York: Guilford Press; 2002.

513. Prochaska JO, DiClemente CC. Transtheoretical therapy: toward a more integrative model of change. *Psychotherapy: Theory, Research and Practice* 1982; **19**:276–288.

514. McLean R. *Recovered, Not Cured: A Journey Through Schizophrenia*. Allen & Unwin; 2005.

515. Saks E. *The Center Cannot Hold: My Journey Through Madness*. Hyperion; 2007.

516. Kemp R, Hayward P, Applewhite G et al. Compliance therapy in psychotic patients: randomised controlled trial. *BMJ* 1996; **312**:315–319.

517. Churchill R, Owen G, Singh S, Hotopf M. *International experiences of using community treatment orders*. London: Department of Health; 2007.

518. Kisely S, Campbell LA, Preston N. Compulsory community and involuntary outpatient treatment for people with severe mental disorders. *Cochrane Database of Systematic Reviews* 2005; **3**:CD004408.

519. Slade M, Amering M, Oades L. Recovery: an international perspective. *Epidemiologia e Psichiatria Sociale* 2008; **17**:128–137.

520. Deegan P, Rapp C, Holter M, Riefer M. A program to support shared decision making in an outpatient psychiatric medication clinic. *Psychiatric Services* 2008; **59**:603–605.

521. Deegan P. The importance of personal medicine. *Scandinavian Journal of Public Health* 2005; **33**:29–35.

522. Meyer T, Broocks A. Therapeutic impact of exercise on psychiatric diseases: guidelines for exercise testing and prescription. *Sports Medicine* 2000; **30**:269–279.

523. Lakhan SE, Vieira KF. Nutritional therapies for mental disorders. *Nutrition Journal* 2008; **7**:2.

524. Gregory RJ, Canning SS, Lee TW, Wise JC. Cognitive bibliotherapy for depression: a meta-analysis. *Professional Psychology: Research and Practice* 2004; **35**:275–280.

525. Deegan P. The lived experience of using psychiatric medication in the recovery process and a shared decision-making program to support it. *Psychiatric Rehabilitation Journal* 2007; **31**:62–69.

526. Icarus Project and Freedom Center. Harm Reduction Guide to Coming Off Psychiatric Drugs. http://theicarusproject.net/HarmReductionGuideComingOffPsychDrugs [2007, cited 2007 Nov. 15].

527. Darton K. *Making Sense of Coming Off Psychiatric Drugs*. London: Mind; 2005.

528. Peter Lehmann (ed). *Coming Off Psychiatric Drugs: Successful Withdrawal from Neuroleptics, Antidepressants, Lithium, Carbamazepine and Tranquilizers*. Shrewsbury: Peter Lehmann Publishing; 2004.

529. Breggin P, Cohen D. *Your Drug May Be Your Problem: How and Why to Stop Taking Psychiatric Medications*. Reading, MA: Perseus Books; 2007.

530. Watkins J. *Healing Schizophrenia: Using Medication Wisely*. Victoria: Michelle Anderson; 2007.

531. Libermann RP. Future directions for research studies and clinical work on recovery from schizophrenia: questions with some answers. *International Review of Psychiatry* 2002; **14**:337–342.

532. Friedman RA. Violence and mental illness – how strong is the link? *New England Journal of Medicine* 2006; **355**:2064–2066.

533. McEvoy SP, Stevenson MR, Woodward M. The contribution of passengers versus mobile phone use to motor vehicle crashes resulting in hospital attendance by the driver. *Accident Analysis & Prevention* 2007; **39**:1170–1176.

534. Coverdale J, Nairn R, Claasen D. Depictions of mental illness in print media: a prospective national sample. *Australian and New Zealand Journal of Psychiatry* 2001; **36**:697–700.

535. Philo G. *Media and Mental Distress*. London: Longman; 1996.

536. Torrey EF. A crisis ignored. *The New York Post* 2003, Oct 28.

537. Turner M, Beresford P. *User Controlled Research. Its meaning and potential*. London: INVOLVE; 2005.

538. Swanson J, Swartz M, Van Dorn R, Volavka J, Monahan J, Stroup TS et al. Comparison of antipsychotic medication effects on reducing violence in people with schizophrenia. *British Journal of Psychiatry* 2008; **193**:37–43.

539. Mind. *New Survey Reveals Un-therapeutic and 'Depressing' Conditions on Psychiatric Wards.* London: Mind; 2000.

540. Mental Health Foundation. *Knowing Our Own Minds. A Survey of How People in Emotional Distress Take Control of Their Lives.* London: Mental Health Foundation; 1997.

541. Onken SJ, Dumont JM, Ridgway P, Dornan DH, Ralph RO. *Mental Health Recovery: What Helps and What Hinders*? Washington DC: National Technical Assistance Center for State Mental Health Planning, National Association of State Mental Health Program Directors; 2002.

542. Swartz M, Swanson J, Hannon M. Does fear of coercion keep people away from mental health treatment? Evidence from a survey of persons with schizophrenia and mental health professionals. *Behavioral Science and the Law* 2003; **21**:459–472.

543. Birchwood M. Early intervention in psychotic relapse: cognitive approaches to detection and management. *Behaviour Change* 1995; **12**:2–9.

544. Birchwood M, Spencer E, McGovern D. Schizophrenia: early warning signs. *Advances in Psychiatric Treatment* 2000; **6**:93–101.

545. Slade M, McCrone P, Kuipers E, Leese M, Cahill S, Parabiaghi A et al. Use of standardised outcome measures in adult mental health services: randomised controlled trial. *British Journal of Psychiatry* 2006; **189**:330–336.

546. Zhu S-H. Number of quit smoking attempts key to success. *Scoop Health* 2007; 6 September.

547. Tracy B. *21 Success Secrets of Self-made Millionaires.* San Francisco, CA: Berrett-Koehler; 2000.

548. Henderson C, Swanson J, Szmukler G, Thornicroft G, Zinkler M. A typology of advance statements in mental health care. *Psychiatric Services* 2008; **59**:63–71.

549. Appelbaum P. Psychiatric advance directives and the treatment of committed patients. *Psychiatric Rehabilitation* 2004; **55**:751–763.

550. Swanson J, Swartz M, Ferron J, Elbogen EB, Van Dorn R. Psychiatric advance directives among public mental health consumers in five U.S. cities: prevalence, demand, and correlates. *Journal of the American Academy of Psychiatry and Law* 2006; **34**:43–57.

551. Srebnik DS, Russo J, Sage J, Peto T, Zick E. Interest in psychiatric advance directives among high users of crisis services and hospitalization. *Psychiatric Services* 2003; **54**:981–986.

552. Amering M, Stastny P, Hopper K. Psychiatric advance directives: qualitative study of informed deliberations by mental health service users. *British Journal of Psychiatry* 2005; **186**:247–252.

553. Swanson J, Swartz M, Ferron J, Elbogen EB, Wagner H, McCauley B et al. Facilitated psychiatric advance directives: a randomized trial of an intervention to foster advance treatment planning among persons with severe mental illness. *American Journal of Psychiatry* 2006; **163**:1943–1951.

554. Scheyett AM, Kim MM, Swanson JW, Swartz MS. Psychiatric advance directives: a tool for consumer empowerment and recovery. *Psychiatric Rehabilitation Journal* 2007; **31**:70–75.

555. Peto T, Srebnik DS, Zick E, Russo J. Support needed to create psychiatric advance directives. *Administration and Policy in Mental Health* 2004; **31**:409–419.

556. O'Connell M, Stein C. Psychiatric advance directives: perspectives of community stakeholders. *Administration and Policy in Mental Health* 2005; **32**:241–265.

557. Atkinson J, Garner H, Gilmour W. Models of advance directive in mental health care: stakeholder views. *Social Psychiatry and Psychiatric Epidemiology* 2004; **39**:673–680.

558. Elbogen EB, Swartz M, Van Dorn R, Swanson J, Kim M, Scheyett AM. Clinical decision-making and views about psychiatric advance directives. *Psychiatric Services* 2006; **57**:350–355.

559. Byng R, Jones R, Leese M, Hamilton B, McCrone P, Craig T. Exploratory cluster randomised controlled trial of shared care development for long-term mental illness. *British Journal of General Practice* 2004; **54**:259–266.

560. Lester H, Allan T, Wilson S, Jowett S, Roberts L. A cluster randomised controlled trial of patient-held medical records for people with schizophrenia receiving shared care. *British Journal of General Practice* 2003; **53**:197–203.

561. Jonikas J, Cook JA, Rosen C, Laris A, Kim JB. A program to reduce utilization of physical restraint in psychiatric inpatient facilities. *Psychiatric Services* 2004; **55**:818–820.

562. Gilburt H, Rose D, Slade M. Service users' experiences of psychiatric hospital admission: a grounded theory approach. *BMC Health Services Research* 2008; **8**:92.

563. Johnson S, Gilburt H, Lloyd-Evans B, Slade M. Acute in-patient psychiatry: residential alternatives to hospital admission. *Psychiatric Bulletin* 2007; **31**:262–264.

564. Meiser-Stedman C, Howard L, Cutting P. Evaluating the effectiveness of a women's crisis house: a prospective observational study. *Psychiatric Bulletin* 2006; **30**:324–326.

565. Boardman A, Hodgson R. Community in-patient units and halfway hospitals. *Advances in Psychiatric Treatment* 2000; **6**:120–127.

566. Marshall M, Crowther RE, Almaraz-Serrano A, Creed F, Sledge W, Kluiter H et al. Systematic reviews of the effectiveness of day care for people with severe mental disorders: 1. *Acute Day Hospitals Versus Admission. Health Technology Assessment* 2001; **5**(21).

567. Johnson S, Needle J, Bindman J, Thornicroft G. *Crisis Resolution and Home Treatment in Mental Health.* Cambridge: Cambridge University Press; 2008.

568. Hoult J. Community care of the acutely mentally ill. *British Journal of Psychiatry* 1986; **149**:137–144.

569. Burns T, Catty J, Watt H, Wright C, Knapp M, Henderson J. International differences in home treatment for mental health problems: results of a systematic review. *British Journal of Psychiatry* 2002; **181**:375–382.

570. Harrison J, Marshall S, Marshall P, Marshall J, Creed F. Day hospital vs. home treatment. A comparison of illness severity and costs. *Social Psychiatry and Psychiatric Epidemiology* 2003; **38**:541–546.

571. Tondora J, Davidson L. *Practice Guidelines for Recovery-Oriented Behavioral Health Care.* Connecticut: Connecticut Department of Mental Health and Addiction Services; 2006.

572. Rose D, Ford R, Lindley P, Gawith L. *In Our Experience: User-Focussed Monitoring of Mental Health Services.* London: Sainsbury Centre for Mental Health; 1998.

573. Priebe S, McCabe R, Bullenkamp J, Hansson L, Lauber C, Martinez-Leal R et al. Structured patient–clinician communication and 1-year outcome in community mental healthcare: cluster randomised controlled trial. *British Journal of Psychiatry* 2007; **191**:420–426.

574. Ellwood P. Outcomes management – a technology of patient experience. *New England Journal of Medicine* 1988; **318**:1549–1556.

575. Margison FR, Barkham M, Evans C, McGrath G, Clark JM, Audin K et al. Measurement and psychotherapy. Evidence-based practice and practice-based evidence. *British Journal of Psychiatry* 2000; **177**:123–130.

576. Davidson L, Tondora J, Lawless MS, O'Connell M, Rowe M. *A Practical Guide to Recovery-Oriented Practice Tools for Transforming Mental Health Care.* Oxford: Oxford University Press; 2009.

577. Russinova Z, Rogers ES, Ellison ML. *Recovery-Promoting Relationships Scale (Manual).* Boston, MA: Center for Psychiatric Rehabilitation; 2006.

578. Slade M. Routine outcome assessment in mental health services. *Psychological Medicine* 2002; **32**:1339–1344.

579. National Institute for Mental Health in England. *Outcomes Measures Implementation Best Practice Guidance.* Leeds: NIMHE; 2005.

580. Kiresuk TJ, Smith A, Cardillo JE. *Goal Attainment Scaling: Applications, Theory and Measurement.* Hillsdale, NJ: Lawrence Erlbaum Associates; 1994.

581. Slade M, Hayward M. Recovery, psychosis and psychiatry: research is better than rhetoric. *Acta Psychiatrica Scandinavica* 2007; **116**:81–83.

582. Sen A. *Development as Freedom.* New York: Knopf; 1999.

583. Dickerson F. Disquieting aspects of the recovery paradigm. *Psychiatric Services* 2006; **57**:647.

584. Peterson D, Pere L, Sheehan N, Surgenor G. *Respect Costs Nothing: a survey of discrimination faced by people with experience of mental illness in Aotearoa New Zealand.* Auckland: Mental health Foundation of New Zealand; 2004.

585. Pinfold V, Thornicroft G, Huxley P, Farmer P. Active ingredients in anti-stigma programmes in mental health. *International Review of Psychiatry* 2005; **17**(2):123–131.

586. Diaz E, Fergusson A, Strauss J. Innovative care for the homeless mentally ill in Bogota, Colombia. In: Jenkins JH, Barrett RJ, eds. *Schizophrenia, Culture, and Subjectivity. The Edge of Experience.* Cambridge: Cambridge University Press; 2004.

587. Department of Health. *From segregation to inclusion: where are we now?* London: National Social Inclusion Programme; 2008.

588. Grills CN, Bass K, Brown DL, Akers A. Empowerment evaluation: building upon a tradition of activism in African-American community. In: Fetterman DM, Kaftarian SJ, Wandersman A, eds. *Empowerment Evaluation: Knowledge and tools for self-assessment and accountability.* Thousand Oaks, CA: Sage; 1996. 123–140.

589. Duncan C, Peterson D. *The Employment Experiences of People with Experience of Mental Illness: Literature Review.* Auckland: Mental Health Foundation of New Zealand; 2007.

590. Twamley EW, Jeste DV, Lehman AF. Vocational rehabilitation in schizophrenia and other psychotic disorders: a literature review and meta-analysis of randomized controlled trials. *Journal of Nervous and Mental Disease* 2003; **191**:515–523.

591. Russinova Z, Wewiorski N, Lyass A, Rogers ES, Massaro JM. Correlates of vocational recovery for persons with schizophrenia. *International Review of Psychiatry* 2002; **14**:303–311.

592. Russinova Z, Bloch P, Lyass A. Patterns of employment among individuals with mental illness in vocational recovery. *Psychosocial Nursing and Mental Health Services* 2007; **45**:48–54.

593. Nairn RG, Coverdale J. People never see us living well: an appraisal of the personal stories about mental illness in a prospective print media sample. *Australian and New Zealand Journal of Psychiatry* 2005; **39**:281–287.

594. Wright A, Harris MG, Wiggers JH, Jorm AF, Cotton SM, Harrigan SM et al. Recognition of depression and psychosis by young Australians and their beliefs about treatment. *Medical Journal of Australia* 2005; **183**:18–23.

595. Lester H, Gask L. Delivering medical care for patients with serious mental illness or promoting a collaborative model of recovery. *British Journal of Psychiatry* 2006; **188**:401–402.

596. Wang PS, Demler O, Kessler RC. Adequacy of treatment for serious mental illness in the United States. *American Journal of Public Health* 2002;(**92**):98.

597. Fisher DB. We've been misled by the drug industry. *Washington Post* 2001, Aug. 19.

598. Watson AC, Corrigan PW. Challenging public stigma: a targeted approach. In: Corrigan PW, ed. *On the Stigma of Mental Illness. Practical Strategies for Research and Social Change.* Washington DC: American Psychological Association; 2005. 281–295.

599. Pettigrew TF, Tropp LR. Does intergroup contact reduce prejudice: recent meta-analytic findings. In: Oskamp S, ed. *Reducing Prejudice and Discrimination.* Kahwah NJ: Erlbaum; 2000. 93–114.

600. Verdoux H, van Os J. Psychotic symptoms in non-clinical populations and the continuum of psychosis. *Schizophrenia Research* 2002; **54**:59–65.

601. Burdekin B. *Report of the national inquiry into the human rights of people with a mental illness.* Canberra: Australian Government Publishing Service; 1993.

602. Mason KHC. *Inquiry under s47 of the Health and Disabilities Services Act 1993 in Respect of Certain Mental Health Services: Report of the Ministerial Inquiry.* Wellington: Ministry of Health; 1996.

603. Davidson L, O'Connell M, Tondora J, Styron T, Kangas K. The top ten concerns about recovery encountered in mental health system transformation. *Psychiatric Services* 2006; **57**:640–645.

604. Shepherd G, Boardman J, Slade M. *Making recovery a reality. Briefing Paper.* London: Sainsbury Centre for Mental Health; 2008.

605. Rissmiller DJ, Rissmiller JH. Evolution of the antipsychiatry movement into mental health consumerism. *Psychiatric Services* 2006; **57**:863–866.

606. Chamberlin J. The ex-patients movement: where we've been and where we're going. *Journal of Mind and Behavior* 1990; **11**:323–336.

607. Oyebode F. Invited Commentary on: The rediscovery of recovery. *Advances in Psychiatric Treatment* 2004; **10**:48–49.

608. Peyser H. What is recovery? A commentary. *Psychiatric Services* 2001; **52**:486–487.

609. Kelly BD, Feeney L. Psychiatry: no longer in dissent. *Psychiatric Bulletin* 2006; **30**:344–345.

610. Jackson C. Service users say they are sick of being used by the NHS. *Mental Health Today* 2003; February:8–9.

611. Petrova M, Dale J, Fulford KWM. Values-based practice in primary care: easing the tension between individual values, ethical principles and best evidence. *British Journal of General Practice* 2006; **56**:703–709.

612. Tennyson AL. *In Memoriam*. 1850.

613. Anthony W, Huckshorn KA. *Principled Leadership in Mental Health Systems and Programs*. Boston: Center for Psychiatric Rehabilitation; 2008.

614. Scottish Recovery Network. *Conference Summary Report: Celebrating and Developing Peer Support in Scotland*. Glasgow: 2005.

615. Kotter JP. *Leading Change*. Boston: Harvard Business School Press; 1996.

616. Rummler G. *Serious performance consulting*. Tampa, FL: Annual conference of the International Society for Performance Improvement; 2004.

617. Farkas M, Ashcraft L, Anthony W. The 3Cs for recovery services. *Behavioral Healthcare* 2008; February:24–26.

618. Sowers WE, Thompson KS. Keystones for collaboration and leadership; issues and recommendations for the transformation of community psychiatry. *American Association of Community Psychiatrists*; 2007.

619. Tondora J, Pocklington S, Osher D, Davidson L. *Implementation of person-centered care and planning: From policy to practice to evaluation*. Washington DC: Substance Abuse and Mental Health Services Administration; 2005.

620. Oades L, Lambert WG, Deane F, Crowe T. *Collaborative Recovery Training Program: Workbook*. Illawarra, NSW: Illawarra Institute for Mental Health: University of Wollongong; 2003.

621. Clear M. Collaborative Recovery Model. *newparadigm: The Australian Journal on Psychosocial Rehabilitation* 2007; June:32–64.

622. O'Hagan M. *Recovery Competencies for New Zealand Mental Health Workers*. Wellington: Mental Health Commission; 2001.

623. Hope R. *The Ten Essential Shared Capabilities – A Framework for the whole of the Mental Health Workforce*. London: Department of Health; 2004.

624. Perkins R. *Making it! An introduction to ideas about recovery for people with mental health problems*. London: South West London and St George's Mental Health NHS Trust; 2007.

625. Green J. *The Recovery Book. Practical help for your journey through mental and emotional distress*. Norwich: Norwich Mind; 2005.

626. Craddock N, Antebi D, Attenburrow M-J, Bailey A et al. Wake-up call for British psychiatry. *British Journal of Psychiatry* 2008; **193**:6–9.

627. Kuhn T. *The Structure of Scientific Revolutions*. Chicago: Chicago University Press; 1962.

628. McKnight J. *The Careless Society: Community and Its Counterfeits*. New York: Basic Books; 1995.

629. Freire P (Trans. Ramos M). *Pedagogy of the Oppressed*. Harmondsworth: Penguin; 1996.

630. Ashcraft L, Anthony W. A story of transformation: an agency fully embraces recovery. *Behavioural Healthcare Tomorrow* 2005; **14**:12–22.

631. Hutchinson DS, Anthony W, Ashcraft L, Johnson E, Dunn EC, Lyass A et al. The personal and vocational impact of training and employing people with psychiatric disabilities as providers. *Psychiatric Rehabilitation Journal* 2006; **29**:205–213.

632. Copeland M, Mead S. *WRAP and Peer Support: A guide to individual, group and program development*. Dummerston, VT: Peach Press; 2003.

633. Dinniss S, Roberts G, Hubbard C, Hounsell J, Webb R. User-led assessment of a recovery service using DREEM. *Psychiatric Bulletin* 2007; **31**:124–127.

634. Amering M, Hofer H, Rath I. The "First Vienna Trialogue" – experiences with a new form of communication between users, relatives and mental health professionals. In: Lefley HP, Johnson DL, eds. *Family Interventions in Mental Illness: International perspectives*. Westport CT: Praeger; 2002.

635. Bock T, Priebe S. Psychosis seminars: an unconventional approach. *Psychiatric Services* 2005; **56**:1441–1443.

Index